ELECTROCARDIOGRAPHIC BODY SURFACE MAPPING

DEVELOPMENTS IN CARDIOVASCULAR MEDICINE

Recent volumes

Maseri A, Marchesi C, Chierchia S, Trivella MG, eds: Coronary care units. 1981. ISBN 90-247-2456-2.
Morganroth J, Moore EN, Dreifus LS, Michelson EL, eds: The evaluation of new antiarrhythmic drugs. 1981. ISBN 90-247-2474-0.
Alboni P: Intraventricular conduction disturbances. 1981. ISBN 90-247-2484-X.
Rijsterborgh H, ed: Echocardiology. 1981. ISBN 90-247-2491-0.
Wagner GS, ed: Myocardial infarction: Measurement and intervention. 1982. ISBN 90-247-2513-5.
Meltzer RS, Roelandt J, eds: Contrast echocardiography. 1982. ISBN 90-247-2531-3.
Amery A, Fagard R, Lijnen R, Staessen J, eds: Hypertensive cardiovascular disease; pathophysiology and treatment. 1982. ISBN 90-247-2534-8.
Bouman LN, Jongsma HJ, eds: Cardiac rate and rhythm. 1982. ISBN 90-247-2626-3.
Morganroth J, Moore EN, eds: The evaluation of beta blocker and calcium antagonist drugs. 1982. ISBN 90-247-2642-5.
Rosenbaum MB, ed: Frontiers of cardiac electrophysiology. 1982. ISBN 90-247-2663-8.
Roelandt J, Hugenholtz PG, eds: Long-term ambulatory electrocardiography. 1982. ISBN 90-247-2664-8.
Adgey AAJ, ed: Acute phase of ischemic heart disease and myocardial infarction. 1982. ISBN 90-247-2675-1.
Hanrath P, Bleifeld W, Souquet, J. eds: Cardiovascular diagnosis by ultrasound. Transesophageal, computerized, contrast, Doppler echocardiography. 1982. ISBN 90-247-2692-1.
Roelandt J, ed: The practice of M-mode and two-dimensional echocardiography. 1983. ISBN 90-247-2745-6.
Meyer J, Schweizer P, Erbel R, eds: Advances in noninvasive cardiology. 1983. ISBN 0-89838-576-8.
Morganroth J, Moore EN, eds: Sudden cardiac death and congestive heart failure: Diagnosis and treatment. 1983. ISBN 0-89838-580-6.
Perry HM, ed: Lifelong management of hypertension. 1983. ISBN 0-89838-582-2.
Jaffe EA, ed: Biology of endothelial cells. 1984. ISBN 0-89838-587-3.
Surawicz B, Reddy CP, Prystowsky EN, eds: Tachycardias. 1984. ISBN 0-89838-588-1.
Spencer MP, ed: Cardiac Doppler diagnosis. 1983. ISBN 0-89838-591-1.
Villarreal H, Sambhi MP, eds: Topics in pathophysiology of hypertension. 1984. ISBN 0-89838-595-4.
Messerli FH, ed: Cardiovascular disease in the elderly. 1984. ISBN 0-89838-596-2.
Simoons ML, Reiber JHC, eds: Nuclear imaging in clinical cardiology. 1984. ISBN 0-89838-599-7.
Ter Keurs HEDJ, Schipperheyn JJ, eds: Cardiac left ventricular hypertrophy. 1983. ISBN 0-89838-612-8.
Sperelakis N, ed: Physiology and pathophysiology of the heart. 1984. ISBN 0-89838-615-2.
Messerli FH, ed: Kidney in essential hypertension. 1984. ISBN 0-89838-616-0.
Sambhi MP, ed: Fundamental fault in hypertension. 1984. ISBN 0-89838-638-1.
Marchesi C, ed: Ambulatory monitoring: Cardiovascular system and allied applications. 1984. ISBN 0-89838-642-X.
Kupper W, MacAlpin RN, Bleifeld W, eds: Coronary tone in ischemic heart disease. 1984. ISBN 0-89838-646-2.
Sperelakis N, Caulfield JB, eds: Calcium antagonists: Mechanisms of action on cardiac muscle and vascular smooth muscle. 1984. ISBN 0-89838-655-1.
Godfraind T, Herman AS, Wellens D, eds: Calcium entry blockers in cardiovascular and cerebral dysfunctions. 1984. ISBN 0-89838-658-6.
Morganroth J, Moore EN, eds: Interventions in the acute phase of myocardial infarction. 1984. ISBN 0-89838-659-4.
Abel FL, Newman WH, eds: Functional aspects of the normal, hypertrophied, and failing heart. 1984. ISBN 0-89838-665-9.
Sideman S, Beyar R, eds: Simulation and imaging of the cardiac system. 1985. ISBN 0-89838-687-X.
Van der Wall E, Lie KI, eds: Recent views on hypertrophic cardiomyopathy. 1985. ISBN 0-89838-694-2.
Beamish RE, Singal PK, Dhalla NS, eds: Stress and heart disease. 1985. ISBN 0-89838-709-4.
Beamish RE, Panagio V, Dhalla NS, eds: Pathogenesis of stress-induced heart disease. 1985. ISBN 0-89838-710-8.
Morganroth J, Moore EN, eds: Cardiac arrhythmias. 1985. ISBN 0-89838-716-7.
Mathes E, ed: Secondary prevention in coronary artery disease and myocardial infarction. 1985. ISBN 0-89838-736-1.
Lowell Stone H, Weglicki WB, eds: Pathology of cardiovascular injury. 1985. ISBN 0-89838-743-4.
Meyer J, Erbel R, Rupprecht HJ, eds: Improvement of myocardial perfusion. 1985. ISBN 0-89838-748-5.
Reiber JHC, Serruys PW, Slager CJ: Quantitative coronary and left ventricular cineangiography. 1986. ISBN 0-89838-760-4.
Fagard RH, Bekaert IE, eds: Sports cardiology. 1986. ISBN 0-89838-782-5.
Reiber JHC, Serruys PW, eds: State of the art in quantitative coronary arteriography. 1986. ISBN 0-89838-804-X.
Serruys PW, Meester GT, eds: Coronary angioplasty: a controlled model for ischemia. 1986. ISBN 0-89838-819-8.
Van der Wall EE, ed: Noninvasive imaging of cardiac metabolism. 1986. ISBN 0-89838-812-0.
Spencer MP, ed: Ultrasonic diagnosis of cerebrovascular disease. 1986. ISBN 0-89838-836-8.
Van Dam RTh, Van Oosterom A, eds: Electrocardiographic body surface mapping. 1986. ISBN 0-89838-834-1.

ELECTROCARDIOGRAPHIC BODY SURFACE MAPPING

Proceedings of the third International Symposium on Body Surface Mapping

edited by

R.Th. VAN DAM
Department of Cardiology
University of Nijmegen
Nijmegen, The Netherlands

A. VAN OOSTEROM
Department of Medical Physics
and Biophysics
University of Nijmegen
Nijmegen, The Netherlands

1986 **MARTINUS NIJHOFF PUBLISHERS**
a member of the KLUWER ACADEMIC PUBLISHERS GROUP
DORDRECHT / BOSTON / LANCASTER

Distributors

for the United States and Canada: Kluwer Academic Publishers, P.O. Box 358, Accord Station, Hingham, MA 02018-0358, USA
for the UK and Ireland: Kluwer Academic Publishers, MTP Press Limited, Falcon House, Queen Square, Lancaster LA1 1RN, UK
for all other countries: Kluwer Academic Publishers Group, Distribution Center, P.O. Box 322, 3300 AH Dordrecht, The Netherlands

Library of Congress Cataloging in Publication Data

International Symposium on Body Surface Mapping
(3rd : 1985 : Nijmegen, Netherlands)
Electrocardiographic body surface mapping.

(Developments in cardiovascular medicine ; 60)
Includes bibliographies and index.
1. Body surface mapping--Congresses. 2. Electrocardiography--Congresses. 3. Heart--Diseases--Diagnosis--Congresses. I. Dam, R. Th. van. II. Title. III. Series: Developments in cardiovascular medicine ; v. 60.
[DNLM: 1. Electrocardiography--congresses.
W1 DE997VME v.60 / WG 140 1633 1985e]
RC683.5.B63157 1985 616.1'207547 86-23499

ISBN-13: 978-94-010-8412-3 e-ISBN-13: 978-94-009-4303-2
DOI: 10.1007/978-94-009-4303-2

PREFACE

This book represents the proceedings of the 3rd International Symposium on Body Surface Mapping (BSM) held at Nijmegen; the Netherlands, from 11th to 13th of June, 1985, under the auspices of the International Council on Electrocardiology.

This meeting brought together a group of international scientists engaged in the field of the study of *electrocardiographic* body surface potentials. Previous meetings of this kind took place at Burlington, Vt; U.S.A. in 1972, organized by Rush and Lepeschkin, and in 1982 at Tokyo organized by Yamada, Harumi and Musha.

The special aims of this 3rd International Symposium were:

- to take stock of recent theoretical, technical, clinical and analytical advances
- to discuss and stimulate future developments with respect to international cooperation
- to discuss promising clinical applications of the BSM technique

A number of scientists engaged in this field had been invited to participate in this meeting, either by presenting a formal, introductory lecture, or by presenting a poster devoted to their more recent work. The invitation list was made up following suggestions of the scientific committee for this meeting, the members of which were:

Prof.Dr. B. Taccardi	(Parma; Italy)
Prof.Dr. F.A. Roberge	(Montreal; Canada)
Prof.Dr. A. van Oosterom	(Nijmegen; The Netherlands).

The organizing committee noted with great satisfaction that almost all people invited were indeed able to attend.

The book includes all invited papers as well as documents related to the posters presented. The editors have confined themselves to making minimal corrections and to arranging the contribution in a coherent way. This coherence is outlined in the chapter INTRODUCTION, which also represents the editors' views on the relevance of the various contributions. The responsibility for the scientific content of the various contributions lies entirely with the authors.

A major part of the symposium was devoted to a discussion on the present "state of the art" and on possible future developments. An extensive summary of this discussion is included in this book.

At the end of the discussion round a new society was founded:

THE INTERNATIONAL SOCIETY ON CARDIAC POTENTIAL MAPPING

The main objectives of this society will be to work towards the standardization of recording- and display methods which will promote the exchange of data and which will stimulate the introduction of mapping techniques for clinical diagnostic applications.

I hope and trust that this book will serve the same purpose.

R.Th. van Dam
Chairman of the
Organizing Committee

ORGANIZATION OF THE 3RD INTERNATIONAL SYMPOSIUM ON BODY SURFACE MAPPING

The symposium was organized by the Department of Cardiology at the University Hospital 'Sint Radboud' Nijmegen, The Netherlands, under the auspices of the International Council on Electrocardiology.

Organizing Committee:

R.Th. van Dam (chairman)
G.J.H. Uijen
Mrs. E. Piersma (secretariat)
W. IJsenbrandt
Mrs. J. Koot (University Congress Office)

Scientific Committee:

Prof. Dr. A. van Oosterom (Nijmegen)
Prof. F.A. Roberge (Montreal)
Prof. B. Taccardi (Parma)

INTERNATIONAL COUNCIL ON ELECTROCARDIOLOGY

President : I. RUTTKAY-NEDECKY, Czechoslovakia

Vice president : R.Th. VAN DAM, The Netherlands

Honorary Members: V. LAUFBERGER, Czechoslovakia; H. PIPBERGER, U.S.A.; O. SCHMITT, U.S.A.

Members : H. ABEL, F.R.G.; P. d'ALCHÉ, France;
R. AMIROV, U.S.S.R.; Z. ANALOCZY, Hungary;
G. ARENESCU, Rumania; A.J. BAYES DE LUNA, Spain;
K. HARUMI, Japan; F. KORNREICH, Belgium;
P. MACFARLANE, United Kingdom. F. DE PADUA, Portugal;
Z. PAVLOV, Bulgaria; J.C. RIOS, U.S.A.;
E. SCHUBERT, G.D.R.; B. TACCARDI, Italy;
H. UEDA, Japan; R. WENGER, Austria;
P. RAUTAKARJU, Canada.

The Symposium has been sponsored by:

Astra
Eli Lilly
Interspace
Knoll
Portanje
Smith Kline
Vitratron

CONTENTS page

INTRODUCTION

A. van Oosterom, R.Th. van Dam

The contributions of the participants to the symposium have been arranged by us in 6 parts.

In part one some papers are included which deal with the general aspects of mapping and with mapping in normals. This part is opened (chapter 1) by a contribution by the founding father of the mapping technique: Prof. B. Taccardi from Parma, Italy, who introduces the mapping techniques and presents his views on "present and future" of electrocardiographic body surface potential mapping. In chapter 2 the main map features of normals of different sex, age and body habitus. Chapter 3 is a contribution of a relatively new group, who discuss the features of the maps in new born normals. In chapter 4 an attempt is made to interprete body surface potentials in terms of the timing of epicardial breakthrough. This illustrates the interest in the mapping technique as an entry to cardiac electrophysiology. Recently several groups have been involved in solving the implied so called "INVERSE PROBLEM", the solution of which would enable one to compute cardiac phenomena from observed surface potentials. More on this topic is included in part 6 of this book.

In part two a number of papers discuss the application of body surface potential mapping to the diagnosis of Myocardial Infarction (M.I.). This includes papers on mapping in the acute stage (chapter 5), the detection of old anterior M.I. (chapter 6), criteria for the quantification of an infarct as deduced from computer simulations (chapter 7), a critical evaluation of usefulness of mapping in M.I. (chapter 8) and a comparison between the diagnostic performance of maps versus that of standard ECG/VCG methods, both read by the cardiologist (chapter 9).

One of the most promising applications of the mapping techniques is the class of conduction abnormalities. Being of an electrical nature the mapping technique is the obvious choice. This category is treated in part three. Two chapters (10 and 11) discuss the application of mapping to solve the riddles posed by the various bundle branch blocks in combination with other cardiac malfunctioning. In the next two chapters (12 and 13) the WPW syndrome is diagnosed by mapping. The cited reference list in these two papers is by no means complete. See e.g. (1) and (2). Ventricular tachycardia is tackled with mapping techniques in chapters 14 and 15. The concept of Wilson's Ventricular Gradient has lead to an analysis of the activation of the heart in terms of time integrals of the signals recorded at the various electrodes. The application of maps of the values of these integrals to the analysis of premature ventricular beats is presented in chapter 16. The final chapter in this group (chapter 17) deals with pseudo-ischemic T waves.

Body surface maps may be derived from different numbers of leads applied to the thorax. Some groups base their maps on as few as 24 electrodes, others use as many as 240. The technical problems involved in recording, storing and displaying the data have now been overcome by advances in the fields of electronics and computer science. This still leaves the problem of how many electrodes should be used, where they should be placed and how the maps should be presented. These problems have been amply discussed during the meeting (see: DISCUSSION). The different approaches that are in use at the moment, and the variety of opinions on this subject may be learned from the papers included in part four. Chapters 18 and 19 present the Parma system, chapters 20 and 21 present comparable approaches towards reaching a common data format which will ultimately facilitate the exchange of data between groups. The problem of display of the recorded maps are treated in chapters 22 and 23.

After the introduction of the Body Surface Map it was hoped that by just looking at the (sequence of) maps the nature of the cardiac disease or disorder would be clear. It has now become very clear that this is by no means true in general. This has called for the support of statistical methods in separating different diagnostic categories. The lack of a sufficiently large data base has inspired the search for appropriate methods for data analysis and data reduction. These approaches are discussed in part 5. The use of orthogonal expansions (principal components, Karhunen Loève expansions, singular vectors) are treated in chapters 24 to

26. All authors seem to be unaware of the work of Damen (3) who was the first one to introduce the Singular Value Decomposition in the field of electrocardiography. Time integration of the observed signals as a means of data reduction is used in chapter 27. In any evaluation of the gain in diagnostic performance which might arise from the larger number of leads in a mapping system as compared to the standard ECG lead systems, the features used in the statistical analysis should be comparable. At least this is claimed in chapter 28. When this principle was applied to a particular diagnostic category no advantage of the additional category could be demonstrated.
One way of expanding body surface maps is to use a polynomial expansion on a cylindrical surface. This is demonstrated in chapter 29. In order to keep the participants close to the more classical clinical practice some experts in the field of VCG had been invited to this "mappers den". Their contributions are contained in chapters 30 and 31.

In the final part: <u>part six</u>, various model studies are presented. Such studies can be classed as either FORWARD, or INVERSE model studies. In FORWARD studies the electrical properties of the heart as an electrical generator are assumed to be known as well as the properties of the surrounding medium in terms of electrical conductivity. This enables the <u>computation</u> of body surface potentials based on these assumptions. INVERSE studies start off on an assumed forward model and concentrate on the problem of deducing the electrical state of the heart from the <u>observed</u> body surface potentials. Chapter 32 gives a very clear introduction to the forward problem in general with a special application to the WPW syndrome. The authors seem to have overlooked some comparable work that has recently appeared in the literature (1,2) as well as some fine work which was done in Halifax (Nova Scotia) as early as 1972 (4). Chapter 33 demonstrates the effect of inhomogeneities in the electrical conductivity in a model composed of (concentric) spheres. The interested reader may be well advised to also consult reference 25 of chapter 33, in which a more realistic geometry is treated. The inverse approach to epicardial potentials is also included in this book. Chapter 34 demonstrates the power of this technique (see also reference 4 of the same chapter 34).
One of the basic forward problems which allows an analytical solution is the case in which the source is a dipole and the volume conductor is a

homogeneous cylinder. Chapter 35 draws the attention to an error in the Okada formula for this case and presents the correct answer. Chapter 36 is another example of a forward study. It uses a propagation model for the spread of activation in a heart composed of numerous units and a homogeneous volume conductor having a realistic geometry. As such this study is comparable to several earlier studies (see e.g. 4,5). The final chapter attempts to use the residual between observed potentials and computed potentials as a means to establish the non-dipolar contribution of the observed body surface potentials, which is in turn used for diagnostic purposes. The implied model of sources and volume conductor is of an extreme symplicity: a dipole in a homogeneous semi-infinite space, at the boundary of which the potentials are compared.

NOMENCLATURE

We would like to use this opportunity to clarify some of the terms used in the material contained in this book and to make some suggestions regarding future nomenclature.

The main topic of this book is the study of the potential distribution at the torso surface generated by the electrical activity of the heart. A map of the potential distribution at any given time instant may be called either a

body surface potential map (BSPM)

or, for short, a

body surface map (BSM).

Clearly, in "BSM" the nature of the map, i.e. that it is a map of the electrical potential values over the torso, and the origin, i.e. being generated by the heart (electrocardiographic), is lost.
A map of any scalar function over a surface may be displayed by a number of techniques (see chapter 23). One possible technique is the use of isofunction lines, in this case being isopotential lines. Other techniques (grey scale, colour displays) are just as easily used these days. This demonstrates (we hope) that the use of the term isopotential map should be abolished completely, it is a map of the body surface potential (distribution) that one is interested in and hence should be called BSM or BSPM.

An even stronger objection should be raised against the multitude of different, very imprecise terms which are used (also in this book) to refer to the map which results from time integration of the potentials (signals) recorded at the electrodes of a mapping system.
Maps of the distribution of the values of these integrals over the body surface may, again, be plotted by using either isofunction (iso-integral) lines or a grey scale, or a colour coding.
Such a map should be called a

time integral map (TIM), or,
integral map (IM) .

Often the timespan over which the integration has been carried out is of importance. In such cases the terms to be used should be

QRS-integral map , or,
QRST-integral map .

The reader is invited to see for him/herself how many different terms are used in this book to refer to a time integral map, or to a QRS(T) integral map and to work out for him/herself why these should be replaced by the terms suggested here.
The very worst in this respect is the term "iso-area map" (to be printed in invisible ink). This is a complete misnomer which causes a lot of confusion by seeming to refer to a map of equal areas (of what?); nonsense! Such maps should be called

integral maps , or,
QRS(T) integral maps .

REFERENCES

1. Macchi E, Bonatti V, di Cola G, Marmiroli D, Musso E, Nicoli F, Stilli D, Taccardi B: A solution of the Inverse Problem in Terms of Single or Multiple Dipoles in a Homogeneous Torso Model. In: Advances in Body Surface Potential Mapping, eds. K. Yamada, K. Harumi, T. Musha. Univ. of Nagoya Press, Nagoya, 1983.
2. Sippens Groenewegen A, Spekhorst HHM, Reek EJ: A quantitative method for the localization of the ventricular pre-excitation area in the WPW syndrome using Singular Value Decomposition. J. Electrocardiology 18/2, 157-168, 1985.

3. Damen AA, van der Kam J: The use of the singular value decomposition in electrocardiology. Med. & Biol. Eng. & Comput. 20, 473-482, 1982.
4. Ritsema van Eck HJ: Digital Computer Simulation of Cardiac excitation and repolarization in man. Thesis. Dalhousie University, Nova Scotia, 1972.
5. Miller WT, Geselowitz DB: Simulation studies of the electrocardiogram: I. The normal heart. Circ. Res. 43/2, 301-315, 1978.

PART 1

N O R M A L S

Chapter 1

PRESENT AND FUTURE OF BODY SURFACE ELECTROCARDIOGRAPHIC MAPPING

B. TACCARDI

1. INTRODUCTION

The spread of excitation through the human atria and ventricles and the subsequent recovery process give rise to a three-dimensional, time-varying distribution of intra- and extra-cardiac bioelectric currents. A three-dimensional potential field is associated with the current distribution. To obtain a complete picture of the cardiac electric field we must measure the potential distribution in the cavities of the heart, on the endocardial surface, in the thickness of the walls, on the epicardial surface, in the extracardiac conducting media and on the surface of the body.

The traditional procedures, which consist of measuring local potential changes at a limited number of sites on the body surface or in the heart, yield only partial information.

2. METHODS

2.1. Procedure and instrumentation for recording and displaying cardiac electric fields.

In recent years considerable advances have been achieved in the mapping of cardiac fields. Instruments have been built in many laboratories, that enable the heart potentials to be recorded and digitized almost simultaneously from up to 256 points. Clinical, mobile instruments are commercially available which record heart potentials from 28 to 128 points. These instruments can be used both in medical wards and at surgery. All the mapping machines essentially perform the same operations. The electric signals recorded from the body surface or from the heart are amplified, sampled, digitized, stored on disc or tape and displayed on line in the form of multiple electrograms for quality control. Further processing yields different types of maps, which are described below.

2.2. Types of maps.

2.2.1. Equipotential contour maps illustrate the instantaneous potential distribution in the area explored. This is achieved by measuring the voltage reached by all the electrocardiograms at one time instant and by writing the values on a table or matrix representing the electrode array. Equipotential lines are then drawn automatically, usually by linear interpolation. The procedure is repeated for every instant during the PQRSTU interval.

2.2.2. Iso-integral contour maps are obtained by computing the time integral of each electro(cardio)gram and by writing the values on a table or matrix. The integration can be extended to the entire QRST interval or to part of it. The further steps of the procedure are as in 2.2.1.

2.2.3. Departure Maps (1) represent the difference between an "average" map relating to a normal population and an individual map under examination. By dividing each local value in the departure map by the relevant standard deviation one obtains the departure index map (2) which shows the areas where the pattern under study significantly differs from the normal average.

2.2.4. Isochrone contour maps depict the sequence of excitation on the heart surface or in the heart walls. They are usually obtained by determining the time of occurrence of the negative peak in the first derivative of the unipolar QRS complex. In other cases they are obtained by plotting the time of occurrence of the spike in the bipolar epicardial, endocardial or intramural electrograms. More recently, attempts have been made to map the sequence of recovery and also the local duration of excitation, on the assumption that the time of occurrence of the positive peak in the first derivative of the unipolar T wave is a good index of local recovery time (3).

3. EXPERIMENTAL AND CLINICAL APPLICATIONS OF ELECTROCARDIOGRAPHIC MAPPING.

3.1. Experimental studies.

During the last two decades the mapping of cardiac fields has become a widely used experimental method. Equipotential, isointegral and isochrone contour maps have been obtained in experimental animals, both in normal conditions and after inducing conduction disturbances or local ischemia. Heart potentials have been mapped in the ventricular cavities, on the endocardial surface, in the thickness of the ventricular walls, on the epicardial surface and in three-dimensional conducting volumes surrounding isolated hearts. These studies have considerably improved our understanding of the cardiac electric field, particularly as regards the anisotropy of the excitation wavefront as a current generator (4,5).

3.2. Electrocardiographic maps in humans.

In humans, intracavitary, endocardial, epicardial and body surface maps are used more and more frequently for diagnostic and research purposes. In this report we will limit the discussion to body surface mapping in humans.

3.2.1. Body Surface Maps in humans. It is widely recognized that body surface maps provide more information on the electrical activity of the heart, both normal and abnormal, than can be obtained from the standard 12 lead electrocardiogram. The diagnostic value of BSMs is due to the fact that when the intracardiac electrical events are altered, significant changes in the surface field often occur in areas which are not sampled by the 12 leads. In other cases, the changes are present in the 12 leads, but their significance becomes apparent only when the local signals are compared with the rest of the field.

3.2.2. Interpretation of B.S.M. For many years, BSMs have been interpreted by visual inspection. The trajectory of maxima and minima on the chest surface, the time and location of their appearance and disappearance and their peak values were used for interpreting potential patterns in terms of intracardiac events and for detecting abnormalities. The above criteria were used to describe maps in normal individuals and heart patients with acute and old myocardial infarction, ischemia, atrial or ventricular enlargements and conduction disturbances. These early investigations showed that BSMs could detect myocardial infarction or ischemia in patients with normal 12 lead ECG, and revealed different types of ventricular hypertrophy, atrial enlargement and local conduction disturbances; however, the papers published between 1960 and 1975 were mostly descriptive and did not assess the sensitivity and specificity of the method (6,7,8,9). During the last decade, attempts have been made to evaluate the diagnostic performance of maps more accurately. To this end, BSMs have been systematically compared with ventriculograms, coronary angiograms, radionuclide imaging etc., to assess the correlation between map data and other independent evidence of heart disease. Moreover, large data bases have been collected, particularly for normal populations (10). This is indispensable for determining the normal variability range of BSM.

Some of the recent studies still utilize the trajectories of maxima and minima as diagnostic parameters. Thus, in 26 out of 32 cases of anterior myocardial infarction with normal ECG, the trajectories of the potential minimum were abnormal and correlated well with the location of the asynergy (11). Similar findings were obtained in 24 cases of inferior myocardial infarction with normal 12 lead ECG (12). In angina patients with normal resting ECG de Ambroggi et al observed a typically abnormal location of the ST minimum in about one half of the patients (13). During exercise tests, BSMs were superior to 12 lead ECG recordings and suggested optimal electrode location for detecting ischemic changes (14). Also, in old myocardial infarction with superimposed ischemia, exercise maps provided significant information on the location of the ischemic areas (15). Finally, the trajectory of the maxima revealed the location of focal right bundle branch block in children after surgical repair of congenital heart diseases (16).

Quantitative analysis has been recently applied to BSM with interesting results. Peak potential values and the integral of the potential function extended to the entire chest surface have been combined in a multivariate statistical analysis to reveal myocardial infarctions, left ventricular hypertrophy and myocardial ischemia in 42 patients with left bundle branch block, while these conditions were undetectable from the 12 lead electrocardiogram (17). The same parameters, combined with the location of the ST minimum, enabled myocardial ischemia to be detected in 80% of angina patients with normal resting ECG (unpublished observation).

Iso-integral contour maps have the advantage of summarizing the map information relating to the entire QRST interval, or parts of this interval, into one map. Iso-integral maps, departure maps and departure index maps have provided information on the location and size of myocardial infarctions (2) and also revealed old myocardial infarctions in patients with normal ECG (18). Right ventricular involvement in acute, inferior myocardial infarction has been detected by means of iso-integral maps relating to the first half of QRS (19).

The number of variables contained in equipotential contour maps or in isoarea maps is too high for statistical analysis. A promising procedure for selecting those variables that have the highest discriminant power has been introduced by Lux et al. and Evans et al. in 1981 (20,21). Every instantaneous map is expressed as a linear combination of 12 fundamental maps (eigenvectors) which are the same for the entire population. Thus, 12 coefficients replace the 192 instantaneous potential values. The 12 waveforms that depict the temporal variation of the 12 coefficients during QRST can also be expressed as linear combinations of 12 (for QRS) plus 6 (for ST-T) fundamental waveforms. In this way any complete sequence of maps relating to the QRST interval can be reconstructed from 216 coefficients (12 x (12 + 6)). This number is still too high for statistical analysis. However, only those coefficients need be considered that exhibit significant between/within groups variance ratios. Also, the selected coefficients may be used to construct "departure" maps whose configuration may help interpreting the abnormal maps in terms of intracardiac electrical events. This approach, combined with the limited lead system developed by the same authors, looks promising for making clinical mapping more practical and workable.

Another promising approach which, however, is not yet ready for clinical use, consists in solving the "inverse problem" for an individual patient (22). By means of appropriate transfer coefficients and regularization procedures it is possible to calculate epicardial maps and epicardial electrograms non invasively from body surface potentials. To this end, the geometry of the torso must be measured and the location of the heart in the chest must be assessed from X ray pictures. The location of pre-excited areas and the site of origin of stimulated beats has been successfully determined with the inverse procedure in a few patients.

4. CONCLUSION AND FUTURE PERSPECTIVES OF BSM.

Body surface maps provide more information on the electrical activity of the heart than can be obtained from the 12 lead ECG. Despite this advantage, BSMs are not yet widely used as a diagnostic tool for the following reasons:

1) Lack of standardization. In all laboratories the basic procedure is the same, but the thoracic area explored is different and the number of electrodes varies between 16 and 256. This prevents comparing results and creating a common data base for statistical evaluation of new material.

2) Equipment. The equipment is comparatively expensive. It often lacks flexibility, which is indispensable for implementing all the new methods for map analysis that continuously appear in the literature. Data exchange with external computers for more sophisticated processing, population studies, etc. is often difficult. Maps are generally obtained on line but in many cases quality control, averaging, graphic display and extraction of data for further analysis are still too slow.

3) Application of electrodes is time-consuming: the spatial coordinates of the electrodes are rarely measured and this prevents applying inverse computations.

4) Analysis of data is not standardized. A number of different criteria are used, which have been discussed in this article. Sensitivity and specificity data are seldom available in the papers published so far.

The above difficulties can be overcome by a cooperative effort of all the research centers involved in body surface mapping. The availability of low-cost, powerful microcomputers with large memories can be a decisive factor in this respect.

Supported in part by grant n. 83.00564.57 of the Italian National Research Council, Special Project on Bioengineering and by a grant of the Ministry of Education to the author.

REFERENCES

1. Flowers NC, Horan LG, Johnson JC: Anterior infarctional changes occurring during mid and late ventricular activation detectable by surface mapping technique. Circulation 54:906, 1976
2. Tonooka J et al: Isointegral analysis of body surface maps for the assessment of location and size of myocardial infarction. Am J Cardiol 52:1174, 1983
3. Millar CK, Kralios FA, Lux RL: Correlation between refractory periods and activation recovery intervals from electrograms; effects of rate and adrenergic interventions. Circulation. In press
4. Corbin LV, Scher AM: The canine heart as an electrocardiographic generator. Circ Res 41:58, 1977
5. Colli-Franzone P et al: Potential fields generated by oblique dipole layers modeling excitation wavefronts in the anisotropic myocardium. Circ Res 51:330, 1982
6. Taccardi B: Distribution of heart potentials on the thoracic surface of normal human subjects. Circ Res 12:341, 1963
7. Taccardi B et al: Characteristic features of surface potential maps during QRS and S-T intervals. In Rush S and Lepeschkin, editors: Body surface mapping of cardiac fields (Adv Cardiol 10, Karger, Basel, 1974)
8. Taccardi B, de Ambroggi L, Viganotti C: Body surface mapping of heart potentials. In Nelson CV and Geselowitz DB, editors: The theoretical basis of electrocardiology, Clarendon Press, Oxford, 1976
9. Blumenschein SD et al: Genesis of body surface potentials in varying types of right ventricular hypertrophy. Circulation 39:917, 1968
10. Green LS et al: Effects of age, sex and body habitus on QRS and ST-T potential maps of 1100 normal subjects. Circulation 71:244, 1985
11. Hirai M et al: Body surface isopotential maps in old anterior myocardial infarction undetectable by 12-lead electrocardiograms. Am Heart J 108:975, 1984
12. Osugi J et al: Body surface isopotential maps in old inferior myocardial infarction undetectable by 12 lead electrocardiogram. J Electrocardiol 17:55, 1984.
13. de Ambroggi L et al: Electromaps during ventricular recovery in angina patients with normal resting ECG. In Abel H, and Pavlov Z, editors: Electrocardiology II. Adv Cardiol 19, Karger Basel, 1977
14. Simoons ML, Block P: Toward the optimal lead system and optimal criteria for exercise electrocardiography. Am J Cardiol 47:1366, 1981
15. Tavazzi L et al: Can body surface mapping improve the diagnostic power of standard electrocardiography in effort ischemia? Symposium on diagnosis of myocardial ischemia in man. Pisa, Abstract No 14, 1985
16. Liebman J et al: The spectrum of right bundle branch block as manifested in electrocardiographic body surface potential maps. J Electrocardiol 17: 329, 1984
17. Musso E et al: Discrimination among different groups of LBBB patients by means of body surface maps, 11th International Congress on electrocardiology, Caen, (Abstract p 108), 1984
18. Bertoni T et al: Body surface potential maps in patients with old myocardial infarction and normal ECG. Time-integral analysis of surface potentials, 11th International Congress on Electrocardiology, Caen, (Abstract p 105), 1984

19. Montague TJ et al: Body surface electrocardiographic mapping in inferior myocardial infarction. Circulation 67:665, 1983
20. Lux RL et al: Redundancy reduction for improved display and analysis of body surface potential maps. I. Spatial compression. Circ Res 49:186, 1981
21. Evans AK et al: Redundancy reduction for improved display and analysis of body surface potential maps II: Temporal compression. Circ Res 49:197, 1981
22. Colli Franzone P et al: A mathematical procedure for solving the inverse potential problem of electrocardiography. Analysis of the time-space accuracy from "in vitro" experimental data. Math Biosc. In press

Chapter 2

FEATURES OF BODY SURFACE POTENTIAL MAPS FROM A LARGE NORMAL POPULATION

L.S. GREEN, R.L. LUX, C.W. HAWS, M.J. BURGESS, J.A. ABILDSKOV

INTRODUCTION

Clinical use of body surface potential maps requires some means of quantitative comparison and classification. Visual inspection of maps is only qualitative and use of models to predict cardiac sources is based on incomplete information that has had limited success in clinical use. In our laboratory, we have developed a method of map analysis that represents map data as a set of temporal and spatial basis functions common to all maps and 216 coefficients unique to each individual map (1,2). These 216 coefficients can be used with common statistical techniques to compare individual maps or groups of maps classified by independent clinical methods. The details of this method of quantitative map analysis are discussed in another chapter. Since the method involves the statistical comparison of map features, it requires definition of the range of potential patterns in a large population of normal subjects. This chapter describes body surface map features of over 800 normal subjects in relation to age, sex and body habitus and is intended to provided the basis for diagnostic studies involving body surface potential mapping.

STUDY POPULATION

Characteristics of the normal population used in this study are shown in table 1. Subjects were classified by sex, age and body habitus. Definitions of body habitus type are shown at the bottom of the table. The criteria were based on tables of height, weight and wrist size. All of the subjects were clinically normal as determined by detailed medical history, physical exam, normal 12 lead ECG and normal blood chemistries. All subjects were normotensive, none had a history of chest pain and none were taking medication at the time of mapping. All maps in this group of subjects were taken using the 32 lead array reported from our laboratory (3,4). Because of the characteristics of the population in our area, all of the subjects were caucasian. All subjects gave informed consent for the mapping procedure. For analysis, maps were grouped by subject age decade and into groups based on subject sex and body habitus.

TABLE 1
BODY HABITUS

Age (yr)	S	A	M	V	No. E	TOTAL SUBJECTS subjects
Male Subjects						
10-19	24	16	2	1	0	43
20-29	53	82	20	7	0	162
30-39	17	54	40	6	0	117
40-49	2	21	14	9	0	46
50-59	3	16	12	1	0	32
60-69	2	10	5	2	0	19
70-79	0	2	2	0	0	4
80-89	1	0	0	0	0	1
						424
Female Subjects						
10-19	16	36	3	1	0	56
20-29	22	81	38	7	0	148
30-39	8	66	26	8	0	108
40-49	2	23	15	5	2	47
50-59	0	14	14	5	1	34
60-69	0	6	8	1	0	15
70-79	1	2	1	0	0	4
80-89	0	0	0	0	0	0
						412

S = slender (10 pounds or more less than ideal weight); A = average weight; M = moderately overweight (+20-40 pounds; V = very overweight (+50-99 pounds); E = extremely overweight (+>100 pounds)

MAP PROCESSING AND ANALYSIS

To identify those map features that were important in discriminating between each pair of map classes, a new technique of map analysis was developed. Since each subject map was accurately represented by 216 parameters as well as common spatial and temporal bases, averages and variances of each of the 216 parameters were calculated to represent the "average map" for each class. Since the 216 parameters were independent, features that were significantly different between any pair of map classes could be identified with the simple t statistic at any chosen level of significance. Difference maps were constructed using only those coefficients of the 216 that were significantly different at the $p<.01$ level and a set of spatial and temporal basis vectors common to all subjects. We have designated this type of map a feature difference map. In this map display, only features that are significant in discriminating between two classes of maps are displayed as a sequence of potential distributions. More importantly, insignificant feature differences are excluded from resulting maps, thus yielding an enhanced display of the important discriminating information. This approach differs from conventional map subtraction techniques in which corresponding frames of time-aligned map sequences are subtracted and express all potential differences, whether significant or not.

FIGURE 1.

Selected frames from an average normal map compiled from all subjects aged 30-39 years. Isopotential lines are 0.1 mV apart during the QRS and 0.05 mV apart during the T wave. This and all subsequent maps are displayed as a cylinder unrolled from the right midaxillary line. Vertical lines superimposed on an electrocardiogram above each map indicate time during the cardiac cycle. The top of the grid is the level of the clavicles and bottom of the grid is the level of the umbilicus.

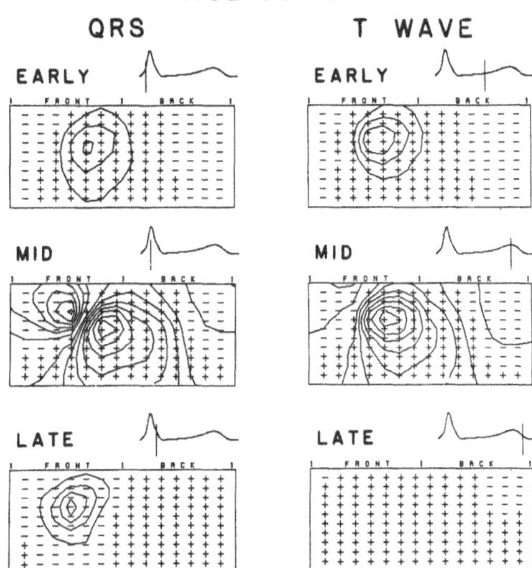

MAP FEATURES RELATED TO AGE, GENDER AND HABITUS

Figure 1 shows map frames from an average map of normal subjects in the decade aged 30-39 years. Frames from the early, mid and late QRS and ST-T wave are shown. Map features were similar to previously published maps of normal subjects. Average map features in the decade aged 10-19 years and the decade aged 20-29 years were similar. As age increased, peak recorded potentials tended to decrease slightly as illustrated in figure 2. Panel A of figure 2 shows a feature difference map obtained by subtracting significant map feature differences of the 20 to 29 year old group from those of the 10 to 19 year old group. Panel B illustrates a feature difference map obtained by subtracting significant map feature differences in the decade aged 30-39 average map from an average map of subjects aged 20-29. Representative frames from early, mid, and late QRS show few differences as indicated by the small number of isopotential lines. These feature difference maps show that the statistically significant difference in maps from age 10 to age 39 is a decrease in peak potentials recorded. Though illustrated only for the QRS, the decrease also occurred in the ST-T potentials. These decreases continued through age 80.

FIGURE 2.

A. A feature difference map constructed by subtracting statistically different map coefficients in subjects aged 20 to 29 from those in subjects aged 10 to 19. B. A similar feature difference map showing average feature differences between the 20 to 29 and 30 to 39 age group. Maps are displayed as in figure 1. The small number of isopotential lines indicates differences are small. These two examples show the gradual decrease in absolute value of recorded potentials with advancing age.

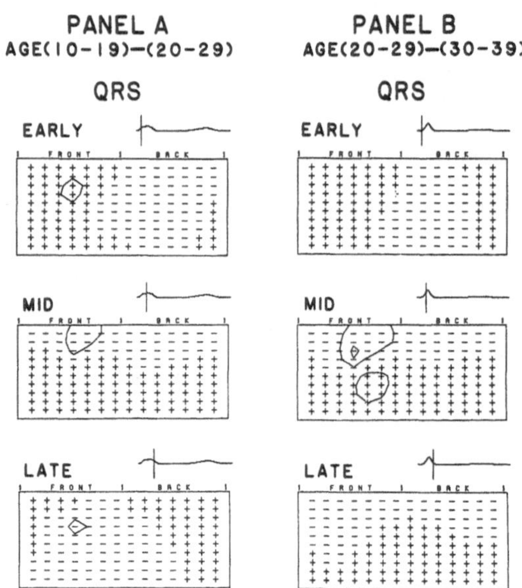

In normal subjects over age 40, two types of potential distributions were recorded which are shown in figure 3. About 2/3 of normal subjects showed a pattern similar to that of maps in younger subjects and these were designated group I. About 1/3 of normal subjects, designated group II, showed a different map pattern in which negative potentials were more widely distributed over the right hemithorax and there was a more vertically oriented null line. Map frames during the first 30 msec of the QRS are shown in figure 3. Gender and body habitus did not determine the pattern of maps in subjects over age 40 but the incidence of the group II pattern increased with age. 27% of subjects in the 50-59 year old group exhibited the group II pattern while 63% of subjects in the 60-69 year old group exhibited this finding. None of the group II subjects had left axis deviation on 12 lead ECG although the average axis of group II subjects was slightly more to the left than group I subjects. This map pattern is consistent with delayed conduction in the left anterior fascicle of the cardiac conduction system and is probably explained by the variable but progressive fibrosis of the intraventricular conduction system documented to occur with advancing age (5).

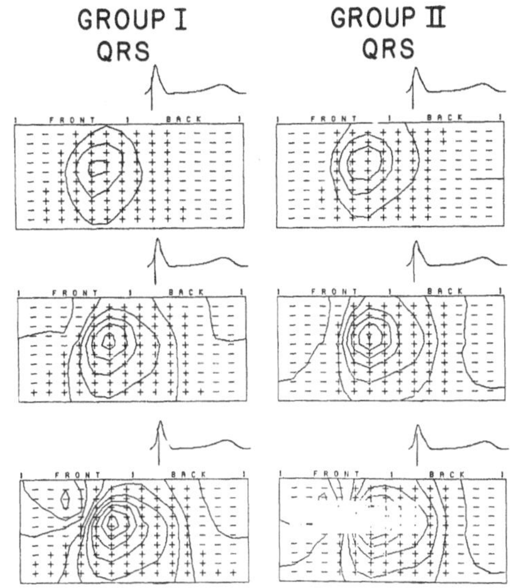

FIGURE 3.

Comparably timed average map frames at 5 msec intervals from early portions of the QRS are shown for two different groups of normal subjects over the age of 40. Group II is distinguished by greater anterior distribution area of negative potentials.

Representative map feature differences due to gender are shown in figure 4. Average maps were constructed for each male and female age group. Since there was nearly equal distribution of slender, medium and obese subjects in each group defined by age and sex, the groups were not further subdivided. Figure 4 shows a feature difference map constructed by subtraction of significantly different map coefficients in the 30 to 39 year old female group from the map coefficients in the 30 to 39 year old male group. There are few feature differences during the QRS but male subjects showed greater amplitude of T potentials. These differences between sexes were similar for all age decades and were apparent on maps for subjects over age 40 as well, irrespective of classification in group I or II. The physiologic basis for higher T potentials in males when there is little difference in QRS potentials is unknown.

FIGURE 4.

Feature difference map constructed by subtraction of statistically different map coefficients in normal female subjects 30 to 39 years old from those in normal male subjects 30 to 39 years old. Lack of isopotential lines during the QRS indicates little difference between maps for the two groups during QRS. T potentials were on average higher in men and this was also true in all other age groups.

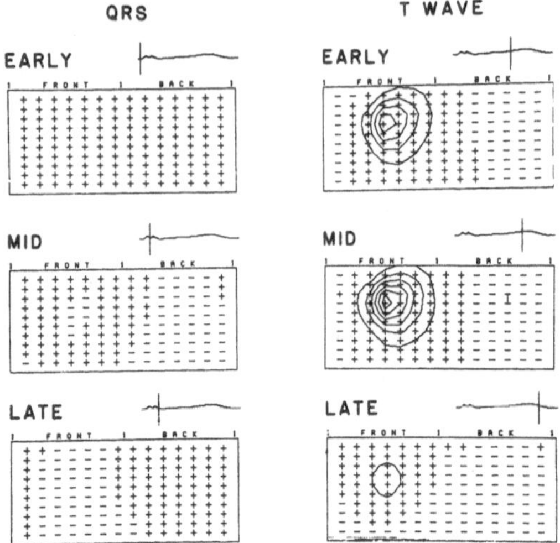

Map feature differences related to body habitus were examined in the same manner as differences due to gender. Figure 5 shows a feature difference map constructed by subtraction of statistically different map coefficients of obese men from slender men aged 30 to 39 years old. The horizontal null line between positive and negative poles is consistant with a more vertically oriented cardiac position in the slender males. T potentials revealed the same pattern during early repolarization with a slight increase in T potentials in the slender group. In female subjects, body habitus had minimal effects on body surface map features.

FIGURE 5.

Feature difference map constructed by subtraction of statistically different map coefficients of slender and obese men 30 to 39 years old. Horizontal null line between positive and negative poles is consistent with a more vertically oriented activation sequence. T potentials are not shown but revealed the same pattern during early repolarization.

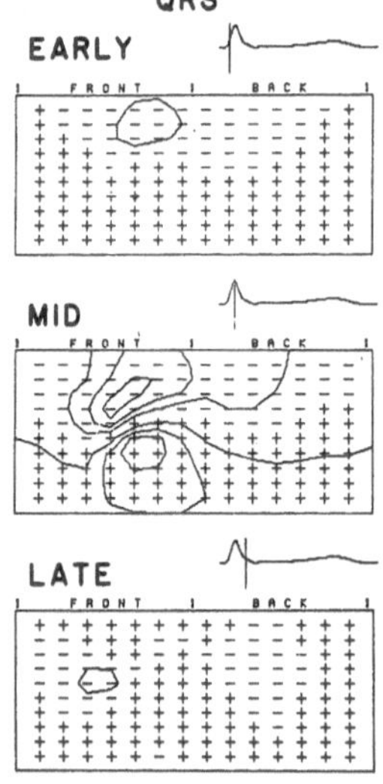

As illustrated in figure 6, locations of peak minimum and peak maximum during ventricular activation were constant for both sexes of all ages and body habitus types. In each age group, peak maximum and peak minimum were higher in males and declined in both sexes with increasing age as already noted.

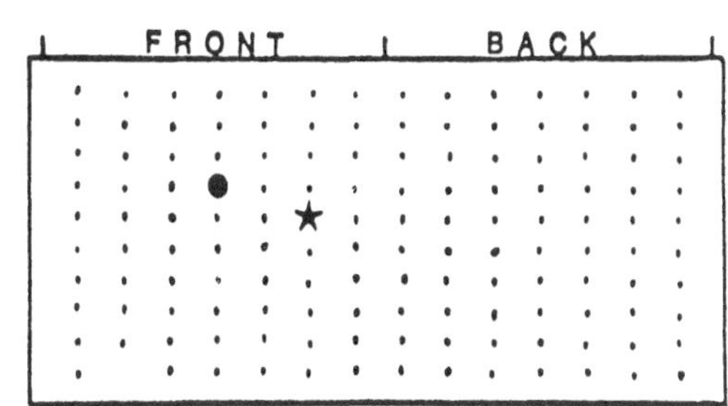

FIGURE 6.

Locations of the peak minimum (circle) and maximum (star)QRS potentials.

ST segment potentials in normal subjects were obtained by averaging the potential recorded at each electrode site for 80 msec after the manually selected end of QRS as determined from the rms voltage vs time curve of the entire map. These values for each electrode site were then averaged for all subjects in each age decade by sex. Figure 7 shows examples of average ST segment potential maps of men and women from the second through the seventh decade. Isopotential lines are displayed in 10 microvolt increments. In each decade, male subjects had higher precordial positive potentials. Female subjects, on average, tended to have more extensive negative potentials recorded during the first 80 msec of the ST segment, especially after age 40. Small negative potentials were recorded over an increasingly larger area of the precordium in women in the fourth and fifth decade. By the seventh decade, the area of negative potentials over the precordium increased in both men and women. All maps were recorded at rest and the significance of these findings in relation to exercise testing is not known.

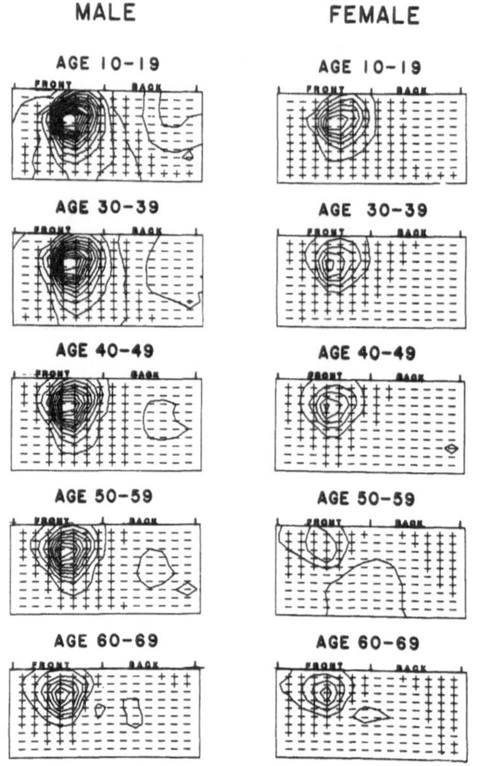

FIGURE 7.

Average ST potential maps for each sex in the age groups indicated. Average ST maps were constructed by averaging ST potential for 80 msec after the J point and then averaging all sites in each sex and age group. Isopotential lines represent 10μV increments. Female subjects over the age of 40 tended to have a greater distribution of precordial negative potentials until age 60 when distribution in male and female subjects was similar.

CLINICAL UTILITY OF MAPPING

The greater information content of body surface potential maps compared to the standard 12 lead electrocardiogram has been demonstrated in a variety of studies (6-13). This apparent advantage has not led to widespread use of the technique in diagnostic cardiology. This is due at least in part to the difficulty of applying the nearly 200 electrodes used in most centers and because of the previous lack of methods for quantitative map analysis. Work from our laboratory (3,4) and from Barr and co-workers (14) has shown that total thoracic distribution of cardiac potentials can be accurately estimated by selected, limited lead arrays of 32 or 24 electrodes. We have also developed a method of map representation that utilizes a set of basis functions common to all maps as well as 216 coefficients unique to each subject map (1,2). This method of map representation permits statistical comparison of the temporal and spatial features of body surface potential maps. Although this method of map representation and comparison is not based on a physiologic model, it does identify map features of discriminating value between groups of subjects categorized by independent means.

The 216 independent coefficients unique to each subject's map can be used to analyze maps at least two ways. One use, described in this chapter, involves grouping of subjects by clinical characteristics by any of a variety of independent means of diagnostic testing. Corresponding map coefficients from all subject maps in a particular diagnostic class are averaged and an average map for that class is constructed. Differences between average maps of different diagnostic classes can then be displayed by subtraction of only those map coefficients that differ to a statistically significant degree and then construction of a feature difference map using those coefficients. Map differences in feature difference maps can then be related to known electrophysiologic differences between the diagnostic groups of subjects. This type of comparison of average maps is somewhat limited by the fact that average maps are based on time normalized data and time alignment errors are possible.

The more important use of the 216 coefficient map descriptors is likely to be the statistical diagnostic classification of individual maps. This technique initially requires the classification of subjects by independent diagnostic testing to establish a training set of maps for each diagnostic group to be considered. Statistically significant map coefficients are identified for each training set that represents a particular cardiac disease under consideration. Coefficients from unclassified maps can then be compared with coefficents of each training set and with coefficients from a broad group of normal subject maps to diagnostically classify the maps. Accuracy of this technique of map classification is limited by the adequate representation of disease characteristics in each training set, the number of diagnostic categories available and adequate representation of all of the characteristics of normal maps. The effects of age, gender and body habitus decribed in this chapter have been presented in terms of average maps. In actual practice, the comparison technique described above requires comparison of an individual map in question with a large number of normal subject maps reflecting all of the effects of age, gender or body habitus as well as with maps reflecting characteristics of cardiac disease.

Our experience during acquisition of this large data base of normals suggests that a very large number of body surface potential maps can be recorded rapidly and quantitatively compared by mostly automated techniques. The recording and analysis system used is practical, however, the clinical diagnostic utility and limitations of this approach must be demonstrated by comparison of the large normal data base with maps from subjects with a variety of specific cardiac diseases defined by independent means.

Table and Figures reprinted by permission of the American Heart Association, Inc from: Green LS, Lux RL, Haws CW, Williams RR, Hunt SC and Burgess MJ: Effects of age, sex, and body habitus on QRS and ST-T potential maps of 1100 normal subjects. Circulation 71:244-253, 1985.

Supported by Program Project grant HL13480, the Nora Eccles Treadwell Foundation, the Richard A. and Nora Eccles Harrison Fund for Cardiovascular Research, and grants HL21088-07 and HL24855-05 from the National Heart, Lung and Blood Institute.

REFERENCES

1. Lux RL, Evans AK, Burgess MJ, Wyatt RF, and Abildskov JA: Redundancy reduction for improved display and analysis of body surface potential maps. I. Spatial Compression. Circ. Res. 49:186, 1981.
2. Evans AK, Lux RL, Burgess MJ, Wyatt RF, and Abildskov JA: Redundancy reduction for improved display and analysis of body surface potential maps. II. Temporal compression. Circ. Res. 49:197, 1981.
3. Lux RL, Burgess MJ, Wyatt RF, Evans AK, Vincent GM, and Abildskov JA: Clinically practical lead systems for improved electrocardiography: Comparison with precordial grids and conventional lead systems. Circulation 59:356, 1979.
4. Abildskov JA, Burgess MJ, Lux RL, Wyatt RF, and Vincent GM: The expression of normal ventricular repolarization in the body surface distribution of T potentials. Circulation 54-6:901, 1976.
5. Regoliosi G, Barone P, Ciarlini P, Guspini A, Macchi E, Musso E, Stilli D, Taccardi B: Interactive procedure for automated averaging of body surface maps. In Yamada K, Harumi K, Musha T, editors: Advances in body surface potential mapping. Nagoya, 1983, The University of Nagoya Press, p. 85.
6. Vincent GM, Abildskov JA, Burgess MJ, Millar K, Lux RL, Wyatt RF: Diagnosis of old inferior myocardial by body surface isopotential mapping. Am. J. Cardiol. 39:510, 1977.
7. Ohta T, Toyama J, Yamada K: Body surface map and vectorcardiographic correlation in old inferior myocardial infarction undetectable by 12 lead electrocardiogram. Circulation 66-II:377 1982.
8. DeAmbroggi L, Taccardi B, Macchi E: Body surface maps of heart potentials, tentative localization of pre-excited areas in forty-two Wolff-Parkinson-White patients. Circulation 54:251, 1976.
9. Yamada K, Toyama J, Wada M, Sugiyama S, Sugenoya J, Toyoshima H, Mizuno Y, Sotahata I, Kobayashi T, Okijima M: Body surface isopotential mapping in Wolff-Parkinson-White syndrome. Noninvasive method to determine the localization of the accessory atrio-ventricular pathway. Am. Heart J. 90:721, 1975.
10. Stilli D, Musso E, Macchi E, Taccardi B, Rolli A, Aurier E, Favaro L and Botti G: Diagnostic value of body surface maps in left bundle-branch block. Adv. Cardiol. 28:36, 1981.
11. Green, LS, Lux RL, Merchant MH, Burgess MJ, Sheinman MM, Vincent GM, Anderson JL, and Abildskov, JA: Identification of patients at risk of ventricular arrhythmias with body surface mapping. Circulation 66-II:377, 1982.
12. Vincent GM, Green LS, Lux RL, Merchant MH, and Abildskov JA: Use of QRST area distributions to predict vulnerability to cardiac death following myocardial infarction. Circulation 68-II:352, 1983.
13. Gardner MJ, Montague TJ, Horacek MB, Cameron DA, Flemington CS, Smith ER: Vulnerability to ventricular dysrhythmia: Assessment by body surface mapping. Circulation 64-IV:328, 1981.
14. Barr RC, Spach MS, Hermann-Giddens GS: Selection of the number and positions of measuring locations for electrocardiography. IEEE Trans Biomed Eng 18:125, 1971

Chapter 3

EVOLUTION OF BODY SURFACE POTENTIALS IN THE HEALTHY NEWBORN DURING THE FIRST WEEK OF LIFE

H. SPEKHORST, A. SIPPENS GROENEWEGEN, R.L. WILENSKY, R. SPAANS

1. INTRODUCTION

During the neonatal period a number of changes occur in the human cardiovascular system as the newborn child adapts to life outside the uterus. Non-invasive registration of the cardiac electrical activity in the early postnatal phase has been described (1-4). The conventional ECG is valuable in studying the neonatal cardiac rate and rhythm (3), a disadvantage of this method is that much of the spatial electrical information is missed. Body Surface Mapping has proven itself superior in this respect, but still very few researchers (1,2) have used this method to investigate the changes in Body Surface Potential (BSP) distribution during the first week of life of the normal newborn. Thus, we performed a qualitative analysis of the QRS Body Surface Maps (BSMs) of healthy neonates, obtained immediately after birth (serie A) and on the 6th or 7th day (serie B). In this study the emphasis lies on the spatial aspects of the BSP distribution during the ventricular activation sequence. Extreme presence, location and migration in three different time phases of the depolarization process (early, mid and late QRS) are the studied parameters.

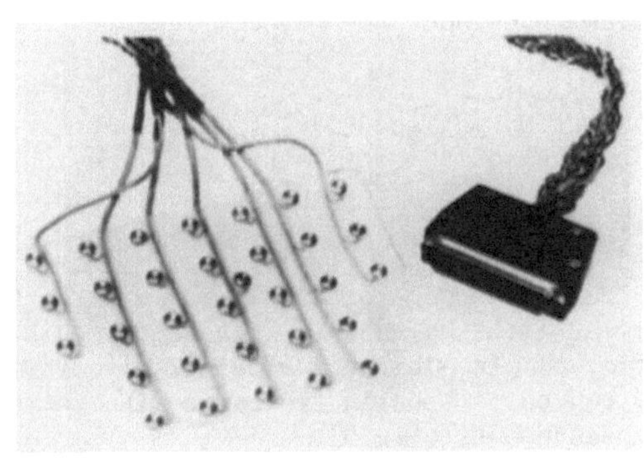

FIGURE 1. The silicon vest containing 32 electrodes.

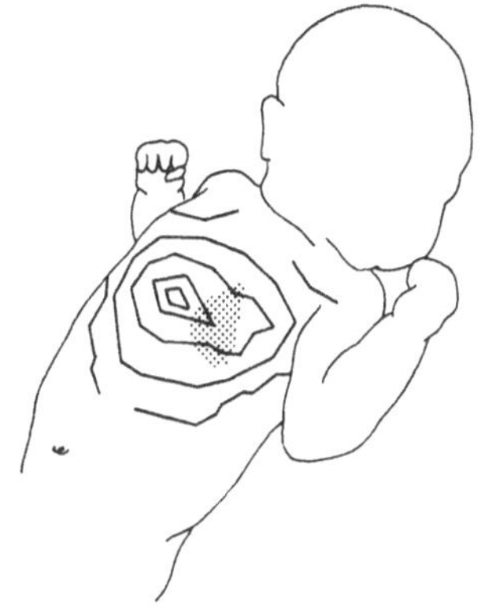

FIGURE 2. The projection of the potential distribution on the anterior thorax of a newborn infant.

2. MATERIALS AND METHODS

2.1. Patients

This study includes 21 healthy mature newborn infants with a birthweight ranging from 2420 to 4275 gram (10 males and 11 females). Physical examination revealed no evidence for heart disease. Parental informed consent was obtained postnatally. For each individual we made two measurements during sinus rhythm. The serie A recordings took place within 12 hours (mean 6h.) of a normal vaginal delivery during which the mother did not receive any medication. The serie B recordings were performed on the 6th day (5 cases) or on the 7th day after birth.

2.2. Data recording and processing

Our equipment consists of a recently described (5) data acquisition system for which we designed a flexible limited lead array suited for neonates (fig.1). The silicon vest containing the 32 uniformly positioned Ag/AgCl electrodes covered the entire anterior thorax and upper abdomen with the left and right midaxillary lines as lateral boundaries (fig.2). The ECG signals were simultaneously recorded with Wilson central terminal as a reference and with a sampling rate of 1000 Hz. Floppy disks were used for data storage. The fast electrode application enabled the recording procedure to be completed within 5 minutes. During measurement the infants were mostly asleep and showed relaxed tidal volume respiration.

After recording, digital noise filtering was performed. When necessary, bad quality signals were rejected and replaced by the mean value of the surrounding lead signals. Baseline adjustment was done by linear interpolation by choosing a point before the P wave and after the T wave. Via a plotting program the BSMs were then reproduced at 1 msec intervals. Equipotential lines were drawn by linear interpolation. Depending on the peak value of the potential extremes in the regarded time instant the amplitude difference between the two equipotential lines varies. Further details can be found in the legend of fig 3.

3. RESULTS

An example of the BSP distribution throughout the QRS complex of serie A and serie B are shown in figure 3 and 4.

3.1. Early QRS

The serie A showed an initial anterior maximum (max) (fig.3a) appearing at the right parasternal, the midsternal or the left parasternal region in 5, 8 and 8 cases respectively. With the serie B recordings the initial max (fig.4a) occurred in the right parasternal, the midsternal and left parasternal region in 1, 8 and 12 cases respectively. During the first week, in 9 cases the initial max moved more leftward, in 10 cases the initial max presented in a similar location, and in 2 cases the initial max appeared more rightward (fig. 6). In addition, a transitory minimum (min) at the lower left axillary region is seen in two cases with serie A and in 10 cases with the serie B measurements (fig.5).

3.2. Mid QRS

The max increased in amplitude and showed an extension towards the lower left axillary area (fig.3b and 4b). Thereafter the main min appeared in the upper left region of the anterior thorax (fig.3b and 4c), both in serie A and in serie B, although the precise location is different (fig.7). In 8 cases the min appears at the same region, in 10 cases the min appears more leftward and in 3 cases more rightward on the anterior thorax.

After the main min had appeared either a pseudopod (fig.3c) or a saddle was found in all cases of serie A. In 12 cases a pseudopod was followed by a saddle, in 5 cases only a pseudopod, and in 4 cases only a saddle was noted. With serie B neither a pseudopod nor a saddle was found in one

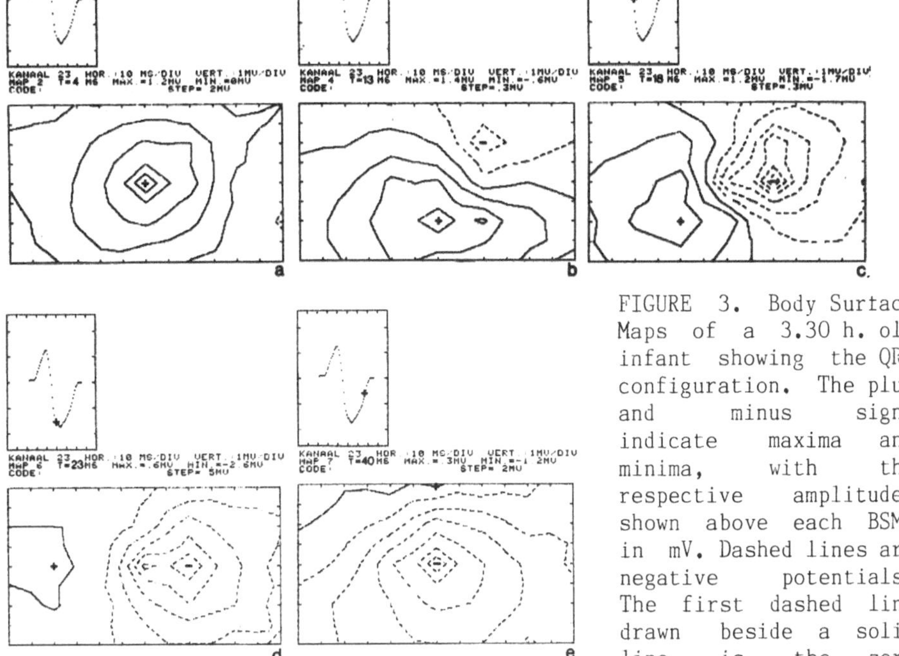

FIGURE 3. Body Surface Maps of a 3.30 h. old infant showing the QRS configuration. The plus and minus signs indicate maxima and minima, with the respective amplitudes shown above each BSM, in mV. Dashed lines are negative potentials. The first dashed line drawn beside a solid line is the zero potential. The step between two equipotential lines, the magnitude of the amplitude difference between two lines, can be seen in the legend above each BSM. The time instant, in which the BSM was determined is indicated in lead (kanaal) 23, a left precordial lead. Note the characteristic migration pattern of the maximum throughout the depolarization sequence.

case, in 13 cases a pseudopod followed by a saddle was evident, in 3 cases only a pseudopod, and in 4 cases only a saddle appeared.

With both series the min increased in voltage and expanded to cover the left anterior thorax while the max moved towards the lower right axillary region (fig.3d and 4d).

3.3. Late QRS

In serie A the max moved to the right subclavicular region in 11 cases forming a terminal max (fig.3e). In 10 cases the max disappeared at the lower right axillary region and subsequently a new terminal max appeared in 7 cases at the right subclavicular region. In 3 cases no terminal max was found. With serie B, in 9 cases the max moved to the right subclavicular region becoming the terminal max. In 12 cases the max disappeared at the lower right axillary region and in 3 cases a new terminal max was noted at the right subclavicular region, and in 2 cases at the lower left axillary region. In 7 cases no terminal max was seen (fig.4f).

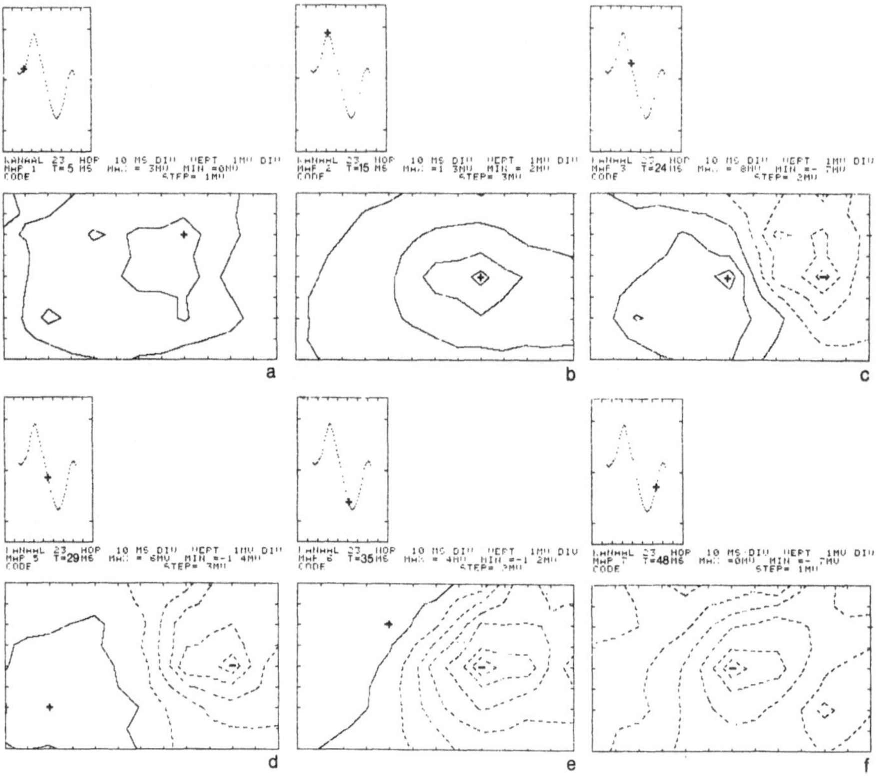

FIGURE 4. The QRS body surface map of the same child as in figure 3, in this case recorded 7 days after birth. Notice the slight differences in extreme position during ventricular excitation.

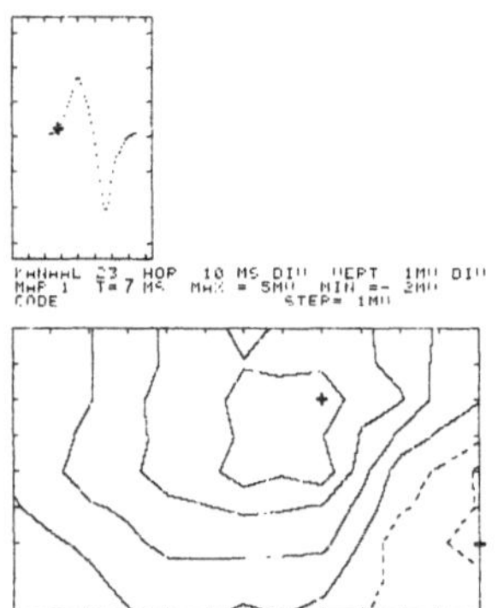

FIGURE 5. A transitory minimum on the early QRS BSM of another infant (time instant 7 msec.), recorded 7 days after birth.

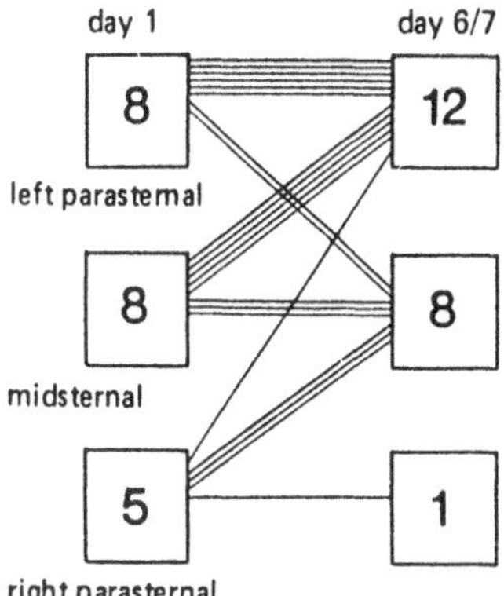

FIGURE 6. Of all 21 infants, the location of the maximum at the onset of the QRS complex, on the first day BSM and on the 6/7th day BSM is illustrated. A more leftward position of the maximum can be observed at the end of the first week.

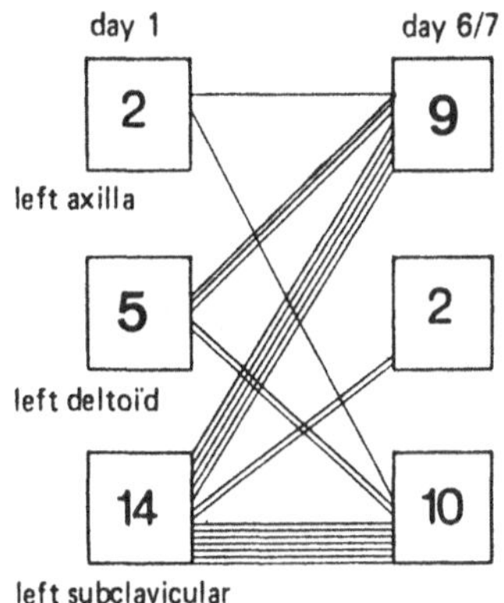

FIGURE 7. The location of the minimum is indicated at its appearance on the first day BSM and on the 6/7th day BSM. At the 6/7th day, the minimum found during ventricular depolarization, tends to appear more often at the left axillary region.

4. DISCUSSION

At birth the elimination of the low resistance placental circulation and subsequent rise in systemic vascular resistance leads to an increasing work load on the left ventricle. The ductus arteriosus and foramen ovale close and although a left to right shunt persists after birth this shunt is markedly decreased at the end of the first week causing a second gradual increase in left ventricular load (6). The hemodynamic changes result in a progressive change from right ventricular preponderance to left ventricular dominance. These changes are in turn reflected in the electrocardiographic changes we have measured. Our results demonstrate that during the first week of life the QRS BSM shows a leftward shift in the appearance of an initial max (fig.6), and a leftward shift in the appearance of the main min (fig.7).

In the healthy newborn child an initial max appears on the anterior thorax thereafter shifting rightward with a min appearing on the left anterior thorax spreading to cover the entire thorax. This agrees with results from Tazawa and Yoshimoto (1) and represents the right ventricular preponderance present at birth. As the left ventricle becomes more dominant the appearance of the initial max moves leftward as shown in figure 6. However, the max still progresses rightward in 6/7 day old neonates indicating that electrocardiographic changes lag behind hemodynamic changes. This supports the findings of Benson and Spach (2). Our results indicate that during the first week of life the appearance of the min moves from the left subclavicular region to the left axillary region. This tendency is in variance to evidence offered by Benson and Spach who showed that towards the end of the first month the appearance of the min moves to the left subclavicular region.

In this study a transitory min appeared twice with the serie A and 10 times with the serie B recordings. Tazawa and Yoshimoto (1) did not observe this transitory min before the fifth day after birth. The reason for this difference is not known but may result from the fact that we used a more extensive electrode grid which also covered both axillary regions. The transitory min corresponds with the Q-deflection described by Walsh (5) who attributed this phenomenon to a temporary pulmonary hypertension seen for some days after birth.

According to an experimental study of Brusca and Rosettani in human fetal hearts (7) final ventricular excitation generally takes place on the diaphragmatic and basal aspects of the right ventricle. Benson and Spach (2) mentioned the early completion of left ventricular depolarization and prolonged depolarization of the right ventricle in newborn infants. Thus the terminal max could well reflect depolarization of these right ventricular sites. Our findings show the presence of a terminal max in 18 cases in serie A and in 12 cases in serie B recordings. We feel that this difference in the occurrence of the terminal max might be due to an improved synchronization of left and right ventricular depolarization towards the end of the first week. The two cases of serie B with a max presenting at the lower left axilla can be attributed to early repolarization.

In summary it can be stated that the electrical status of the heart undergoes a more gradual development during the first week of life, in contrast to the profound alterations in cardiac hemodynamics occurring immediately after birth. This gradual electrocardiographic development is reflected in the evolution of the body surface potential distribution showing a pattern of right ventricular preponderance which is still present at the end of the first week but has become less pronounced.

<u>Acknowledgements</u>: We would like to thank Professor A.J. Dunning, Professor T.G. Losekoot, E.J. Reek, C.E. Grimbergen and P. Broekhuijsen for their help and support in the realization of this study.

REFERENCES

1. Tazawa H and Yoshimoto C: Electrocardiographic Potential Distribution in Newborn Infants from 12 Hours to 8 Days after birth. Am Heart J 78: 292-305, 1969.
2. Benson DW and Spach MS: Evolution of QRS and ST-T-wave Body Surface Potential Distributions During the First Year of Life. Circulation 65: 1247-1258, 1982.
3. Southall DP, Richards J, Mitchell P, Brown DJ, Johnston PGB and Shinebourne EA: Study of Cardiac Rhythm in Healthy Newborn Infants. Brit Heart J 43: 14-20, 1980.
4. Walsh SZ: The Electrocardiogram During the First Week of Life. Brit Heart J 25: 784-794, 1963.
5. Reek EJ, Grimbergen CE, and van Oosterom A: A Low Cost 64 Channel Data Acquisition System for Bedside Registration of Body Surface Maps. In: Advances in electrocardiology, P. d'Alché, ed.; Centre de Publications de l'Université de Caen, 112-114, 1985.
6. Rudolph AM: The Changes in the Circulation After Birth. Their Importance in Congenital Heart Disease. Circulation 41: 343-359, 1970.
7. Brusca A and Rosettani E: Activation of the Human Fetal Heart. Am Heart J 86: 79-87, 1973.

Chapter 4

RECOGNITION OF EPICARDIAL BREAKTHROUGH BY BODY SURFACE ISO-POTENTIAL MAPPING

T. OHTA, S. USUI, M. HIRAI, J. TOYAMA, K. YAMADA

1. INTRODUCTION

An advantage of body surface isopotential maps is the detection of the breakthrough of the activation front into the right ventricular epicardium. Previous recognition of this breakthrough phenomenon has been based solely on specific spatial potential distributions including niche or breakthrough minimum. However, it is speculated that abrupt potential changes will occur around the time of epicardial breakthrough on the body surface region where the niche or breakthrough minimum appears. It is also possible that addition of temporal information to the previous spatial analysis will achieve more clear recognition of the breakthrough phenomenon. Present study demonstrates a new method for this purpose using both spatial and temporal information on cardiac electrical events.

2. METHOD

Body surface isopotential maps were recorded in 10 normal subjects according to the method reported previously. Briefly, 87 unipolar electrocardiograms (ECGs) were recorded simultaneously with reference to Wilson's central terminal using a new mapping system (HPM-6500). These ECG data were digitized by A/D converter at a sampling interval of 1 msec, and processed by a microcomputer to make maps every one msec throughout ventricular activation. Serial isopotential maps were analyzed visually, and the time and location of breakthrough phenomenon were speculated.

Temporal information of the breakthrough phenomenon was examined as follows. For each lead point, the envelope wave form of the first derivative wave form of the ECG was obtained based on the first derivative and its Hilbert transformed wave forms, and then isoenvelope maps indicating the distribution of envelope value were made for each instant of QRS. Isoenvelope maps were compared with isopotential maps, and the electrophysiological basis of the isoenvelope maps were examined.

3. RESULTS AND DISCUSSION

Figure 1 shows isopotential maps (left), isoenvelope maps (middle), and difference maps (right) between isopotential and isoenvelope maps at 20, 30, and 40 msec from the onset of QRS. The isopotential map at 30 msec is characterized by a niche phenomenon (protrusion of negative area into positive area) as indicated by an arrow. The isoenvelope map at the instant showed 2 peaks corresponding to the niche and the maximum (peak of positive potential) in the isopotential map. The peak corresponding to the niche was considered to be caused by an abrupt potential change in the niche area, and another peak was speculated to result from high potentials at the maximum. Difference map was made by subtracting isoenvelope map from isopotential map at the same instant of QRS.

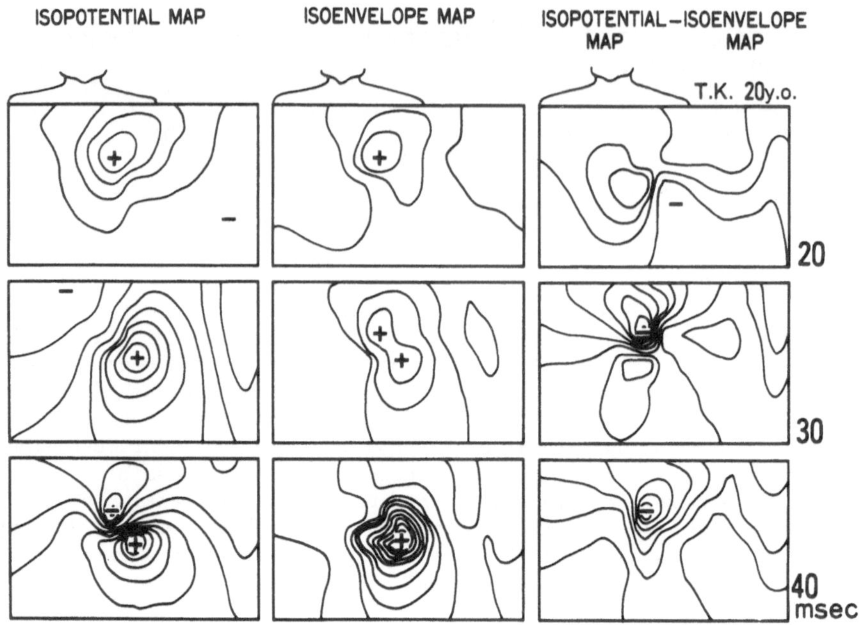

FIGURE 1. Isopotential maps (left), isoenvelope maps (middle), and difference maps (right) at various instants of QRS.

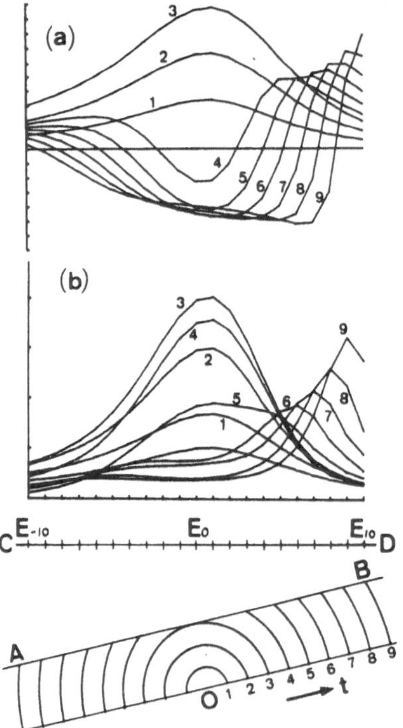

FIGURE 2. A simple two-dimensional simulation study.

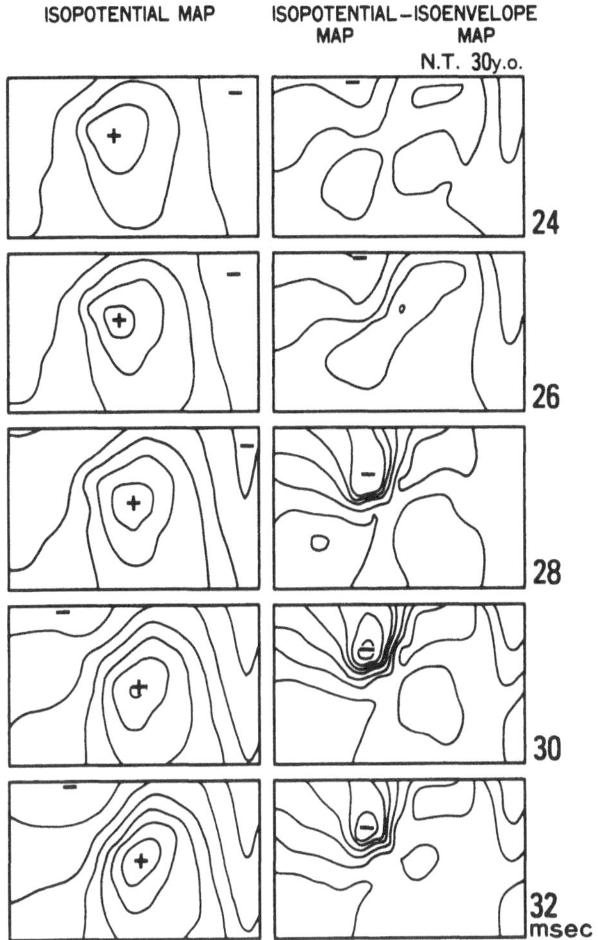

FIGURE 3. Isopotential and difference maps in a normal adult.

The sink of the difference map was considered to extract the peak of isopotential map due to abrupt potential change. In order to confirm this speculation, a simple two-dimensional simulation study was performed (figure 2). A-B represents the epicardial surface and C-D the chest surface. The activation front propagated circularly from point 0. Chest surface potentials were calculated according to the solid angle theory. Isopotential maps and isoenvelope maps at instants 1-9 were shown in (a) and (b), respectively. In isopotential maps, potentials at surface point E_o increased at instants 1-3, but abruptly decreased at instant 4 when epicardial breakthrough occurred. In isoenvelope maps, however, values of point E_o remained high even at instant 4. The finding was in agreement with our speculation that the peaks in the isoenvelop map resulted from abrupt potential changes or high potentials.

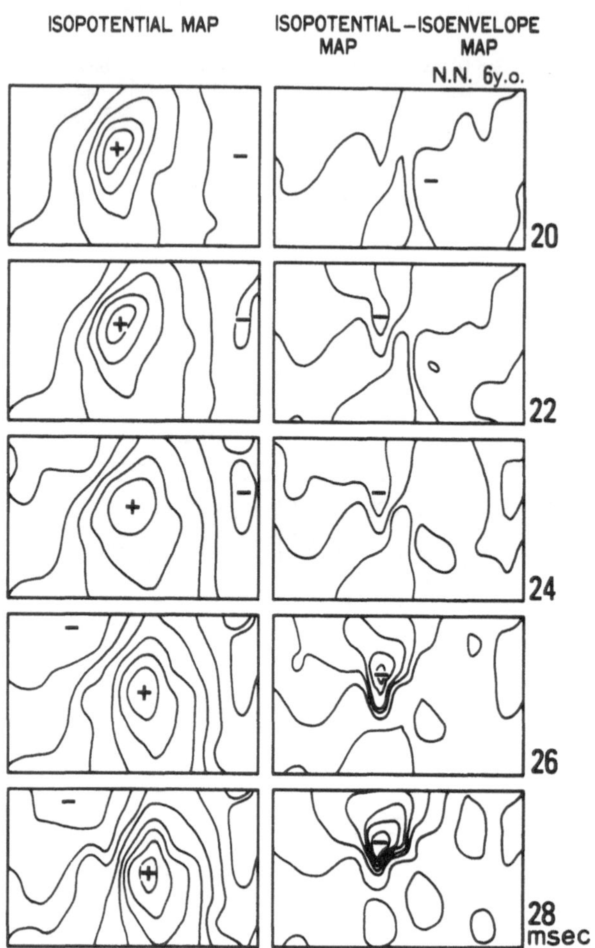

FIGURE 4. Isopotential and difference maps in a normal child.

Figure 3 indicates isopotential maps and the difference maps in a normal adult. Isopotential maps showed smooth-contoured isopotential lines on the anterior chest. It was difficult to determine the time and location of the epicardial breakthrough with the isopotential maps. However, the difference maps showed clearly the sink of value on the anterior chest from 28 msec of QRS, indicating the occurrence of the breakthrough phenomenon.

Figure 4 indicates maps in a normal child. The isopotential maps showed niche-like phenomena at 24 and 28 msec indicated by the arrows. It was difficult to determine which niche-like phenomenon indicates the breakthrough. However, the isoenvelope map clearly indicated a sink at 24 msec, and this sink became greater after the instant.

In conclusion, temporal as well as spatial information is important for better recognition of the epicardial breakthrough with body surface isopotential mapping.

PART 2

MYOCARDIAL INFARCTION

Chapter 5

ISOPOTENTIAL MAPPING IN ACUTE MYOCARDIAL INFARCTION

D.M. MIRVIS

Electrocardiographic patterns are standard markers of acute myocardial infarction. In this review, we shall 1] explore the potential values of the electrocardiogram in evaluation of patients with acute myocardial infarction, 2] identify reasons why body surface isopotential mapping may be of added value, 3] summarize our applications of these mapping methods, and 4] comment upon the limitations of isopotential mapping efforts undertaken to this date. By doing so, we shall attempt to delineate the appropriate position of body surface mapping methods in the study of acute myocardial infarction.

1. VALUES AND LIMITATIONS OF THE ELECTROCARDIOGRAM

Two categories of applications for the ECG in the study of myocardial infarction may be defined - anatomic considerations and functional considerations. The former attempts to detect the presence of infarction and to quantitate its location and size, while the latter efforts seek to define functional or arrhythmogenic properties of the anatomically defined disorder. In each case, a significant value for a quantitative electrocardiographic measure would exist. Such an instrument would provide a noninvasive, safe and reproducible measure using commonly available equipment. These characteristics are unique to ECG approaches.

Anatomic studies have been most prevalent to date. However, the use of the standard, 12-lead ECG has had limited success in all areas. First, the routine ECG is of limited sensitivity in detecting myocardial infarction during normal and particularly during abnormal ventricular activation. Raunio et al (1), for example, detected QRS changes diagnostic of infarction in only 65% of patients with acute and in 71% of those with old transmural lesions. Other studies have correlated the ECG with ventriculographic evidence of prior infarction. Several studies have reported incidences of nondiagnostic ECGs of up to 32% in the presence of regional akinesis, dyskinesis, or frank aneurysm formation (2). These data illustrate the limited sensitivity of the standard ECG for detecting prior myocardial infarction using either pathologic or functional comparisons.

Determination of the location and anatomic extent of infarction is a second role for electrocardiography. Pathologic studies (3,4) have documented that the ECG often underestimates the extent of infarction, and that when a lesion in a specific site is recognized, there is likely to be necrosis in other areas as well. As reported by Sullivan et al (3), the precise ECG location was confirmed at necropsy in only 15% of cases.

The last anatomic consideration is that of infarct size. Such a measure derived from the ECG would provide a predictor of morbidity and mortality using readily applied, noninvasive and reproducible methods. Efforts using computed sums of S-T segment or R wave amplitudes met with mixed but generally disappointing results. Development of a QRS scoring system (5) has, however, renewed interest in an ECG approach to lesion sizing. Such a score, computed from 18 QRS variables, is significantly correlated with infarct size in both anterior and posterior infarctions. Thus, there is revived interest in and hope for an electrocardiographic sizing scheme.

Applications of the standard electrocardiogram to assess functional consequences of infarction are virtually nonexistent. Efforts have typically relied upon the known interaction of infarct location and size with arrhythmogenic status.

2. VALUES OF BODY SURFACE ISOPOTENTIAL MAPPING

Body surface mapping techniques have five established advantages over other ECG approaches. First, because of large areas of the thorax from which potentials are registered, body surface mapping permits detection of diagnostically important information not transmitted to the usually studied left precordial zones. Such information has been detected with right and left ventricular hypertrophy, as well as with myocardial infarction (6).

Second, surface mapping permits study of the spatial as well as the intensity and temporal components of ECG signals. A single isopotential map depicts voltages at all thoracic sites at one instant during a cardiac cycle. This emphasis on the location - intensity relationship provides spatial resolution not found in the usual ECG, which stresses time-intensity interactions. These spatial factors are of major importance, as a given voltage at one torso site may be derived from an infinite number of total body potential distributions. Examination of a sequence of maps then adds temporal resolution.

Third, body surface mapping permits regional cardiac examination. The ability to relate surface and epimyocardial events has been succinctly summarized by Wilson et al (7), stating that unipolar precordial leads "are in reality semi-direct leads from the... ventricular surface, capable within certain limits of serving the same purposes as direct leads from... the exposed heart".

Ample evidence has been presented supporting this conclusion. Experimental studies have correlated surface patterns with epicardial and intramural excitation sequences during normal and ectopic beats, and with the location of induced lesions, including cautery, coronary ligation, myocardial ischemia, and pacing (8-10). Clinical studies have likewise related surface patterns to epicardial events in patients with right ventricular hypertrophy and pre-excitation syndromes (11,12).

Fourth, isopotential mapping allows evaluation of equivalent cardiac generator properties. Such assessment is important because, as summarized by Geselowitz (13), "the problem of relating the surface potentials to an equivalent generator is simpler than relating them to actual sources", as not enough data are currently known to treat the actual problem precisely. In addition, several studies from our laboratory have demonstrated the physiologic relevance of such intermediate steps in tracking cardiac excitation and in localizing experimental lesions (14).

Last, techniques to assess functional states have more recently been developed. Arrhythmogenic states are characterized by a greater than normal regional dispersion of refractory periods (15). The mechanism of generation of the T wave is likewise dependent upon differences in ventricular recovery times (16). Hence, it may be expected that ECG measurements based upon recovery properties may be of value in assessing arrhythmogenic states.

3. APPLICATIONS TO ACUTE INFARCTION

Many studies from several laboratories have begun to apply these advantages to the aforementioned electrocardiographic problems of acute infarction. In this review, we shall focus on our own work, but only because of our familiarity with it.

Each of the anatomic and functional applications may be considered. First, efforts to detect and to localize the acute lesions may be described. We initially studied patients within 48 hours of acute infarction to define the spatial distribution of S-T segment potentials (17). In patients with anterior lesions, positive potentials dominated, with a maximum located on the anterior torso. In contrast, the isopotential distributions from subjects with an inferior infarctions, positive potentials were displaced to the inferior torso margins, with an abnormal minimum located on the left anterior, superior chest wall. These descriptive studies demonstrated that 1] isopotential mapping was technically feasible during the acute phases of myocardial infarction, and 2] lesions in different locations had different spatial patterns of repolarization potentials.

To further refine the attempt, we computed equivalent dipole locations and moments using surface integration methods based upon the Gabor-Nelson equations (18). Our previous work (19) with an isolated rabbit heart preparation demonstrated 1] that dipole ranging methods could accurately localize highly dipolar epicardial lesions, and 2] that injury currents of the type to be studied were quantitatively highly dipolar. Thus, a dipole ranging method was appropriate.

Two findings were apparent. First, the locations of the S-T dipoles in the two subsets were different. That from the patients with an anterior lesion was located superior and to the left of that of the inferior infarction dipole. This is consonant with the positions of the two lesions in the chest.

Second, the orientations of the dipoles differed in ways consistent with an endocardial to epicardial orientation, that is, the known orientation of injury current vectors. Thus, the anterior dipole was directed leftward and anteriorly, whereas the inferior lesion dipole was directed inferiorly and posteriorly. These findings demonstrate that dipole ranging methods, based upon isopotential surface mapping techniques, can provide physiologically relevant information for localization of ischemic lesions.

One last study investigated the spatial distribution of frequency content of electrocardiographic signals (20). Because waveforms recorded from different sites have different configurations, we reasoned that the frequency content of these signals may likewise vary from site to site. To test this hypothesis, we subjected ECG data recorded during the QRS complex from isolated rabbit hearts to Fourier analysis.

A clear spatial distribution of frequency content was observed. An area of high harmonic content was seen in control conditions overlying the basal left ventricle. After ligation of the anterior interventricular artery, this peak shifted location to overly the anterior left ventricular surface, that is, the location of the infarction. This translocation may be due to wavefront fractionation by the infarction, and may therefore be useful in localizing otherwise undetectable lesions.

The third area in which mapping may provide useful information is in the sizing of the ischemic lesion. Our initial efforts at determining infarct size from surface potential data utilized an isolated rabbit heart preparation (19). Hearts were suspended in a spherical chamber and ECG potentials were recorded from thirty-two torso electrodes. The anterior descending artery was ligated to produce acute infarction, and Evans blue dye was then infused through the aortic root to delineate the unperfused area. This area was then correlated with the dipole moment computed form potentials sensed forty milliseconds into the S-T segment. Results demonstrated a good relation between anatomic and electrical measurements, with a correlation coefficient of 0.82.

One limitation of using dipole moment to measure lesion size is the creation of extradipolar forces as dipolar sources are spead over a surface. Thus, a lesion of significant size would have quadripolar, octapolar, etc, forces as well as dipolar ones. These extradipolar terms may be used to directly measure the size of the lesion. To test this hypothesis, we simulated an ischemic lesion as a planar, uniform disc placed within a bounded, uniform volume conductor (21). Disc radius was vared from 0.5 to 1.5 cm. Dipoles of equal moment, oriented perpendicular to the disc plane, were radially and evenly located. Surface potentials were computed and were fit to a moving dipole-octapole generator model. The octapole term was selected because of its physiologic relevance, being related, as shown by Brody and others, to the size of the rim bounding the lesion.

For all disc diameters used, the inversely computed disc radius was within 0.01 cm of the known radius when the lesion was centric. As eccentricites increased, the errors increased. At an eccentricity of 0.5 or greater, a negative diameter was calculated. Thus, this approach, while theoretically based, is limited in application.

Last, interesting but preliminary data are available defining the functional, that is, arrhythmogenic, properties of acute myocardial infarction. Major emphasis has been placed upon the Q-T interval and QRST area distributions. We have explored the utility of each of these measures. First, we examined the spatial distribution of the Q-T interval in normal persons and in subjects with acute infarction (22). In normal subjects, the Q-T interval duration was spatially distributed in a characteristic manner. Q-T intervals were shortest on the right inferior torso and longest over the left lateral chest. These data correspond to recorded differences in refractory period or monophasic action potentials.

This normal pattern was compared to those in patients with acute anterior or inferior infarction. In each infarct set, the distribution of long Q-T intervals shifted to a position to overly the supposed infarct location. This redistribution occurred without an absolute increase in mean Q-T intervals. These results illustrate the ability of mapping techniques to depict normal and abnormal deviations in recovery times. Because these regional differences may be arrhythmogenic, a more complete assessment of this variable may be useful in identifying clinical states at risk of sudden death.

Most recently, we have begun to explore the correlation between isoarea distributions and acute, post-infarction ventricular arrhythmias. ECG measurements from 84 torso electrodes were processed to compute QRST root-mean-square area and QRST isoarea field dipolarity using the Karhounen-Loeve expansion method (Figure 1). After acute circumflex artery occlusion, QRST area rose promptly, followed by a reduction in dipolarity that corresponded with the falling phase of QRST area.

Ventricular ectopy after acute occlusion occurs in two phases - one 5-7 minutes after occlusion and the second approximately 20 minutes after occlusion (23). Changes in areas and dipolarity correlated well with this phenomenon. The early phase ectopy occurs when QRST area is maximal, while the latter phase ectopy occurs when dipolarity is lowest during the period of rapid change in QRST area. Thus, these pilot data suggest a significant temporal relation between body surface measures of recovery properties and post-occlusion ectopy.

4. LIMITATIONS OF MAPPING STUDIES

Although these studies indicate theoretical as well as practical advantages of surface mapping techniques, general clinical application may be hampered by any of several problems. First, most mapping systems require complex and expensive computerized hardware and software systems. New microprocessor - based approaches should considerably reduce hardware costs and increase availability. Commercially available units, including software that is almost "turn-key", have become available in several countries.

Second, the requirement for hundreds of leads imposes concerns about patient comfort and technician time, as well as about the shear volume of data to be managed. Development of new lead systems using only 20-30 electrodes, with few or none to be placed on the back of critically ill patients, should overcome many of these concerns as well as significantly reducing hardware costs.

Third, underlying these hardware issues is the lack of standardization of methods. How many leads in what positions are to be used? What sampling rate is minimally or optimally acceptable? What display format should be used? A related obstacle to widespread clinical application is generated by the differences in display format between the standard ECG and the isopotential map. Although the two forms are interconvertible and both may be approached by a pattern - recognition model, the display differences present a perceived if not a real stumbling block.

Another conceptual concern is the usual semiqualitative, subjective approach to map study. Most studies rely upon determination of extrema number and position, as well as location of low level contours, to define map characteristics. Although semiquantitative methods have been developed, problems exist. Departure mapping, depicting the difference of one map from the statistically - determined normal range, has probably been the most widely used method. It does not consider abnormal time sequences of patterns, each of which, when considered in isolation, is "within normal limits". Subtraction mapping, depicting the difference between two individual patterns before and after an event, requires the optimal but generally unavailable "control" data set.

Development of methods such as those based upon numerical expansion techniques may provide a true quantitative system for map study. By defining spatial information in a manageable number of terms, they reduce data set size. Of particular note is their ability to include temporal as well as spatial variations and comparison.

A last concern is the need for comprehensive, controlled applications. Comparison of mapping to standard ECG suffers from the lack of anything resembling a "gold standard". The limits of the standard ECG are well known. Validation of surface mapping methods by pathologic data is optimal, but difficult to do. The major, large scale pathology - ECG correlation studies reported in past decades have not been undertaken.

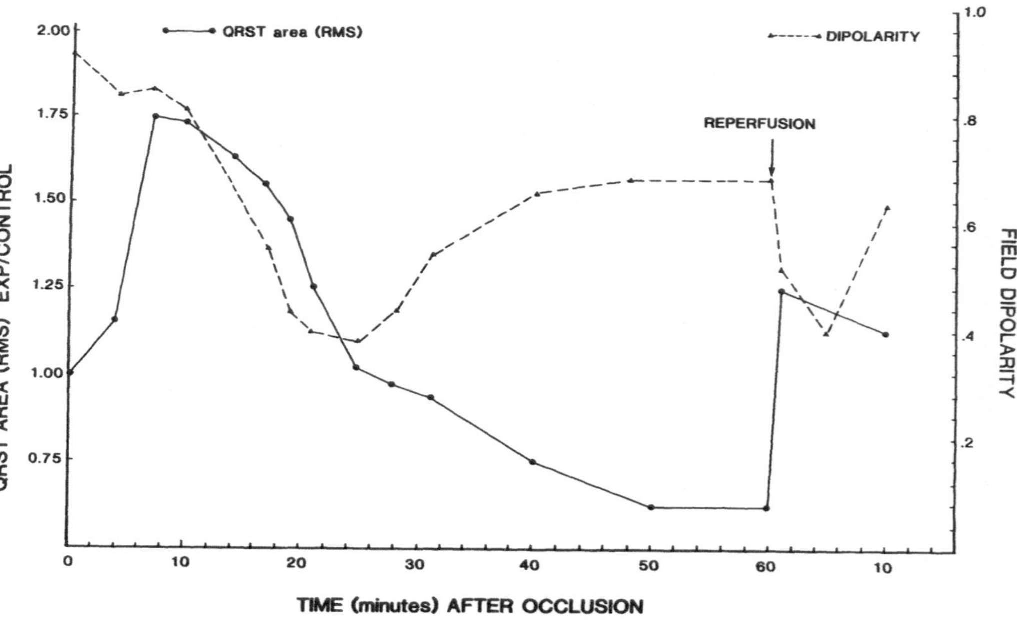

FIGURE 1:

Plots of root-mean-square (RMS) QRST area (left axis) and computed QRST dipolarity (right axis) before and after occlusion and after reperfusion of the left circumflex artery.

Invasive or noninvasive correlations using angiography, radionuclide imaging and/or echocardiography should, however, provide reasonable substitutes.

Thus, obstacles do exist. But the combination of new technology, and continued research, when coupled with a clinical need, should provide reasonable assurances for progress and ultimate success.

5. REFERENCES

1. Raunio H, Rissanen V, Romppanen T, et al: Changes in the QRS complex and ST segment in transmural and subendocardial infarction. Am Heart J 98:170, 1971.
2. Arkin BM, Hueter DC, Ryan TJ: Predictive value of electrocardiographic patterns in localizing left ventricular asynergy in coronary artery disease. Am Heart J 97:453, 1979.
3. Sullivan W, Vlodaver Z, Tuna N, et al: Correlation of electrocardiographic and pathologic findings in healed myocardial infarction. Am J Cardiol 42:724, 1978.
4. Roberts WC, Gardin JM: Location of myocardial infarcts: A confusion of terms and definitions. Am J Cardiol 42:868, 1978.
5. Palmeri ST, Harrison DG, Cobb FR, et al: A QRS scaring system for assessing left ventricular function after myocardial infarction. New Eng J Med 306:4,1982.
6. Spach MS, Barr RC, Blumenschein SD, Boineau JP: Clinical implications of isopotential surface maps. Ann Intern Med 69:919, 1968.
7. Wilson FN, Johnston FD, Rosenbaum FF, et al: The precordial electrocardiogram. Am Heart J 27:19, 1944.
8. Mirvis DM, Keller FW, Ideker RE, et al: Detection and localization of multiple epicardial electrical generators by a two-dipole ranging technique. Circ Res 41:351, 1977.
9. McLaughlin VW, Flowers NC, Horan LG, Killam HAW: Surface potential contributions from discrete elements of ventricular wall. Am J Cardiol 34:302, 1974.
10. Abildskov JA, Burgess MJ, Lux RL, Wyatt RF: Experimental evidence for regional cardiac influence in body surface isopotential maps of dogs. Circ Res 38:386, 1976.
11. Blumenschein SD, Spach MS, Boineau JP, et al: Genesis of body surface potentials in varying types of right ventricular hypertrophy. Circulation 38:917, 1968.
12. DeAmbroggi L, Tacardi B, Macchi E: Body surface maps of heat potentials: Tentative localization of pre-excitation areas in forty-two Wolff-Parkinson-White patients. Circulation 54:251, 1976.
13. Geselowitz D: The concept of an equivalent cardiac generator. Biomed Sci Instrumentation 1:325, 1963.
14. Ideker RE, Bandura JP, Cox JW, Jr., et al: Path and significance of heart vector migration during QRS and ST-T complexes of ectopic beats in isolated perfused rabbit hearts. Circ Res 41:558, 1977.
15. Han J, Moe GK: Nonuniform recovery of excitability in ventricular muscle. Circ Res 14:44, 1964.
16. Burgess MJ, Harumi K, Abildskov JA: Application of a thearetic T wave model to experimentally induced T wave abnormalities. Circulation 34:669, 1966.
17. Mirvis DM: Body surface distributions of repolarization forces during acute myocardial infarction. I. Isopotential and isoarea mapping. Circulation 62:878, 1980.

18. Mirvis DM, Holbrook MA: Body surface distributions of repolarization potentials after acute myocardial infarction. III. Dipole ranging in subjects and in patients with acute myocardial infarction. J Electrocardiol 14:387, 1981.
19. Mirvis DM, Keller FW, Ideker RE, et al: Equivalent generator properties of acute ischemic lesions in the isolated rabbit heart. Circ Res 42:767, 1978.
20. Nichols, TL, Mirvis DM: Frequency content of the electrocardiogram. Spatial features and effects of myocardial infarction. J Electrocardiol 18:185, 1985.
21. Mirvis DM and Larsen RA: Experimental evaluation of a moving dipole-octapole pair equivalent cardiac generator. J Electrocardiol 12:169, 1979.
22. Mirvis DM: Spatial variation of Q-T intervals in normal persons and in patients with acute myocardial infarction. J Am Coll Cardiol 5:625, 1985.
23. Kaplinsky E, Ogawa S, Balke CW, Dreifus LS: Two periods of early ventricular arrhythmias in the canine myocardial infarction model. Circulation 60:397, 1979.

Chapter 6

BODY SURFACE ISOPOTENTIAL MAPS IN OLD ANTERIOR MYOCARDIAL INFARCTION UNDETECTABLE BY 12 LEAD ELECTROCARDIOGRAMS

T. OHTA, M. HIRAI, J. TOYAMA, K. YAMADA

1. INTRODUCTION

The 12 lead electrocardiogram is one of the most important methods for the diagnosis of myocardial infarction. However, the abnormal Q wave indicating the presence of infarction sometimes disappears in the late phase of infarction(1). Also, it sometimes appears in cases without myocardial infarction.

On the other hand, the clinical usefulness of body surface isopotential maps has been reported(2-12). Our previous studies suggest the advantage of maps in detecting the location and extent of myocardial infarction with abnormal Q waves(9, 10). However, there have been few reports in which body surface maps were examined for patients with old myocardial infarction undetectable by 12 lead electrocardiograms(3-5,12).

In the present study, we examined body surface maps of old anterior myocardial infaction with and without electrocardiographic findings of infarction at the time of their inclusion in this study.

2. PROCEDURE

2.1. Patients

From consecutive cases who underwent left ventriculography(LVG) and coronary arteriography(CAG) in Anjo Kosei Hospital, the following 3 groups were selected for this study.

1. Normal subjects (n= 30).
2. Old anterior myocardial infarction without evident electrocardiographic findings of infarction (n= 32).
3. Old anterior myocardial infarction with evident electrocardiographic finding of infarction (n= 30).

The normal subjects came to the hospital with a complaint of atypical chest pain or palpitation. But they proved to be normal after extensive examination including cardiac catheterization. The infarction groups had evident history of acute myocardial infarction confirmed by the typical chest pain, serum enzyme changes and electrocardiographic changes. Their CAGs showed significant narrowings of luminal area of more than 75% in the left anterior descending coronary arteries. The electrocardiographic finding of anterior infarction was defined as Q and QS pattern in the anteroseptal and anterolateral sites in the modified Minnesota Code criteria(13).

2.2. Cardiac Catheterization

Left ventriculography was performed in the 30 degrees right anterior oblique(RAO) and 60 degrees left anterior oblique(LAO) projection after sublingual administration of nitroglycerin (0.3 mg) and recorded at 30 frames/sec on 35 mm Kodak Shellburst film using a Philips 6 inch image intensifier system (Cardiodiagnost). Left ventricular asynergy was analyzed quantitatively according to the reporting system of the American Heart Association evaluated for coronary artery disease(14). Coronary arteriography was performed by Sones' technique and significant obstruction was defined as a 75% or greater reduction in cross sectional area of the coronary artery. Evaluation was performed by 2 observers who had no knowlege of clinical data including body surface maps.

2.3. Body Surface Isopotential Maps

Body surface isopotential maps were recorded within 1 week prior to cardiac catheterization. Since we have already reported the details concerning the method of data acquisition and processing, it will be described only briefly in the present paper(15). Unipolar electrocardiograms were recorded simultaneously from 87 lead points on the chest surface (59 and 28 lead points on the anterior and poaterior chest, respectively) with reference to Wilson's central terminal using a new body surface mapping system developed in our institute (HPM-5100 or HPM-6500, Chunich Denshi Co. Ltd.). These electrocardiographic data were scanned by multiplexers, digitized by A/D converters at a rate of 1000 samples/sec and processed by a microcomputer to make maps every 1 msec through ventricular activation. The onset of ventricular activation was determined as follows. Approximate time of onset of QRS was determined visually using lead II of 12 lead electroardiograms. Root mean square values of the 87 electrocardiograms were plotted at 1 ms intervals around the approximate time of onset. The exact point of onset of ventricular activation was determined as the first of 5 successive increases in the root mean square value within the approximate onset interval.

Figure 1 shows the 87 lead points in a grated system we are using for body surface mapping. Vertical lines A, I and E indicate the right midaxillary, left midaxillary and midsternal lines, respectively. Horizontal lines 4 and 6 indicate the 5th and 2nd intercostal lines. Large open circles show the precordial lead points of the 12 lead electrocardiograms.

2.4. Statistics

The position of the minimum was compared for the infarction and normal group at 5 msec intervals from the onset of QRS during ventricular activation. Statistical analysis was assessed using a t test.

3. RESULT

3.1. Normal Group

Thirty subjects in the normal group showed similar map findings with respect to the positional change of minimum in the early phase of QRS. Figure 2 shows left ventriculograms, 12 lead electrocardiograms and body surface isopotential maps in a typical case of normal subjects. Left ventriculograms were presented for the RAO and LAO projections and showed normal contraction. The 12 lead electrocardiograms were also normal. Maps are presented on the right for 5, 10, 15, 20, 25 and 30 msec from the onset of QRS. The left and right halves of the map frame indicate the anterior and posterior chest, respectively. Maximum is shown by +, and minimum by -. Isopotential lines are drawn an interval of 0.2 mV. At 5 msec from the onset of QRS, a minimum appeared on the left back. The minimum remained on the back during 10 to 20 msec, then moved gradually to the right and was located in the upper portion of the anterior chest at 25 and 30 msec. Thus, the minimum was mostly located on the back in the early phase (5-20 msec) of QRS in normal subjects.

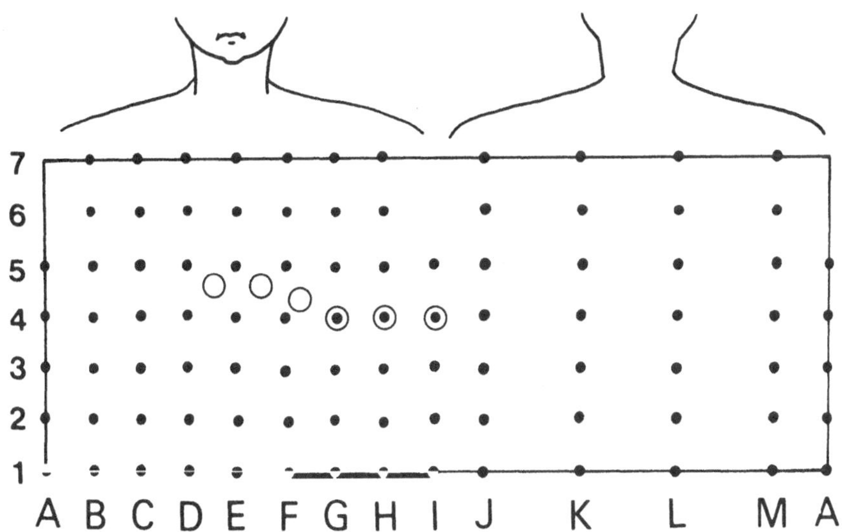

Figure 1. Eighty-seven lead points for body surface mapping

3.2. Infarction Group with Abnormal Q wave

Twenty-eight of the 32 patients in the infarction group with abnormal Q wave showed asynergy in the anterior segments (anterobasal, anterolateral, apical or septal segments) of the left ventriculograms. The remaining 4 patients, who exhibited no asynergy in any segment at the time of cardiac catheterization, showed a positional change of minimum quite similar to that in normal subject. Therefore, 2 typical cases belonging to the 2 subgroups will be presented hereafter.

Figure 3 shows left ventriculograms, 12 lead electrocardiograms and body surface maps in a typical case. The left ventriculogram revealed akinesis in the septal segment and hypokinesis in the anterolateral and apical segments. Coronary arteriograms showed 75% luminal area stenosis in the proximal portion of the left anterior descending coronary artery. The 12 lead electrocardiograms showed embryonic r wave in the right precordial lead, but did not satisfy the criteria for anterior infarction in the modified Minnesota Code. Body surface maps are presented on the right. At 5 msec, a minimum was located on the right anterior chest and remained on the anterior chest through 30 msec. Thus, body surface maps in this subgroup differed from those in the normal group in that the minimum was observed on the anterior chest in the early phase (5-20 msec) of QRS.

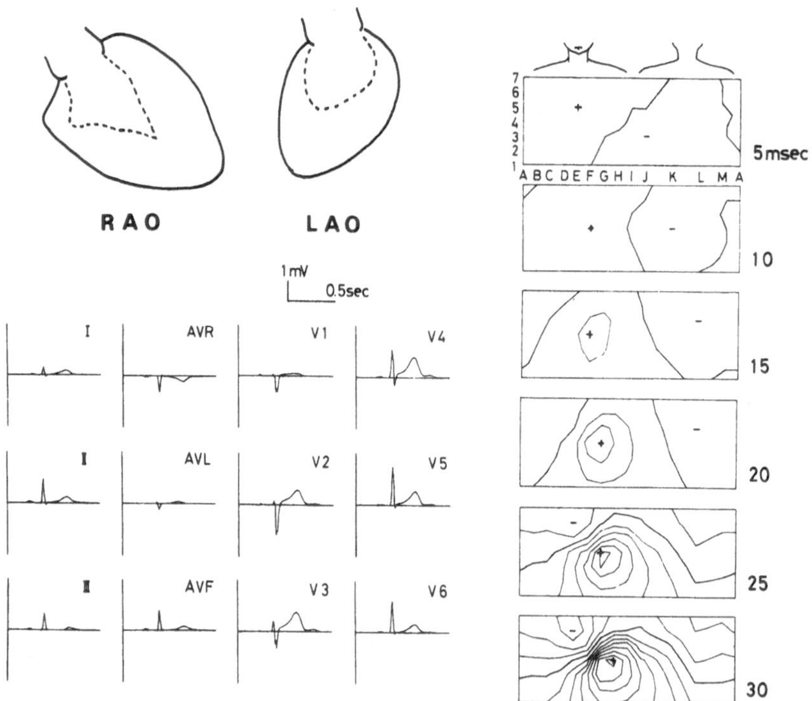

Figure 2. Body surface maps in a normal subject

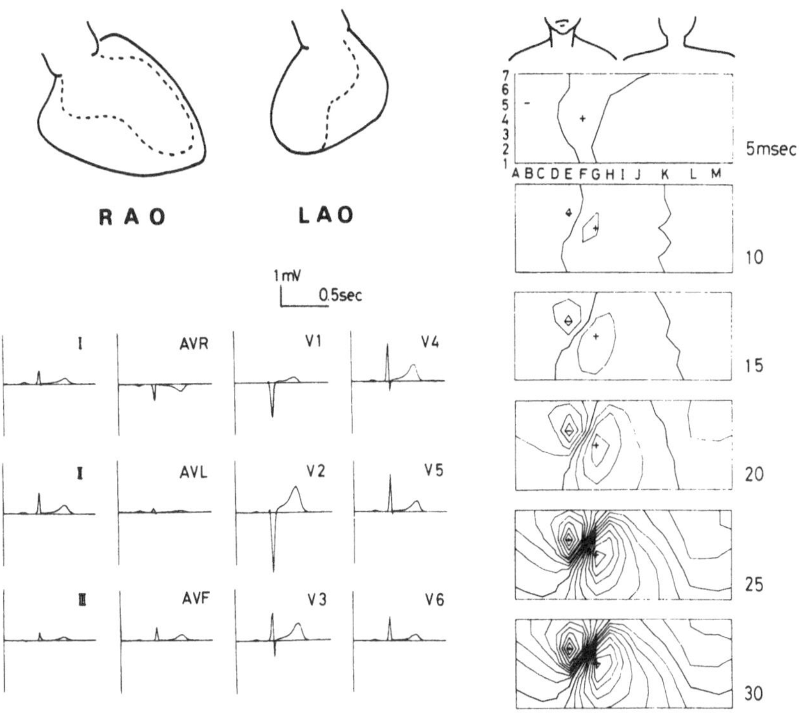

Figure 3. Body surface maps in an infarction case with ventricular asynergy but without abnormal Q wave

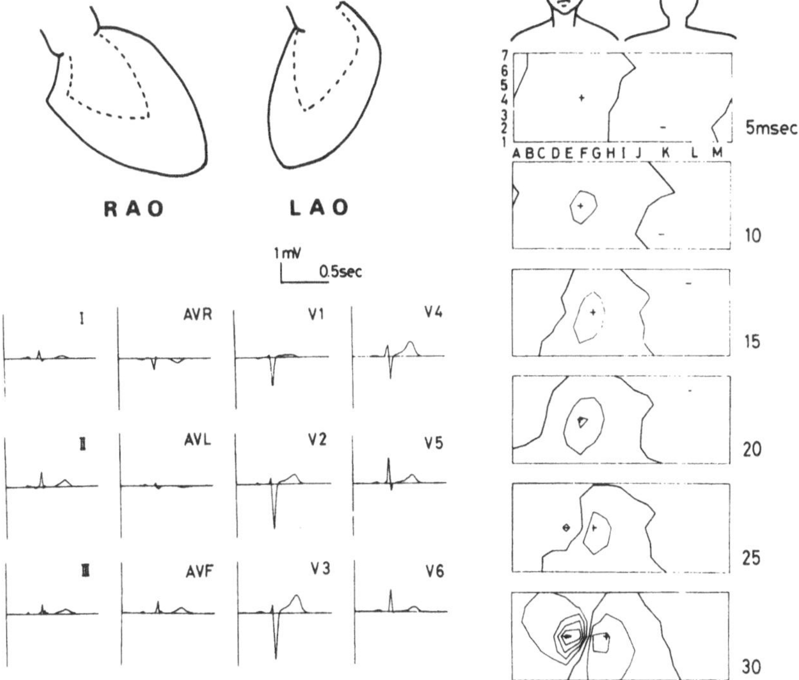

Figure 4. Body surface maps in an infarction case without ventricualr asynergy and abnormal Q wave

Figure 4 shows a typical case who had evident history of anterior infarction but whose left ventriculograms showed no asynergy at the time of cardiac catheterization. The infarction was confirmed by the typical chest pain, serum enzyme changes and electrocardiographic manifestations in the acute phase of infarction. However, 12 lead electrocardiograms returned to normal and left ventriculograms revealed no asynergy at the time of cardiac catheterization. In the body surface maps, a minimum remained on the back during 5 to20 msec, moved to the right and was located on the anterior chest at 25 and 30 msec. This finding was quite similar to those for normal subjects.

3.3. Infarction Group with Abnormal Q wave

All of 30 patients in the infarction group with abnormal Q wave exhibited similar surface map finding.

Figure 5 shows left ventriculograms, 12 lead electrocardiograms and body surface maps in a typical case. The left ventriculogram revealed akinesis in the septal, anterolateral and apical segments. CAGs showed total occlusion in the proximal portion of the left anterior descending coronary artery. The 12 electrocardiogram showed QS pattern in V1-V4, and satisfied the criteria for anterior infarction in the modified Minnesota Code. Body surface maps showed a minimum on the anterior chest during 5 to 30 msec. Thus, body surface maps in old anterior infarction

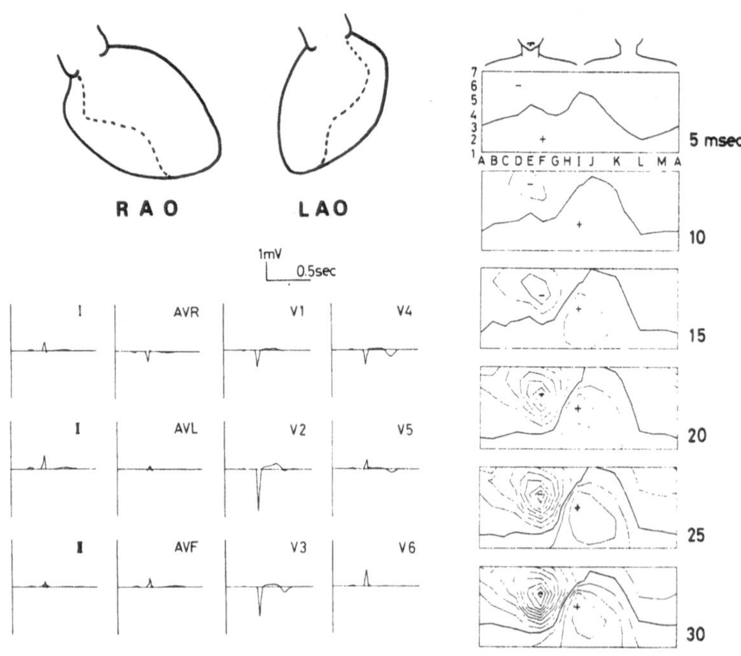

Figure 5. Body surface maps in an infarction case with ventricular asynergy and abnoemal Q wave

with abnormal Q wave was characterized by a minimum remaining on the anterior chest in the early phase of QRS.

3.4. Comparison of Minimum in Normal Group and Infarction Groups with and without abnormal Q wave

Figure 6 summarizes position of minimum at 5,10,15,20 and 25 msec in 30 normal subjects, 32 patients with and 30 patients without abnormal Q wave. The left column represents the position of minimum for the 92 cases in the 3 groups. The right column represents the mean position and standard deviation for the 3 groups. Open circle, closed circle and cross indicate normal subjects, patients without abnormal Q wave and patients with abnormal Q wave, respectively. The normal and infarction groups showed a significant difference with respect to the mean position of minimum at 5, 10, 15, 20 and 25 msec with a p value of less than 0.001 (right). Furthermore, the position of minimum at 15 msec was best for screening the normal and infarction groups (left). If we define the criteria that the minimum at 15 msec appearing on lines A and J or more anteriorly suggests the presence of old anterior infarction, the criteria showed a sensitivity of 81% and a specificity of 97% in the materials of this study. It was interesting that 4 out of the 6 false negative cases diagnosed by the map criteria were patients (as shown in Figure 4) with clinical evidence of infarction but without ventricular asynergy.

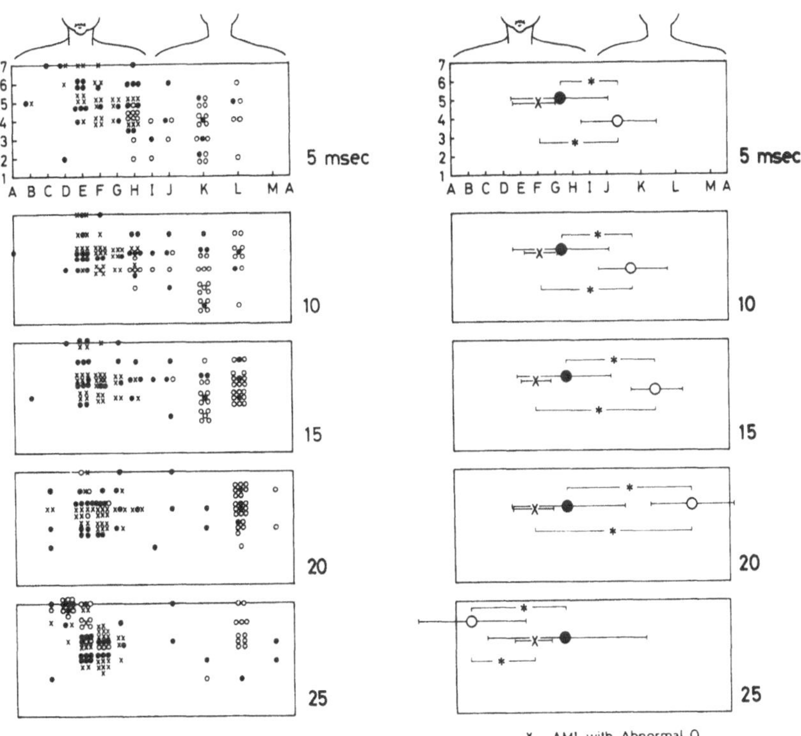

Figure 6. Comparison of position of minimum in the 3 groups

Diagnostic accuracy of Frank lead vector cardiograms were also examined in the materials. Vectorcardiographic criteria by Chou et al.(17) exhibited a sensitivity of 28% and a specificity of 100%.

4. DISCUSSION

4.1. Body Surface Maps in Normal Subjects

Taccardi recorded body surface maps of 44 normal subjects and examined the positional changes of minima(16). At the onset of ventricular excitation, a minimum was located in the lower portion on the left thoracic wall or in the dorsal region. The minimum migrated dorsally towards the right shoulder, and then appeared anteriorly in the right clavicular area. Thereafter, the minimum migrated to the midsternal area or a new minimum appeared in the midsternal region until the mid phase. The movement of the minimum in the early phase of QRS in a normal subject shown in Figure 2 was quite similar to that described by Taccardi.

4.2. Body Surface Maps in Anterior Infarction

Patients with clinical evidence of anterior infarction differed from normal subjects with respect to the position of minimum in the early phase of QRS. The minimum was located on the anterior chest in patients with anterior infarction, while on the back in normal subjects. Abnormally located minimum in patients with antrior infarction was considered to reflect loss of electromotive forces due to myocardial infarction. In patients with clinical evidence of infarction but without ventricular asynergy, however, the minimum was located on the back, and this finding was similar to that in normal subjects. It was considered that in these patients the myocardial mass affected by infarction was quite small and consequently body surface maps showed nearly normal findings.

In our recent study, we examined body surface maps of patients with electrocardiographic finding of infarction but without clinical evidence of infarction. Figure 6 shows 12 lead electrocardiograms and body surface maps of a typical case. The 12 lead electrocardiograms showed QS pattern in leads V1 and V2, and suggested the presence of anterior infarction. However, body surface maps showed a minimum on the back in the early phase of infarction. This finding is quite similar to that in normal subjects.

4.3. Conclusions

The present study showed that patients with evidence of anterior infarction but without electrocardiographic findings of anterior infarction could be clearly distinguished from normal subjects by the position of the minimum at 15 msec from the onset of QRS. The minimum is a finding only available from body surface isopotential maps. This suggests the highly specific usefulness of body surface maps in diagnosing the presence or absence of old anterior myocardial infarction.

REFERENCES

1. Kalbfleish JM, Shadaksharappa KS, Conrad LL, Sarkar NK: Disappearearance of the Q-deflection following myocardial infarction. Am Heart J 76:193, 1968.
2. Boineau JP, Blumenschein SD, Spach MS, Sabiston DC: Relationship between ventricular depolarizaton and electrocardiogram in myocardial infarction. J Electrocardiol 1(2):233, 1968.
3. Flowers NC, Horan LG, Johnson JC: Anterior infarctional change occurring during mid and late ventricular activation detectable by surface mappong techniques. Circulation 54:906, 1976.
4. Flowers NC, Horan LG, Sohi GS, Hand RC, Johnson JC: New vidence for inferoposterior myocardial infarction on surface potential mapping. Am J Cardiol 38:576, 1976.
5. Vincent GM, Abildskov JA, Burgess MJ, Miller K, Lux RL, Wyatt RF: Diagnosis of old inferior myocardial infarctoin by body surface isopotential mapping. Am J Cardiol 39:510, 1977.
6. Yamada K, Toyama J, Sugenoya J, Wada M, Sugiyama S: Body surface isopotential maps. Clinical application to the diagnosis of myocardial infarction. Jpn Heart J 19: 28, 1978.
7. Hayashi H, Watanabe Y, Ishikawa T, Wada M, Uematsu H, Inagaki H: Diagnostic value of body surface map in myocardial infarction. Jpn Circ J 44:197, 1980.
8. Essen RV, Merx W, Doerr R, Effert S, Sily J, Rau G: QRS mapping in the elevation of acute anterior myocardial infarction. Circulation 62:266, 1980.
9. Ohta T, Toyama J, Osugi J, Kinoshita A, Isomura S, Takatsu F, Ishikawa H, Nagaya T, Yamada K: Correlation between body surface isopotential maps and left ventriculograms in patients with old anterior myocardial infarction. Jpn Heart J 22:747, 1981.
10. Toyama S, Suzuki K, Koyama M, Yoshino k, Fujimoto K: The body surface isopotential mapping of the QRS wave in myocardial infarction. J Electrocardiol 15:241, 1982.
11. Ohta T, Kinoshita A, Ohsugi J, Isomura S, Takatsu F, Ishikawa H, Toyama J, Nagaya T, Yamada K: Correlation between body surface isopotential maps and left ventriculogram in patients with old inferoposterior myocardisl infarction. Am Heart j 104:1262, 1982.
12. Ohta T, Toyama J, Yamada K: Body surface map and vectorcardiographic correlation in old inferior myocardial infarction undetectable by 12 lead electrocardiogram. Circulation 66 (suppl II): II-376, 1982.
13. AHA The Coronary Drug Project: Design, methods and baseline results. Appendix D, ECG recording codes. Circulation 47 (suppl I): I-39, 1973.
14. Austen WG, Edward JE, Frye RL, Gensini GG, Gott VL, Griffith LSC, Mcgoon DC, Murphy ML, Roe BB: AHA Committee Report: A reporting system on patients

evaluated for coronary artery disease. Circulation 51:5. 1975.

15. Toyama J, Ohta T, Yamada K: Newly developed surface mapping system for clinical use. In Yamada K, Harumi K, Musha T, editors: Advances in body surface potential mapping. Nagoya, 1983, The University of Nagoya Press. p 125.

16. Taccardi B, De Ambroggi L, Viganotti C: Body surface mapping of heart potentials. In Nelson CV, Geselowitz DB, editors: The theoretical basis of electrocardiology London, 1976, Oxford University Press, p 436.

17. Chou TC, Helm RA, Kaplan S: Clinical Vectorcardiography. New York, 1974, Grune & Stratton, Inc, p 229.

Chapter 7

BODY SURFACE MAP CRITERIA FOR QUANTITATING INFARCT AS DERIVED FROM COMPUTER SIMULATIONS

R.H. STARTT/SELVESTER, J.C. SOLOMON, R.B. PEARSON

INTRODUCTION

The computer simulation of the total body surface Electrocardiogram (ECG) developed by us contains detailed geometry of the torso, lungs, intracardiac blood mass, and anatomy of the heart and purkinje conduction system (1). The simulation also contains a mathematic model of the electromotive surface (2) that is made to propogate through the normal, hypertrophied or infarcted heart geometry so as to produce 12 lead ECGs, Vectorcardiograms (VCGs) and ECG body surface maps (BSMs) that are typical of normals, right ventricular hypertrophy (RVH), LVH or classic MIs. Simulation of typical surface ECGs of the various conduction abnormalities are produced by appopriate modification of the Purkinje input to the ventricular propagation simulation. The model was built to conform to measured torso geometry and electric properties and to electrophysiology, and anatomy of normal, infarcted, and hypertrophied hearts. Thus it contained all the first order variables known to effect the body surface ECG or BSM.

The simulation was used to model the detailed activation and BSM ECG changes, of myocardial infarct in the distribution of each of the 3 main coronary arteries. These were then incorporated into ECG, VCG, and BSM criteria for infarct size and location (3). In collaboration with us, the 12 lead ECG criteria were validated by Ideker, Wagner, et al (4,5), showing good correlation with quantitative planimetric pathology in subjects without hypertrophy or conduction defects and with first infarcts in each of the 3 main locations. The poorest correlation occurred with small infarcts, especially those on the postero(lateral) wall. This correlation was improved in recent preliminary studies, as yet unreported, when extra leads on the back were included, suggesting that BSMs which contain added information might result in more resolution for location in any individual patient and less variability in the quantitation of MI size.

ELECTROPHYSIOLOGICAL AND ANATOMIC CONSIDERATIONS

The purpose of this communication is to discuss the use of the simulation to develop specific BSM criteria for improving the localization and quantitation of MI. In a previous report (6) we have shown that local segments of LV myocardium project their electric signals with variable attenuation to local regions of the body surface. For the purpose of this discussion the 12 segment LV subdivision adopted by the committee on regional LV nomenclature of the 8th annual Engineering Foundation Conference on Automated ECG Diagnosis will be used (see Figure 1). This segmental subdivision is based on dividing the LV through its long axis into quadrants circumferentially using the middle of the septum as a reference point as proposed by Ideker (5). Two planes at right angles to each other are passed through the long axis of the LV producing the 4 quadrants. The LV is further divided from apex to base into 3 regions, apical, middle, and basal by passing 2 planes through the LV at right angles to its long axis so as to divide the long axis into 3 equal parts. This divides the LV into 12 segments of approximately equal volume: The anterior or septal wall of the LV with 3 equal subdivisions, apical, middle, and basal, and clockwise around the long axis as viewed from the apex into the (antero)superior, postero(lateral),

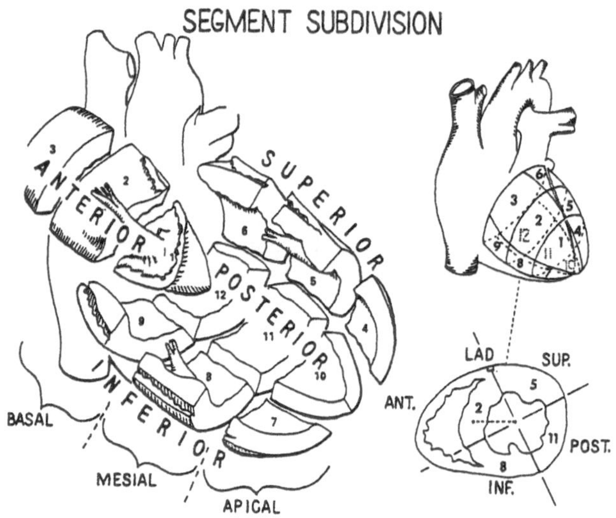

FIGURE 1. The center of the septum as seen in cross sections of the heart taken parallel to the AV groove (lower right diagram) is used as a reference. A line is passed through this point and the long axis of the LV as shown. Two planes at right angles to each other are passed through the long axis, one of which is placed at an angle of 22.5 degrees to the line described above. This divides the LV into quadrants along the long axis. Two more planes pass through the LV at right angles to the long axis and dividing it into equal thirds produces the 12 segment subdivision shown above (described in more detail in the text.

and inferior walls, each with the three equal apex-to-base subdivisions. This particular subdivision has the advantage not only of dividing the LV into segments of approximately uniform size, but along lines that conform rather closely to the coronary artery blood supply. The anterior (septal) and superior walls are perfused by the left anterior descending coronary artery, the posterior wall by the circumflex, and the inferior wall by the posterior descending, usually a branch of the right coronary artery. The apical segments of the latter 2 walls are supplied to a variable extent from the left anterior descending. It follows from the considerations above that the ECG changes of regional ischemia and or infarction due to occlusive coronary disease in any of these arteries has a specific local or regional distribution to the body surface and can be expected to produce isolated ECG BSM changes specific for the segment or artery involved.

As regards the development of the criteria for quantitation of MI from the surface ECG changes, the results of the simulations, which were based on measured torso geometry, cardiac anatomy, activation sequences, and electric properties, are discussed in detail in the papers referred to above, but for clarity certain aspects will be reviewed here. Unit dipoles placed at the centroid of each of the 12 LV segments described above usually produced isolated local potential distributions for the positive potentials. On the other hand, a large overlap of the negative potential distributions was produced with little local specificity. Those regions of the heart close to the torso surface produced large and sharply localized positive potential distributions while, predictably, based on the solid angle theorem, those posterior regions deep in the chest with activation fronts passing through them in a posterior direction produced low amplitude positive potentials on the back with a broader base of distribution and less separation between posterior wall segments. These general relationships, and the lower limits of normal for a small number of normal subjects are shown in figures 2 and 3.

The propagation velocity of the excitation wavefronts in the LV of man and the strength of the electromotive surface are rather uniform from endocardium to epicardium. Thus the percent of amplitude change of QRS on the body surface is not significantly different for the same sized small local infarct (15-20 mm across and 4-5 mm thick) whether it is located in the subendocardium, in the mural myocardium or in the subepicardial region, nor are there significant differences for lesions located from apex to base. Small infarcts of this size do not produce classic Q waves unless they are very strategically located in the subendocardium. This accounts for the widely held opinion that subendocardial infarcts do not produce classic Q wave abnormalities. Larger infarcts involving less than 50% of the transmural thickness of the LV wall will usually produce abnormal Q waves if they are located in the subendocardium in the mid or apical areas of the heart, but not if they are located in the basal regions that are activated in the latter half of the QRS. Even very large transmural infarcts of the posterolateral base of the LV, which depolarizes from 40-90 ms in most people, cannot produce an abnormality in the first half of the QRS, ie. a 30-40 ms Q wave.

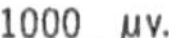

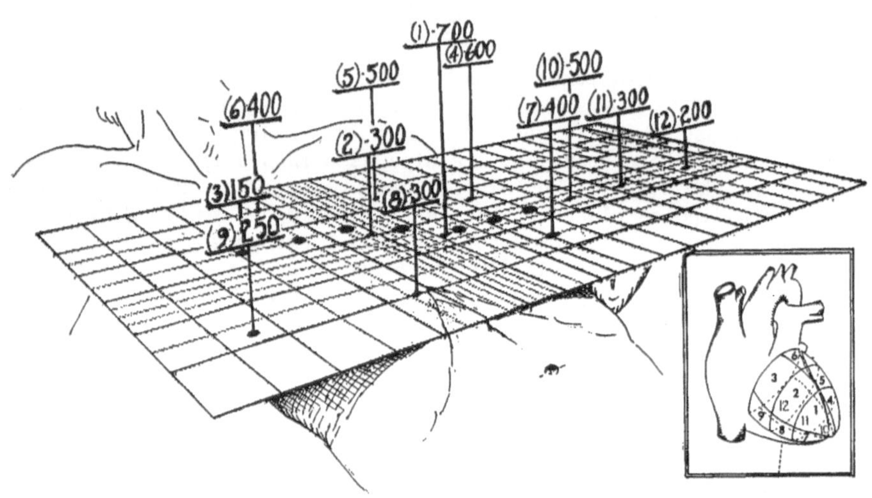

FIGURE 2. A perspective plot of the BSM is shown viewed from the subjects right side and at a 30° elevation. The individual vertical lines define the local regional peak distribution and the relative strength of a unit dipole at the centroid of each of the 12 LV segments shown in the insert lower right. The number on the crossbar at the top of each line is the lower bound of normal of peak positive potential at the same BSM location for a small normal sample.

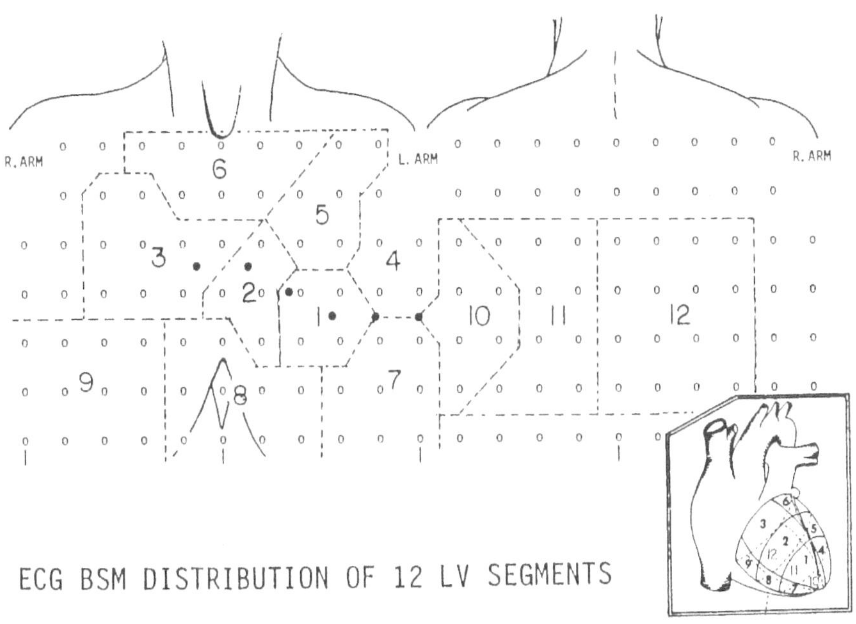

FIGURE 3. The distribution shown is specifically chosen so that each region of the body surface is equivalent to one of the 12 LV segments, each of near the same volume. In this uniform grid, for example, anteroapical segment 1 which is close to the anterior wall is represented by 4 electrodes sites in the left anterior precordium, as is the mid-septal segment 2. The middle and basal Posterior segments 11 and 12, which are deeper in the chest, with posterior directed activation fronts, are represented by 10 and 16 leads respectively. In signal processed low noise BSMs, each of the 12 segments is equally represented by this system.

Numerical experiments a number of years ago with the simulation (1), and later verification with quantitative planometric pathology studies (5), have shown that MIs in the subendocardium in the mid to apical regions of the heart produce initial (Q wave) changes and, if over 30-40 mm in diameter, usually produce abnormally wide Q waves. The same sized lesions in the midwall of the apical or mid regions of the LV will produce mid-QRS changes, ie loss of R, notched R, and when located in the subendocardium or the midwall of the vasal regions activated late, will produce late R or S wave changes or the appearance of abnormal r' waves. A number of recent papers have again called attention to mid and late QRS changes produced by MI. These observations point out the built-in anatomic and physiologic limitation of any 12 lead ECG, VCG, or BSM criteria that depend only on initial R wave or 30-40 ms Q wave criteria such as "Q wave Transmural MI", "Q area BSMs" etc. Since virtually all regions of the LV are subject to infarction it follows that all portions of the QRS from onset to offset can show significant loss of normal vectors. Criteria limited to initial QRS changes can be expected to be insensitive for the diagnosis of MI in general as has been shown in a number of anatomic pathologic studies.

In summary, the anatomic and physiological considerations discussed above lead to the following conclusion: When the 12 regions of the LV as defined above are activated from the endocardium of the LV to epicardium, as they are in normal conduction, and any abnormal conduction except complete left bundle branch block, each of the 12 will project a local distribution of positive potential on the body surface. The sum of potential over time for each BSM region is a function of the electrical integrity of the specific LV segment.

NORMAL VARIABILITY CONSIDERATIONS AND QUANTITATIVE BSM INFARCT CRITERIA

With recent advances in technology it is now reasonable to consider routine recording and automated processing of a high fidelity Electrocardiogram (ECG) of some 16-64 simultaneous leads. The various reduction schemes such as those proposed in this meeting and by a number of groups in the recent literature make it clear that most if not all the potentially diagnostic information in the 200 point BSMs can be captured from this number of leads. The regional considerations from the total body ECG simulations discussed in this paper argue strongly for the inclusion of at least 4 or 5 leads on the back in such a reduced lead set. The well known differences in amplitude and duration of the surface ECG as a function of age, race, and sex makes it mandatory to begin now to plan for the development of a comprehensive normal database stratified by these variables. Myocardial infarction is a disease in developed countries that effects predominantly older males. It follows then that, for the purpose of developing specificity and sensitivity studies using the proposed BSM criteria for quantating infarcts, the most urgent population of normals needed is the middle aged white male group. The design of such a database should be flexible and expandable to make optimum use of a rapidly changing technology, and a number of commercial systems.

At the recent(1984) International Engineering Foundation Conference at Easton, MD on Computerized ECG, IX, the need for a comprehensive normal ECG data base using current multilead simultaneous recording and data processing technology was seen by most of investigators reporting there as a number one priority if we are to make serious headway in the criteria enhancement task highlighted by many at the meeting. One of the most direct ways to improve sensitivity and specificity of any ECG criteria is to compare the specific patient to the age/race/sex group to which he belongs, this instead of comparing the individual adult subject to all adult normals (of all ages, races and both sexes) as now done by all generally available automated computer analysis programs. The job of such a comprehensive normal data base has seemed overwhelming.

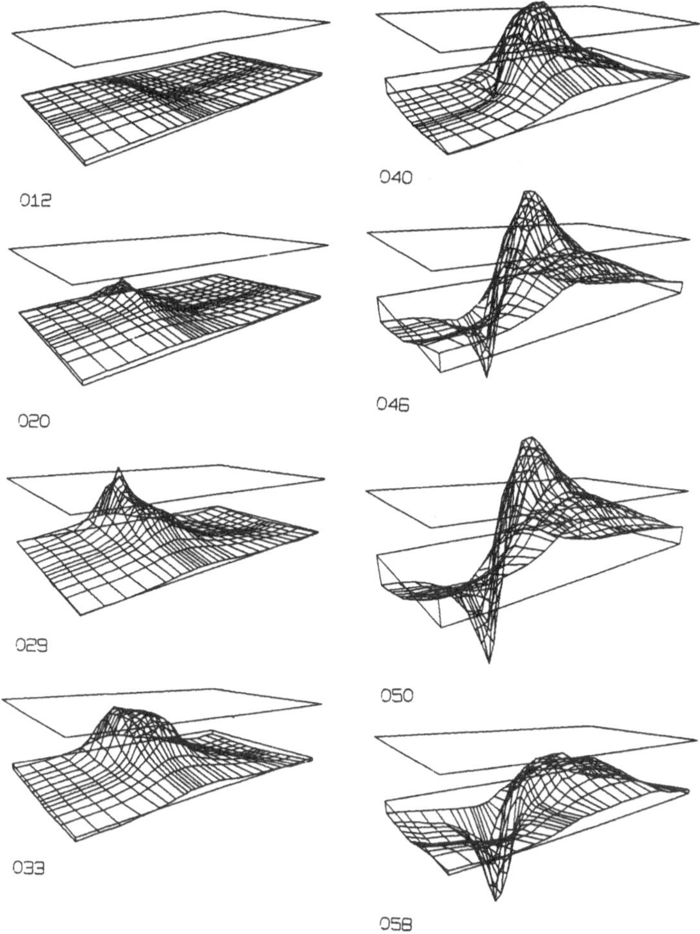

FIGURE 4. Perspective plots of a 190 lead ECG body surface map (BSM) of a normal 22 yr old white female that is typical of those recorded by us to date. Two reference planes are shown in addition to the grid of recording sites. The lower one is set at Zero, the upper one at 500 uv. The initial mound of positive potential produced by the septum and adjacent LV walls is evident on the 12 and 20 ms plots. The latter also exhibits a sharply localized peak from the nearby RV excitation that is just beginning and becomes more prominent on the 29 ms plot. By the 33 ms frame, this sharp peak drops off rapidly as RV breakthrough occurs. A somewhat broader based peak is developing to the left of the initial mound as the LV apex depolarizes. A much broader and low amplitude plateau is also just beginning on the left back from the posterior apex and mid wall excitation. These two latter regions become more developed in the next 3 frames reaching a peak at 46 ms just before LV apical breakthrough. In the meanwhile a large negative well is developing over het mid upper and right chest along with a broad based mound over the entire back from the basal posterior wall excitation which persists with little change at 58 ms after the sharp drop of left chest potentials at LV apical breakthrough.

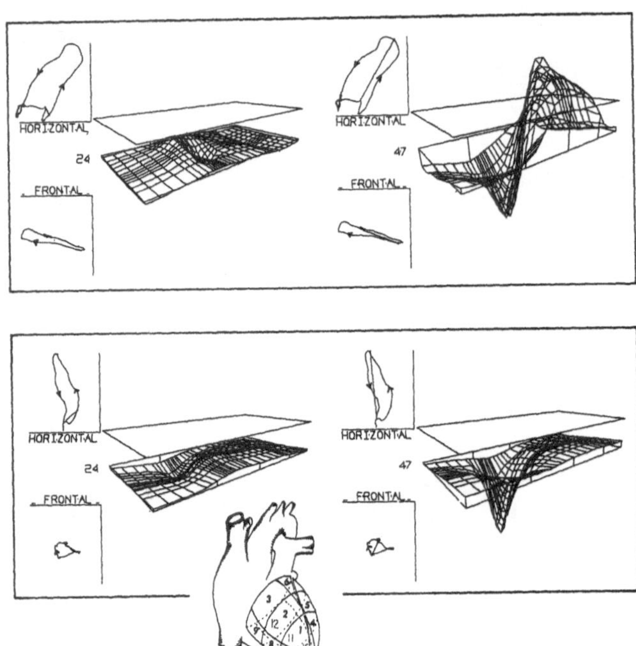

FIGURE 5. The top panel above is a perspective plot at 24 and 47 ms from a 56 yr old white male with a 12 lead ECG and VCG that was read as showing QRS changes of Right Bundle Branch Block and a small anteroapical MI, which was found at biplane angiography along with total occlusion of the LAD coronary artery. A review of the typical normal BSM to the left, and the regional BSM distribution of the 12 LV segments in Fig 3, as compared to the map potential distribution at 24 and 47 ms above reveal the following: Seg.1 shows significant loss in both time plots; Seg.2 shows minimal losses, as do Segs.4 and 7; inferior segs.8 and 9, (antero)superior segs.5 and 6, and postero(lateral) 10, 11, and 12 were all normal in amplitude and distribution. In all there was a loss of BSM positive potentials representing a total of 1.5 seg. or 12% of the LV. This estimate of LV MI was consistant with the ejection fraction of 55% found at angiography.

The bottom panel is from a 48 yr old white male whose 12 lead ECG demonstrated a right axis shift and a large anterior MI, with loss of R but no abnormal Q waves in left precordial leads. The perspective plot, at the same time points as the top panel, shows absence of potential in the distribution of anterior (septal) and superior segs.1, 2, 3, 4, 5, and 6, (seg.6 BSM distribution did show positive potentials after the 47 msec plot shown here). There is minimal loss of positive potential from the inferior wall apical seg.7, but normal potential from segs.8 and 9. The posterior wall apical seg.10, also shows a significant loss, but mid and basal segs.11 and 12 are within normal limits. In all, BSM losses equivalent to 40% LV were found in the LAD coronary distribution. The patient had proximal LAD occlusion, a large anterior superior akinetic segment and an ejection fraction of 35% at left heart angiography.

Assuming only 4 racial groups (Bl, Wh, NA, Or) for starters, and 7 decades (20-89 yrs), and assuming 500 in each cell, which is a reasonable number according to statisticians, the careful qualification and tabulation of non-ECG data (Hist, PE, Xray, and Lab as a minimum) on 28,000 subjects is required. The most time consuming and difficult task here is the human one of recruiting this number of subjects and documenting by non-ECG criteria that they have a very low probability of having heart disease or other conditions known to influence the ECG waveforms. A proposed set of criteria for the definition of normal by non-ECG criteria that was agreed upon by a group of cardiologists at a recent Marquette users meeting is presented in an addendum to this paper for the consideration of those who might be thinking about expanding the 12 lead data base being developed by this group to include body surface maps. In the prospective validation of the BSM criteria for quantitation of regional infarction presented here, this is a very important early step.

SUMMARY AND CONCLUSIONS

The computer simulation of the cardiac electric fields in an inhomogeneous torso from a propagation model that includes realistic heart and torso geometry and electric resistivities has been used to develop a set of QRS body surface map (BSM) criteria for MI in each of 12 regions of the left ventricle for patients in normal conduction and with fascicular blocks. These criteria are based on well established electrophysiological and anatomic principles. Review of BSMs in patients with visible akinesis on biplane ventriculograms suggests that the promising quantitation achieved with the 12 lead ECG MI size scoring system can be significantly improved using the BSM criteria proposed here. Detailed retrosepctive studies of normal subjects and patients with single local infarcts well defined by biplane ventriculograms seem warranted to establish the limits of resolution of these criteria. Such studies would establish the sensitivity, specificity, and diagnostic accuracy of the proposed criteria for quantitating regional infarct in 12 LV segments. The success in earlier studies with the QRS Scoring system for infarct size, which are a set of criteria based on the same simulation, indicate that this approach may be fruitful.

REFERENCES

1. Selvester RH, Solomon JC, Gillespie TL: Digital computer model of a total body ECG surface map. Male torso with lungs. Circ 38: 684-90, 1968.
2. Solomon JC, Selvester RH: Simulation of measured activation sequence in the human heart. Am Ht J 85: 518-524, April 1973.
3. Selvester RH: Criteria for atrial enlargement and infarct size. Conference proceedings Computerized Interpretation of the Electrocardiogram, Cooper, J, ed, HEW and Engineering Foundation, 83-100, 1975.
4. Palmeri ST, Harrison DG, Cobb FR, Morris KG, Harrell FE, Ideker RE, Selvester RH, Wagner GS: A QRS scoring system for assessing left ventricular function after myocardial infarction. N Eng Jour Med 306, 1, 4-9, 1982.
5. Ward RM, White RD, Ideker RE, Hindman NB, Alonso DR, Bishop SP, Bloor CM, Fallon JT, Gotlieb GJ, Hackel DB, Hutchins GM, Phillips HR, Reimer KA, Roark SF, Rochlani SP, Rogers WJ, Ruth WK, Savage RM, Weiss JL, Selvester RH, Wagner GS: Evaluation of a QRS scoring system for estimating Myocardial infarct size. IV. Correlation with quantitative anatomic findings for posterolateral infarcts. Am J Cardiol 53: 706. 1984.
6. Selvester RH, Gillespie TL: Simulated ECG surface map's sensitivity to local segments of myocardium. Proc, VT Conf Body Surface Mapping of Cardiac Fields. Adv in Cardiol Vol 10, Lepeschkin, Rush, Eds Karger, Basel, 1974.

Addendum: A COMPREHENSIVE MARQUETTE 12SL ECG NORMAL DATA BASE

The following group of Marquette Users at the invitation of Ian Rowlandson of the Program Development Group at Marquette met at Isla Morata in 1984, and agreed to conduct a pilot study of the acquisition of a Normal ECG Database:

Rory Childers, Edward Curtis, Antiono De Leon, Kenneth Haisty, Lawrence Jackson, Ralph Lazzara, Charles Moore, Ronald Selvester, and Robert Warner.

This group agreed on the following definition of normal and quality controls:

PURPOSE: To develop comprehensive normal adult ECG database with the Marquette 8 lead system that is stratified by age in decades, race, and sex, ie: white, black, native american, and other. It is expected that ultimately this database can be generalized to the population at large. To get a statistically solid number of normal subjects (the statisticians recommend 500) in each of the 56 cells of this stratified database, we target the acquisition of ECGs from some 30,000 subjects. To make this task tractable a multicenter pilot study group of Marquette users has been formed. When the bugs have been ironed out in the quality control of the acquisition, central archiving, and sharing of this database, it is planned to expand the pilot study group to include any of the Marquette users willing to provide the local supervision of quality control of the data acquisition and normal subject validation in return for having access to the larger comprehensive stratified ECG database.

CLINICAL CRITERIA FOR NORMAL:

1. Negative History as acquired by a certified observer, generally an internist or cardiologist; eg, no history of disease of Heart or any Organ System known to effect the cardiopulmonary or vascular systems.
2. Not taking drugs known to effect the cardiopulmonary vascular systems.
3. Normal Cardiopulmonary and Vascular P.E. as acquired by a certified observer, generally an internist or cardiologist; ie, BP 140/90, no Clicks, Pathological Murmurs, Abnormal Heart Sounds, Abnormal Lung Findings, Peripheral Vascular or Carotid disease. No Skeletal or Neuromuscular abnormalities known to effect the cardiovascular or cardiopulmonary systems.

*4. Normal Clinical Laboratory Data, ie, CBC, Electrolytes, CA, BUN, Creat, Chol, and FBS.

*5. Normal PA Chest X-ray.

* Not required for routine screening of apparently healthy subjects not actively seeking medical care.

Desirable for possible sub-sets of normal:

a. Normal Cath, Echo, Autopsy, etc.
b. Risk factors, ie, Smoking (pkg-yrs), Positive Family History of cardiovascular disease in one or more immediate family members beginning before the age of 55. (Hyperlipidemia, Diabetes, and High BP are exclusions above).

QUALITY CONTROL CONSIDERATIONS: High level coordination must be set in place to keep all participants on track as to definition of demographic normal groups, collection, collation and analysis of data, decisions re data to be included, etc. The quality control must come from within the users group. The ECG Criteria Development Group at Marquette cannot be expected to be objective and firm in excluding the data of one of its customers. A 3 man Ad Hoc Monitoring Committee of users, one each from the west coast, mid US, and east coast is proposed as the working quality control group. The decision that some set of data does not meet the quality control standards of the whole group must come from this monitoring committee. Guidelines for quality controls are:

1. ECG Data Acquisition:
   a. Patient supine.
   b. Trained ECG Technician.
   c. ECG recorded with the digital multilead (12SL) system.
   d. Spot checking of technician (including lead location) at least once a week by a certified observer (certified by the local investigator). Lead Locations will be that specified on the current MAC II cart.
   e. The ECG machines used in this data mission will be calibrated as to frequency response, and gain every 2 weeks by a method that will be defined by Marquette before any data gathering is started. If either is out of specifications by more than 2% the data from the previous 2 weeks will be repeated with the properly calibrated instrumentation or discarded.
2. Data from each participating institution will be reviewed as it comes in by the archiving team in the ECG Program development section at Marquette. This data will be forwarded on a regular basis, usually once a month, to each of the local disc files of the 3 man Ad Hoc Data Monitoring Committee of Users. At least 4 times a year, the data will be reviewed in a 1-2 day shirt-sleeve working session by this 3 man monitoring committee and the Marquette ECG Program development group.
3. All participating Institutions with statistically wider variance in any specific cell or in lumped groups than the average of the group will be reviewed and the data discussed with the responsible investigator to ascertain the possible reasons. If the 3 man monitoring committee decides that the quality control in any given institution cannot, for any number of reasons that may well be out of the control of the local investigator, be brought up to the standards set in the pilot study users group, that data will not be included in the main database.
4. The members of the data monitoring committee, will visit the institutions in their region at least twice a year to reviewstrategies, discuss problems, spot check quality control procedures first hand, and make some assessment of how well the mission is meeting the needs of the individual investigator.
5. The pilot study group will meet one day early at the Annual Marquette Users Group Meeting to review strategies, discuss possible changes in protocols, and to consider widening the pilot study group to include more of the interested users.

REFERENCES

1. Windsor T (ed): The electrocardiographic textbook, The American Heart Association, Inc, New York, 1956.
2. Simonson E: Differentiation between normal and abnormal in Electrocardiography, C V Mosby Co, St. Louis, 1961.
3. Draper HW, Peffer CJ, Stallman FW, Pipberger HV: The corrected orthogonal electrocardiogram and vectorcardiogram in 510 normal men. Circ, 20: 853, 1964.

Chapter 8

BODY SURFACE MAPPING: CONTRIBUTION AND LIMITS FOR THE DIAGNOSIS OF RIGHT VENTRICULAR MYOCARDIAL INFARCTION IN PATIENTS WITH POSTERIOR, INFERIOR OR DEEP SEPTAL LEFT VENTRICULAR MYOCARDIAL INFARCTION

P. BLOCK, E. NYSSEN, J. CORNELIS, L. HUYGHENS, A. BOSSUYT, D. DEMOOR, Y. TAEMANS, X. VERDICKT, PH. DEWILDE

I. Introduction.

In this paper we report our experience with the body surface potential mapping techniques for the diagnosis of right ventricular myocardial infarction (RVMI) in patients with acute posterior, inferior or deep septal myocardial infarction (PIDSMI). In particular we looked wether this technique would be more performant than the conventional and easier to assess E.C.G. criteria such as proposed by Candell Riera (↗ ST in V4R). The radionuclide ventriculography was taken as reference.

II. Methodology.

II.1. Body Surface Potential Maps. (BSPM)

The BSPM were obtained from 60 points located at the anterior thoracic region. They were recorded during the first 12 to 72 hours after the onset of the pain (most often within the first 24 hours). The technical aspects were already extensively described previously (1-3).

II.2. Diagnosis of the acute MI.

This diagnosis rests on typical history, increase of the "specific" heart enzymes and typical anomalies on the 12 leads E.C.G.

II.3. Location of the acute MI.

The assessment of the location of the acute MI was done on the anterior and LAO 45 degrees views of an equilibrium gated angiography of the heart chambers after application of a temporal Fourier transform for the visualization of the regional wall motion.
The posterior, inferior and deep septal location of the MI was assessed on the basis of a decreased amplitude together with a phase delay at the site of the PL, I or DS region of the left ventricle (LV) (4-7).
For the diagnosis of RVMI the same criteria were used but with the anomalies located at the apex or the free wall of the RV.

II.4. Hemodynamic criteria.

The hemodynamic diagnosis of RVMI rests on the presence of at least one of the following criteria, (8-10) eventually after volume loading if hypovolemia was present.

-disproportionate increase of RAP to PCWP
-abnormal RVP wave with no compliant pattern
-sign of Kussmaul (↗ RVDP in inspiration)

III. POPULATION

The learning group consisted in 60 patients with acute PIDSMI, most of them had a true IMI : 35 (58.5 %) with PIDSMI alone; 25 (41.5 %) + RVMI according to the radionuclide ventriculography.

The control group consisted in 62 patients : 37 (59.5 %) with PIDSMI alone, 25 (40.5 %) + RVMI.

IV. RESULTS

IV.1. The best discriminating instants on the BSPM as regards the differentiation between PIDSMI with and without RVMI, were the beginning and end of QRS and S-T (first 2 1/8th and 7th 1/8 QRS, 2 first 1/8th S-T)

IV.2. The "characteristic" patterns of the BSPM of the patients with PIDSMI with and without RVMI were already previously reported. (3-11) The characteristic patterns of ST and T are shown in Fig.1.

Fig. 1. SCHEMATIC DISPLAY OF THE CHARACTERISTIC PATTERNS OF THE BSPM OF S-T AND T OF PATIENTS WITH LVMI WITH AND WITHOUT RVMI

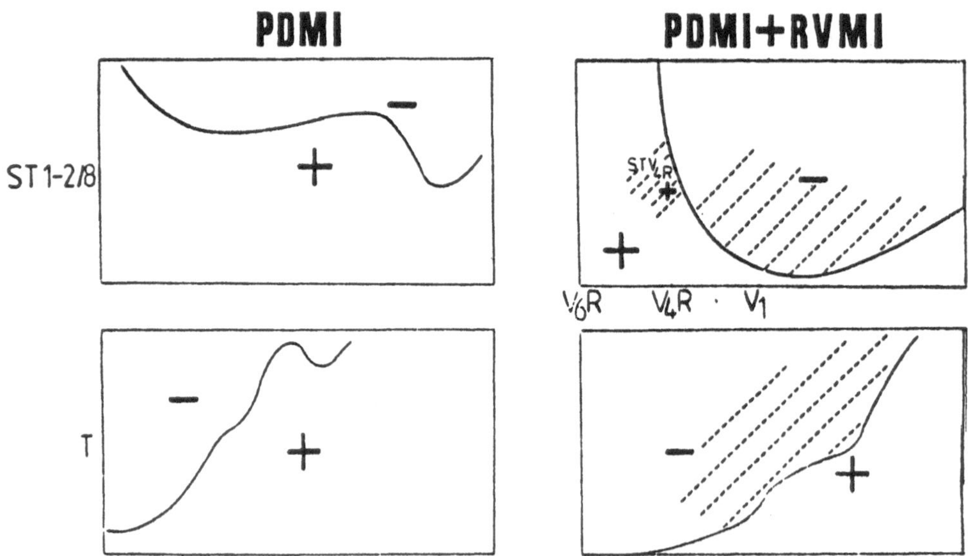

The results obtained in the control group with these "characteristic" patterns of the BSPM of QRS (1st 1/8th) and ST (1st 1/8th) are shown in table I.

Table I: RESULTS OBTAINED IN THE CONTROL GROUP WITH THE SCHEMATIC "CHARACTERISTIC" PATTERNS OF THE BSPM OF QRS (1 st 1/8th) AND S-T (1 st 1/8th) OF THE PATIENTS WITH AND WITHOUT RVMI AND DEFINED ON THE LEARNING GROUP (L).

LVMI Location	PIDSMI		PIDSMI + RVMI	
	QRS1	S-T1	QRS1	S-T1
IMI	13/17 (76%)	12/17 (70%)	6/10 (60%)	8/10 (80%)
PMI	0/5	1/5	1/2	1/2
DSMI	0/2	1/2	1/1	0/1
IPMI	3/9	3/9	0/8	4/8
PDSMI	0/4	0/4	0/4	1/4
Total	16/37 (45%)	17/37 (47%)	8/25 (32%)	14/25 (56%)

The results were very satisfying for the patients with true IMI but disappointing for all the other subgroups of LVMI examined. Therefore we tried to define more specific "characteristic" BSPM patterns for each of these subgroups of LVMI separately. The results obtained on the control group with this new more specific "characteristic" BSPM patterns are shown in table II.

Table II: DIAGNOSTIC PERFORMANCE YIELDED WITH THE NEW SCHEMATIC "CHARACTERISTIC" PATTERNS OF THE BSPM OF QRS-T (SAME INSTANT AS IN TABLE I) DEFINID AND TESTED ON THE CONTROL GROUP.

LVMI Location	PIDSMI		PIDSMI + RVMI	
	QRS1	S-T1	QRS1	S-T1
IMI	13/17 (76%)	12/17 (70%)	6/10 (60%)	8/10 (80%)
PMI	3/5 (60%)	3/5 (60%)	1/2 (50%)	2/2 (100%)
DSMI	1/2 (50%)	1/2 (50%)	1/1 (100%)	1/1 (100%)
IPMI	7/9 (78%)	6/9 (68%)	$0/7^x$ (0%)	4/8 (50%)
PDSMI	1/4 (25%)	2/4 (50%)	$0/4^x$ (25%)	2/4 (50%)
Total	25/37 (69%)	24/37 (65%)	8/25 (32%)	17/25 (68%)

^{x}: no ≠ between LVMI with and without RVMI

No improvement was obtained with these new criteria in the subgroup of patients with true MI, but a slight to moderate improvement was obtained in the other subgroups (mainly PMI, IPMI) with in comparison with the previous criteria a total gain in diagnostic performance (DP) for all the subgroups together of 20% (67% instead 56%, $p < .05$).
Criterion ST/V4R > 50uV gave however slightly higher DP (72%) due to a better DP in the patients with PMI.

These criteria gave the best results in the subgroup of patients analyzed in the very acute stage (first 24 hours) of PIDSMI with hemodynamic evidence of RVMI. In this subgroup the results yieled with the BSPM of ST were even superior to those obtained with ST/V4R (sens SPM: 77% instead 66% with ST/V4R).

V. Discussion.

The following difficulties have to be taken into account for the interpretation of the results:

- There exists various types of LVMI resulting from the thrombosis of the RCA and/or the a.CX with different BSPM patterns.
- The exact localisation of the various types of LVMI is not always easy to assess on the basis of the radionuclide ventriculography (mainly for true IMI, PMI).
- The diagnosis of RVMI is not easy: what criteria should be used ?
  :The hemodynamic data ? Only 18/34 of the suspected RVMI had at the same time + hemodynamic criteria while 2/32 LVMI without radionuclide evidence of RVMI had hemodynamic criteria data suggestive for RVMI.
  :The radionuclide criteria as used in this study ? We should however remember that RVMI often shows a more patchy pattern, with less dyskinesy than it is the case with LVMI. Furthermore LVMI can be more or less extended and to various sites (apical, free wall, both).
  :Finally radionuclide data do not easily discriminate acute MI from ischemia. As both may be present in RCA thrombosis and can produce dyssynergy, we compared the images at day 1, 7 end 12.

These difficulties, pitfalls and also the fact that most often the BSPM were recorded between 12 and 36 hours after onset of the chest pain, probably explain the rather disappointing results we obtained by means of the ECG criteria. It has to be noted that the results were better for the patients with true IMI, PMI and IPMI with or without RVMI (mean DP 70%). The results were still better in the patients with hemodynamic criteria of RVMI. Therefore it may be that the ECG techniques are less sensitive than the radionuclide techniques but better related with the hemodynamic repercussion of RVMI and so probably with the extent of RVMI.

REFERENCES

1. Wartman WB, Hellerstein HK. The incidence of heart disease in 2000 consecutive autopsies. Ann Int. Med. 1948, 28: 41.

2. Wackers Ed, Lie KI, Soloke FB, Res J, Van der Schoot J, Durrez D. Prevalence of right ventricular involvement in inferior wall infarction assessed with myocardial imaging with Tl-210 and Tc 99 m PYP - Am J. Cardiol. 1978; 19: 358.

3. Cohn J.N. Guina NH, Broder MI, Limas CJ. Right ventricular infarction. Clinical and hemodynamic features. Am. J. Cardiol. 1974; 33: 209.

4. Cohn J.N. Right ventricular infarction revisited. Am. J. Cardiol. 1979; 43: 666.

5. Montague T.J., Smith E.R., Spencer C.A., Johnstone D.E., Dalande DL, Bessando R.M., Gardner M.O., Anderson R.N., Horacek M.B. Body surface electrocardiographic mapping in inferior myocardial infarction. Manifestation of left and right ventricular involvement. Circulation 1983, 67: 655.

6. Candell-Riera J., Figueras J., Valle V., Alvarey L, Guttierez L, Cortadellas J., Cinca J, Salas A., Rius J. Right ventricular infarction relation ship between ST-segment elevation in V4R and hemodynamic, scintigraphic and

echocardiographic findings in patients with acute inferior myocardial infarction. Am. Heart J. 1981; 101 : 281.

7. Geft PL, Shah PK, Rodriguez L, Hulse SH, Maddahi J, Berman DS, Gary W. ST elevation in leads V1 tot V5 may be caused by right coronary artery occlusion and acute right ventricular infarction. Am. J. Cardiol. 1984; 53 : 991.

8. Block P., Lenaers A., Dewilde Ph., Tiberghein I., Smets Ph., Kornreich F. Diagnostic value of surface mapping recordings registered at rest and during exercise. In Computer in Cardiology. Publ. Serv. IEEE-NY 1977 : 89.

9. Block P., Tiberghein J.,Raadschelders I, Lenaers A, Kornreich F., Steenhaut O.
A 128 Channel electrocardiographic data acquisition system. In Proc. Med. Int. Eur. 1978; 78 : 521.

10. Block P., Nyssen E., Cornelis J., Dewilde Ph., Demoor D., Taeymans Y., De Meirleir K., Huyghens L., Bossuyt A., Kornreich F. Improved interpretation of ECG surface potential maps. Its usefulness for diagnosis of right ventricular myocardial infarction. In the applications of Computers in Cardiology : State of the Art and New Perspectives. G. Martin Quetglas et al. Elsevier Sc. Publ. B.V. (North-Holland) 1984 : 65.

11. Block P., Nyssen E., Cornelis J. et al. Contribution of the ECG surface potentials to the diagnosis of LV myocardial infarction with and without right ventricular myocardial infarction. In Proc. Working Conf. on Computer ECG Analysis - Towards Standardization - Ed. J.L. Willems, J.H. Van Bemmel and C. Zywietz - North Holland Publ. Ndl - 1985(accepted for publication)

Chapter 9

THE DIAGNOSTIC PERFORMANCES OF VISUAL EXAMINATION OF BSM AND OF ECG/VCG IN THE IDENTIFICATION OF CHRONICALLY INFARCTED LEFT VENTRICULAR SEGMENTS

R.Th. VAN DAM, P.C. ROOSE, P. ARNAUD, C. BROHET

1. INTRODUCTION

Since in Body Surface Mapping the complete information on the surface potentials caused by the heart's action is sampled, this method a priori can be expected to yield a diagnostic power which is superior to that of conventional electrocardiography or vectorcardiography. These conventional methods use only a part of the available information, reduced respectively to a collection of wave forms or to the strength and direction of a single dipole in time. There is abundant evidence that supports this hypothesis (see discussion section). It is questionable whether the method of visual inspection, routinely applied by the majority of clinicians to "bedside" electrocardiographic tracings will suffice to establish an exact diagnosis in all cases. It is for this reason, that computerprograms for the interpretation of both ECG and VCG have been developed which are applied routinely in several diagnostic centers.

The present pilot study was undertaken in order to compare the detailed performance of BSM with that of ECG and VCG as attained by simple visual inspection of body surface maps. The diagnostic category for this comparison was chosen to be the segmental distribution of chronic infarcts in the left ventricle.

2. METHODS.

Single beat signals, recorded with our 64-channel mapping system from 41 subjects with the diagnosis of chronic myocardial infarction were processed into sequential isopotential maps, at 4 ms time intervals. From the same data, standard 12-lead electrocardiograms and vectorcardiograms (modified Frank system) were generated.

These records have been submitted - unmarked and in random order - to 4 different observers for visual inspection and diagnostic interpretation regarding the ventricular segments, involved in the infarction.

The following diagnostic criteria were used:

- body surface maps: "Q-zone" criteria, regarding development and area of negative potentials during the first 30 ms of QRS, as published before (1);
- ECG: NYHA-criteria;
- VCG: criteria of the observers as derived from quantitative vectorcardiography. The scores of both observers have been averaged for the comparison with BSM and ECG.

The resulting detailed diagnoses on the presumed sites of the infarctions at the different ventricular segments have been compared with well-documented evidence of left ventricular asynergy obtained in this case by echo- or ventriculography. Segments of dyskinesis, akinesis or severe hypokinesis were interpreted as being sites of infarction. Descriptions of asynergy had to be divided for some segments; for example "posterolateral" was split into "posterior" and "lateral".

3. RESULTS

Table 1 contains the diagnostic performances of the three electrocardiographic methods for the different left ventricular asynergic segments that were obtained in this pilot study. Of the three methods, the BSM-technique shows the highest sensitivity for septal, lateral and posterior locations of the observed asynergy which is considered to be related to the presence of chronic myocardial infarction, even though just the Q-zone criteria are used in the interpretation of the maps. Relatively low scores were obtained in the anterior segment.

In general, higher diagnostic scores for BSM were obtained in segments with akinesis or dyskinesis than in hypokinetic segments. The recognition from maps of infarctions that are located in the inferior segment is approximately equal to that from ECG and VCG, and that of anterior segment infarction is somewhat less. The diagnostic scores for anterior and for inferior segment infarction were found to be high for all three methods in "pure" cases in which no infarction in the opposite part of the left ventricle was present; see table 2.

In contrast, in the presence of both anterior and inferior asynergy, the diagnostic scores for all three methods appear to be markedly lower as regards the recognition of inferior wall infarction, as is shown in table 3, whereas the diagnosis of anterior segment infarction appears not to be affected in this small number of observations.

TABLE 1. Diagnostic performance for asynergic left ventricular segments in 41 patients with chronic myocardial infarction.

Segment	Number of asynergic segments		BSM	ECG	VCG
Anterior	17	sensitivity	72%	89%	83%
		specificity	86%	68%	83%
Septal	14	sensitivity	93%	79%	46%
		specificity	85%	88%	98%
Lateral	20	sensitivity	55%	45%	45%
		specificity	80%	75%	90%
Inferior	19	sensitivity	74%	79%	63%
		specificity	91%	86%	86%
Posterior	16	sensitivity	37%	23%	28%
		specificity	87%	96%	96%
Apex	12	sensitivity	17%	17%	--
		specificity	86%	89%	--
Basal	10	sensitivity	60%	20%	--
		specificity	93%	90%	--
Total	109				

TABLE 2. Diagnostic performance for - non opposed - anterior and inferior segments

	number of segments		BSM	ECG	VCG
Anterior without inferior infarction	11	sensitivity	100%	82%	92%
Inferior without anterior infarction	14	sensitivity	85%	85%	71%

TABLE 3. Positive diagnostic scores in combined anterior and inferior wall infarction.

	number of segments	BSM	ECG	VCG
Anterior (with inferior)	6	5	5	5
Inferior (with anterior)	5	3	3	2

DISCUSSION

Our results indicate that BSM may yield some degree of improvement in diagnostic recognition of the presence of chronic infarction in the septal, posterior, basal and lateral portions of the left ventricle, as compared to electrocardiographic and vectorcardiographic methods.
The obvious limitations of this study consist of: its limitation to visual interpretation, the use of criteria for abnormal early negativity only, and the comparison with data on left ventricular asynergy.
This study was mainly limited to visual judgement for two reasons. Firstly, we meant to explore the diagnostic possibilities of BSM in a relatively simple fashion. Secondly, in considering the clinical diagnostic application of mapping, the first choice would be the visual inspection of the obtained maps in a way which is similar to the bedside interpretation of electrocardiograms. The results presented demonstrate that this is indeed possible. The gain in diagnostic performance appears to be modest.

In this study we did not yet analyse the abnormalities in the development of positive potentials that may contribute to the recognition of infarctions, particularly those that are situated in the posterior segment. As the initial negativity seen in other locations is small or absent in posterior infarctions, because of the relatively late occurrence of normal activation in this area, the sensitivity of the "Q-area" criteria is necessarily low for this segment.

Abnormal early negativity may also be absent in intramural or subendocardial infarctions of the "non-Q" type. This may explain the relatively low diagnostic scores in hypokinetic areas, and advocates the diagnostic analysis of positive potentials appearing during QRS.
The most controversial issue is the evaluation of diagnostic interpretations by means of data on left ventricular asynergy as an index to the localisation of chronic infarctions. They only are indirectly related to the perfusion disturbances that lead to infarction. In our experience, the best correlation between asynergy and diagnostic localisation by all three electrocardiographic records was observed for segments of akinesis or dyskinesis (100 and 75%, respectively) and the lowest for hypokinetic segments (57%). Also a subjective factor and some degree of observer error in the data on kinetic disturbances as determined by echo- or ventriculography cannot be ruled out. This e.g. may be suggested by the fact that in some patients all electrocardiographic interpreters agreed on the presence of a chronic infarction in a given segment, whereas no abnormal contractile pattern was described for that location.
In spite of these limitations, the results of this pilot study do indicate, that BSM may be of use for the clinical diagnosis of chronic infarctions. We expect that a larger data basis on this topic will confirm the findings in this study.

REFERENCES

1. Dam RTh van, Heringa A, Uijen GJH, Pol AJ van de, Poel J van der, Spierenburg HAM, Lim LSL.
Interpretation of body surface maps of combined infarctions based on kinetics analysis.
in: Electrocardiology '83, Ed. I. Ruttkay-Nedecky and P. Macfarlane, Amsterdam, Excerpta Medica, 1984., pp. 177-181.

PART 3

CONDUCTION DISTURBANCES

Chapter 10

BODY SURFACE POTENTIAL MAPPING IN CONDUCTION ABNORMALITIES

J. LIEBMAN

INTRODUCTION

The pathology, pathophysiology, mechanisms and diagnostic parameters related to ventricular conduction abnormalities have been studied for more than half a century. But in the past decade, newer experimental data, as well as improved surface techniques, have revealed that the field is once again in its infancy.[1-3] One of the most important areas of work was by Dr. Mauricio Rosenbaum[1-3], who attempted to make specific electrocardiographic conduction defect diagnoses based upon specific anatomical abnormalities. Although his techniques did not allow complete success, his classification of abnormalities has proved to be very useful. We have modified his 11 point schema into a 17 point classification.

SUGGESTED MODIFIED ROSENBAUM CLASSIFICATION

1. Advanced RBBB (proximal)
2. Advanced RBBB (distal)
3. Partial RBBB
4. Terminal right ventricular conduction delay
5. Advanced LBBB (proximal)(predivisional)
6. Partial LBBB
7. Left anterior division block
8. Abnormally superior vector
9. Left posterior division block
10. Divisional LBBB, or simultaneous left anterior and left posterior division block
11. RBBB with left anterior division block
12. RBBB with left posterior division block
13. LBBB with an abnormally superior vector
14. LBBB with left posterior division block
15. Advanced bilateral bundle branch block, or simultaneous block in both proximal bundle branches.
16. Advanced trifascicular block (simultaneous block in the proximal right bundle branch plus each of the two divisions of the left bundle branch).
17. Functional "bundle branch block" associated with premature beats, tachycardias and bradycardias

In this presentation, all 17 types of ventricular conduction abnormalities will not be discussed. Only those conduction abnormalities for which body surface potential mapping (BSPM) has given important insights will be included, and,whenever possible, knowledge related to both pathology and pathophysiology will be related to the body surface mapping data.

ADVANCED RIGHT BUNDLE BRANCH BLOCK

The term "complete right bundle branch block" is now known to be a misnomer[4], for there is considerable variation in the degree of completeness of the block from patient to patient despite standard criteria being met. (It makes little sense to describe one electrocardiogram with a diagnosis of complete right bundle branch block as being more "complete" than another with a diagnosis of complete right bundle branch block.) In addition, it is known that lesions distal to the proximal right bundle can produce ECG's which on standard ECG or with vectorcardiographic display also meet the standard criteria. Consequently, in the interests of accuracy, a more appropriate term was necessary; thus the phrase advanced right bundle branch block[4].

In a recent BSPM study of 37 children[5], the spectrum of right bundle branch block was described in a series of patients most of whom had had surgery. These 37 included a group of 20, previously presented, all of whom with tetralogy of Fallot, and all having had extensive ventriculotomy, aggressive infundibulectomy with construction of a right ventricular outflow tract patch extending across the pulmonary valve ring, and all with a patch over the large ventricular septal defect. Electrophysiological studies in seven of the 20 hemodynamic catheterizations performed indicated that the right bundle branch block was distal in six. The BSPM methodology was as previously described with 180 electrodes, enclosed in a vest, no electrode paste, and a color display[6].

Characteristic features were found in all maps. Accompanying the maps is a magnitude function, a scalar representation of the natural values from all 180 electrodes. In advanced RBBB there are four distinctive portions in the QRS magnitude function, each associated with specific findings on the BSPM as documented in the color maps in the recent publication. Initial activation (part 1) is similar to that of the normal. Part 2 is also rapidly inscribed, with very important differences from normal in that there is no evidence for epicardial right ventricular breakthrough; but near the end of part 2, the beginning of evidence for left ventricular breakthrough is invariable. This breakthrough is manifested by an indentation (notch) in the positive region near the anterior axillary line, which is usually from above,but could be from below, and which rapidly expands to divide the maximum into two distinct maxima. In the very brief part 3, the posterior maximum quickly decreases in potential and area whereas the anterior maximum moves to the right, increasing in potential and area. In the very prolonged part 4, the single maximum (or two closely spaced maxima) very slowly progresses to the right and superior, ending with one maximum. The single minimum is left and inferior. The ST segment maps are usually strikingly similar to those of the late portion of part 4 of the QRS, except that the positive and negative regions are now interchanged.

For further details, including quantifications as well as pictures of actual maps, the reader is referred to the original papers[5,7]; but certain measurements as compared to normal are of interest:

1. The time of peak voltage arising from presumed left ventricular activity (35.0 ± 5.2 ms), in advanced RBBB is not different from that of the peak magnitude of the leftward anterior (or posterior) maximum in the normal (37.7 ± 5.2 ms), although the maximal peak to peak magnitude (2410 ± 738 μv) is much less than in the normal (4667 ±1230 μv).

2. The time of left ventricular breakthrough (not recognized in the normal, where right ventricular breakthrough begins at 24.4 ± 4.2 ms) is 40.4 ± 9.4 ms.

3. Evidence for recognition of activation of the right ventricle is at 42.2 ± 9.6 ms (not recognized in the normal).

4. The peak magnitude of the presumed right ventricle is at 94.3 ms with the peak to peak magnitude 3340 ± 1013.7 μv (not recognized in the normal).

5. The right ventricle maximum arrives superior at 101.4 ± 22.0 ms.

6. The right ventricle ends with maximum right anterior superior at 143.4 ± 17.3 ms (duration QRS) with normal duration 76.6 ± 5.6 ms.

7. The peak magnitude of ST-T is 1809 ± 580.2 μv (normal 1180 ± 82.0 μv) and occurred at 309.8 ± 34 ms (normal 276.2 ± 36.3 ms).

8. The duration of QRS-T is 406.1 ± 56.3 ms (normal 351.8 ± 24.9 ms).

It is generally agreed that ventricular activation in advanced RBBB begins normally on the left side of the septum, and that much of the left ventricular activation is completed before right ventricular activation begins. The time to traverse the septum is longer than normal, with activation of the right ventricle beginning on a broad front extending from the septum[8,9,10,11]. Our data indicate that the left ventricle is activated normally, with peak magnitude at the normal time and place (although in the normal the peak maximum is sometimes posterior). The explanation as to why the peak magnitude (2415 μv) is <u>less</u> than the normal (4709 μv) is not evident. The presumed beginning of left ventricular breakthrough (40 ms) was always <u>after</u> the time of peak magnitude of the maximum reflecting left ventricular activation, and always immediately preceded the appearance of a second separate maximum, more to the right and anterior. This second maximum is always high in the inferior left quadrant, and is believed to reflect the initial activation of the right ventricle after the long and slow left-to-right traversal through the septum. From then on, movement of the positive region superiorly and to the right takes a long time, averaging 101 ms until completion. This length of time is greater than that of the entire QRS, so that obviously conduction through the right ventricle in advanced RBBB is very different from that in the normal[11,12]. Myerburg[12,13] has stressed that impulses in the right ventricle appear to be able to enter or leave the conducting system only at longitudinal terminations (a general rule of the system). The BSPM during ST-T is also very different from normal, reflecting a sequence of repolarization that is largely determined by the activation sequence. The morphology was close to a mirror image (similar shape but inverse polarity) to that during late QRS, and the average peak to peak magnitude of the T was 1809 uv compared to the normal of 1180 μv. Studies of right ventricular activation in advanced RBBB demonstrate a slow continuous cell to cell activation in the apex to base direction[11]. Therefore, the very long transventricular propagation time far outweighs the smaller intramural differences in action potential duration that normally play an important role in T wave formation[14,15,16]. The result is a sequence of repolarization that follows the depolarization sequence, but with inverse polarity.

There were nine other children with BSPM and a diagnosis of advanced RBBB, but who demonstrated important differences. None had tetralogy of Fallot, although all had VSD, often with either pulmonic stenosis or previous pulmonary artery band. In two of the nine, the VSD was closed via the atrial route, and of the remaining seven with ventriculotomy, two had VSD closure with direct suture. In none was there any evidence for epicardial right ventricular breakthrough, but although the QRS duration was wide (132 ms) it was 10% less than in the previously discussed group (with a lot of variation). The shortening of QRS occurred during parts 3 and 4 of the magnitude function, but in some, the maps were virtually indistinguishable. In terms of timing major events, the only differences, on the average, were after activation reached the right ventricle. The time of attainment of maximal right ventricular potential was at 86.2 ms compared to 94.3 ms; the time the maximum reached superior was 96.5 ms compared to 101.4 ms; and the duration of right ventricular activation was 85.8 ms compared to 101.2 ms.

Other papers where BSPM has been utilized in the study of right bundle branch block have also been of particular interest[17,18,19].

PARTIAL RIGHT BUNDLE BRANCH BLOCK

The term partial right bundle branch block (partial RBBB) is utilized instead of incomplete right bundle branch block (even though the phrases are probably synonymous), because of the implications involved in the previous use of the diagnosis of incomplete right bundle branch block. Virtually all standard textbooks make the diagnosis wheneven there is an rsr' or rsR' in lead V1, even though all that is represented is that the terminal rightward projection of the QRS crosses the line perpendicular to the lead vector for lead V1. The actual diagnosis may be: Normal, RVH, RVH with terminal right conduction delay, normal with terminal right conduction delay, or incomplete (partial) right bundle branch block. Therefore, in the interest of both preventing confusion and accurate terminology, it seemed more appropriate to create the new term of partial right bundle branch block[4].

In a recent study comparing partial RBBB with RVH and terminal right conduction delay[20,21,22], 11 children with partial RBBB had BSPM's with quantifications as described for advanced RBBB. Six had had surgery, three had tetralogy of Fallot (the surgery being as described above in patients who developed advanced RBBB), and three for large ventricular septal defect (VSD) involving ventriculotomy and patch closure of the VSD. Of the other six, two had VSD with surgery and three were hemodynamically normal.

For the actual pictures of the maps and detailed measurements, the reader is referred to the original paper[20], but certain measurements are of interest:

1. Time of peak LV voltage(34.8 ± 6.7 ms)
2. Time of LV breakthrough (7 of 11)(35.1 ± 5.9 ms)
3. Time of RV activation (41.8 ± 8.5 ms)
4. Time of RV peak magnitude (58.9 ± 14.4 ms)(magnitude 2733.5 ± 984.2 μv)
5. Time of end of RV (duration QRS) (92.9 ± 15.5 ms)
6. Time of peak magnitude ST & T (285.2 ± 15.8 ms)(mgnitude 1001.2 ± 342.8 μv)
7. Duration QRS-T (343.1 ± 17.9 ms)

In no patient (as in advanced RBBB) was there evidence for epicardial right ventricular breakthrough, although in 7 of the 11 children clearcut evidence for left ventricular breakthrough was recognized, similar to that in advanced RBBB. Although the duration of QRS and ST-T were increased, there were children where the measurements were within normal limits. The first three measurements were the same as in advanced RBBB, but then the duration of activation of the right ventricle was considerably less than in advanced RBBB. Furthermore, the peak magnitudes of RV and ST-T were significantly less than in advanced RBBB and for ST-T was no different from that in the normal child of similar age. The variations in the various right ventricular measurements were considerable, just as in advanced RBBB, consistent with the wide spectrum. Although the total QRS-T duration is greater than normal the positions of the maximum and minimum were not different from normal. (This is in contradistinction from that of advanced RBBB, where the polarity of the maximum and minimum is reversed.) It must be presumed, although not proven, that in partial RBBB right ventricular activation is that of a fusion. Activation is via the septum from the left ventricle as well as via the right bundle itself. For detailed discussion of the presumed type of activation, the previously cited paper is recommended[20]. However, it is likely that in partial RBBB, conduction in the right ventricle is that of a fusion. Activation is likely to be partially from the right ventricle, utilizing Purkinje (although late), and partially from the left ventricle, across the septum, as in advanced RBBB.

RIGHT VENTRICULAR HYPERTROPHY (RVH) WITH TERMINAL RIGHT CONDUCTION DELAY

In the recent study the 11 patients with partial RBBB were compared with 13 patients proven to have atrial septal defect of the secundum bype. All eventually had surgery. The reader is referred to the original papers for more detail as well as pictures of the maps, but, as with partial RBBB, certain measurements are of interest:

1. Time of peak LV voltage (29.9 ± 4.6 m)
2. Time of epicardial RV breakthrough (29.7 ± 3.5 ms)
3. Time of RV activation (34.3 ± 4.2 ms)
4. Time of RV peak magnitude (49.9 ± 8.2 ms)(magnitude 2604.6 ± 725.2 μv)
5. Time of end of RV (duration QRS) (82.5 ± 8.4 ms)
6. Time of peak magnitude ST-T (262.5 ± 21.4 ms) (Magnitude 1095.1 ± 244.9 μv)
7. Duration QRS-T (340.2 ± 19.91 ms)

The duration of QRS was significantly less than that in partial RBBB although slightly greater than in the normal (76.9 ms). The time of the peak magnitude of ST-T was also less than in partial RBBB, but the total duration of QRS-T and the peak magnitude of ST-T were the same in both groups. The time at which the right ventricle is recognized to begin activity is slightly earlier in ASD (34.3 ms) than in partial RBBB (41.6 ms), but the length of time till the end of the recognized RV activity is the same (48.2 ms for ASD; 50.9 ms for partial RBBB). A key difference in the two groups, however, is that epicardial right ventricular breakthrough is present in RVH with terminal right conduction delay (more to the left and superior) and <u>not</u> present in partial RBBB. This reflects a fundamental difference in the manner in which the right ventricle is activated. In advanced RBBB, the right ventricle is activated purely by cell to cell conduction from the left ventricle across the septum. In the normal and in RVH with terminal right conduction delay, activation is via the right bundle branch system, including the Purkinje network. In partial RBBB, as previously stated, it seems likely that activation of the right ventricle is that of a fusion.

ENDOCARDIAL CUSHION DEFECT (Atrioventricular Septal Defect)

This congenital anomaly is very varied in its severity, ranging from a small ostium primum type atrial septal defect with or without deficiency in the anteromedial leaflet of the mitral valve to a complete atrioventricular canal with huge atrial and ventricular defects in continuity. Deficiency of the medial portions of both AV valves and continuity of a primitive AV valve leaflet through the atrioventricular defect are part of the complete form. But, no matter what the severity, there is virtually always a conduction defect manifested on the electrocardiogram by an initial inferior vector followed by most of the rest of the vector loop being superior[4,23,24,25]. Unless there is a great deal of concomitant RVH, the direction of QRS inscription is counterclockwise. The electrocardiogram appears identical to that seen when the left anterior branch of the left bundle is cut. Yet, at autopsy, all that has been recognized is perhaps minimal displacement of the left anterior branch to the left and inferior. Burchell's epicardial studies indicated early activation of the posterior-lateral wall of the left ventricle, with delay in excitation of the anterior interventricular groove[26]. Durrer studied epicardial excitation at surgery and found that the posteriorbasal section of the left ventricle was activated very early[27]. In their canine experiments, if the posterobasal left ventricle was excited early, an abnormally superior vector was created. It is now known that although the left posterior branch of the left ventricle initiates activation, the left anterior branch of the left ventricle is responsible for the normal initial activation up the septum. If the left anterior branch is cut or there is the type of conduction abnormality associated with endocardial cushion defects, initial activation is directed inferior rather than the normal superior.

The one extensive BSPM study on endocardial cushion defects, by Spach and his group[28], demonstrated early activation more to the left and inferior than normal, with rapid migration toward the left shoulder. After a period with multiple maxima over the anterior and posterior chest, a prominent minimum developed over the inferior left laterial chest and enlarged superiorly. Finally, for a prolonged period, two maxima, one more superior than the other, remained for a prolonged period as the inferior maximum disappeared. It seems likely that conduction is traveling up the left anterior branch of the left bundle,but the reason why is obscure.

The entire subject needs extensive and varied investigation.

LEFT BUNDLE BRANCH BLOCK

Less is known about the etiology of left bundle branch block than right bundle branch block. Most left bundle branch block (LBBB) is related to left ventricular disease[29]. In children, there are rare cases of congenital left bundle branch block and at all ages surgery within the left ventricular outflow is known to cause left bundle branch block, presumably from damage to the proximal bundle. Distal LBBB has also been postulated, but there is as yet little evidence.

Grant and Dodge, in a brillant paper on the mechanisms of QRS prolongation in man[30], predicted not only that in advanced LBBB there was an alteration in the sequence of activation but there was an additional alteration in the mode of excitation. They postulated that once activation reached the left ventricle, conduction was via fiber to fiber not utilizing the Purkinje system. But, specific surgical studies in animals and humans are sparse as are electrophysiological studies in general. It is likely that activation begins from the right side via the septal branch of the right bundle and via the endocardium of the free walls by way of the moderator band. Activation in the right ventricle is normal, and then after a slow traversal of the septum, there is even slower cell to cell conduction across the left ventricle, possibly beginning in the area of the posterobasal left ventricle,then extending laterally, and, according to van Dam[8], anterolaterally. According to Becker[31],in dogs it could begin in either the posterobasal or anterior septal area, before extending laterally.

Preda and his group have done extensive studies of LBBB utilizing BSPM[32,33,34]. They divided their maps into three time phases, phase I being the normal activation of QRS seen in normal adults including evidence for right ventricular breakthrough. In phase II, which began after 50 ms, there was a broad anterior minimum, increasing in potential and area, together with two distinct maxima, on the back and on the left lower border of the anterior chest wall. The maxima slowly moved left laterally and after 100 ms (phase III) there was development of a new maximum mid sternally with gradual augmentation in voltage and area. Dr. Preda has postulated that there is important anterobasal activation in most patients with LBBB when there is no infarction. Of importance, also, is that when this late anterior activation does not occur, anterior myocardial infarction can be diagnosed in addition to **LBBB**. Other papers,of particular interest, where the BSPM has been utilized in the study of LBBB include those of Stilli[25] and Sohi[36].

WOLFF-PARKINSON-WHITE SYNDROME, WITH FUSION

The WPW syndrome provides a very special type of conduction abnormality. The bypass tract enters a portion of right or left ventricle and initiates slow cell to cell conduction toward the other ventricle. Later, at variable times, from patient to patient, conduction through the atrioventricular node initiates conduction through regular pathways, so that there is a fusion. The BSPM has been documented to be extremely accurate in isolating the location of the bypass tract by early QRS excitation, although the group at Duke[37] has believed that the location of the repolarization wave was even more reliable. In so doing, all now agree that there are seven or eight specific locations for bypass tract conduction[39] and,in the opinion of many, the BSPM may be even more accurate than is the electrophysiological study with the cardiac catheter.

Of particular interest is the documentation with BSPM of clear-cut fusion involving epicardial right ventricular breakthrough, a phenomenon that can occur only via conduction through the Purkinje system to the endocardium, followed by endocardial to epicardial activation.

The following is a BSPM of a 12 year old girl with a presumed posterior left ventricular bypass tract. (The child has had no arrhythmias, and has had neither catheterization nor surgery.) In Fig. 1, early QRS activation (with a typical strong minimum) is evident at the posterior spine. In Fig. 2, by 42 ms the minimum had expanded in area and increased in magnitude. In Fig. 3, at 54 ms, in the strong maximum, near the sternum, there is the beginning of a notch to the right superior, in the typical position for epicardial right ventricular breakthrough. In Fig. 4, the notch gradually expands as a minimum, a large pseudopod, into the maximum. It is very evident that activation has occurred utilizing the AV node and the Purkinje system. In Fig. 5, two maxima are evident. The large anterior left maximum has been activated from the left ventricle, and, presumably as well, by cell to cell conduction across the septum to the right ventricle. The smaller maximum, right anterior superior, is the last to be depolarized (Fig. 6), and has been activated via the normal conduction system. Therefore, a fusion beat has been detailed, and clearly recognized in the body surface potential map.

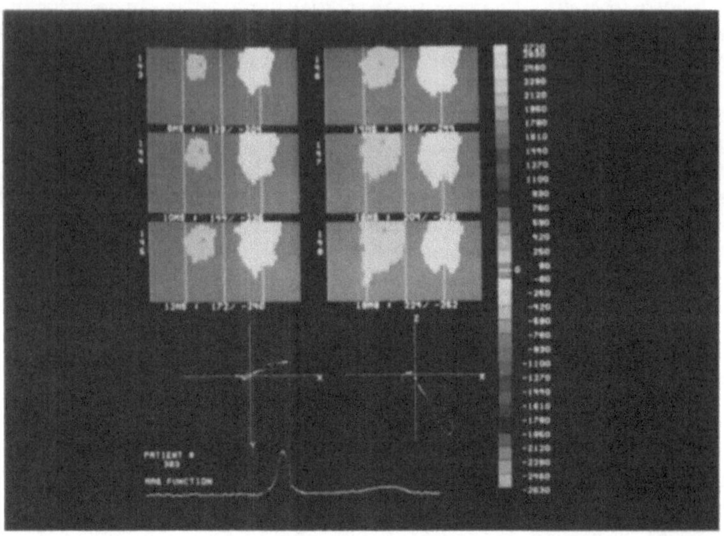

Fig. 1 - 6. Body Surface Potential Map (QRS),in color, of a
FIGURES 1 - 6. Body Surface Potential Map (QRS), in color, of a 12 year old female. Each frame is recorded at 2 ms intervals. The frontal plane (XY) and horizontal plane XZ) Frank system vectorcardiograms are included, as is a magnitude function, the total of the natural values from all 180 electrodes. In each ECG of the magnitude function and VCG's, the red dots indicate the BSPM position in time. In each frame, the two sections on the patient's right are from the anterior chest, first right, then left, separated by the sternum. The next two frames are from the posterior chest, first left, then right. The five vertical lines in order, from patient's right, are right axillary line, sternum, left axillary line, spine, and right axillary line. Thus the maps envelop the chest, anteriorly and posteriorly, from clavical to a line just above the navel. For more details, the reader is referred to references 5 and 6 (J. Electrocardiol. 17:329, 1984, and J.Electrocardiol. 14:249, 1981.

FIGURE 1. The BSPM frames (from 6 to 18 ms) are in the delta wave. The initial "minimum" was straight posterior and still there, consistent with the bypass tract being in the posterior left ventricle.

FIGURE 2. The BSPM frames (from 32 to 42 ms) are past the delta wave, and the minimum and maximum remain in the same position (as they were from 20 to 30 ms). They have expanded in area and increased greatly

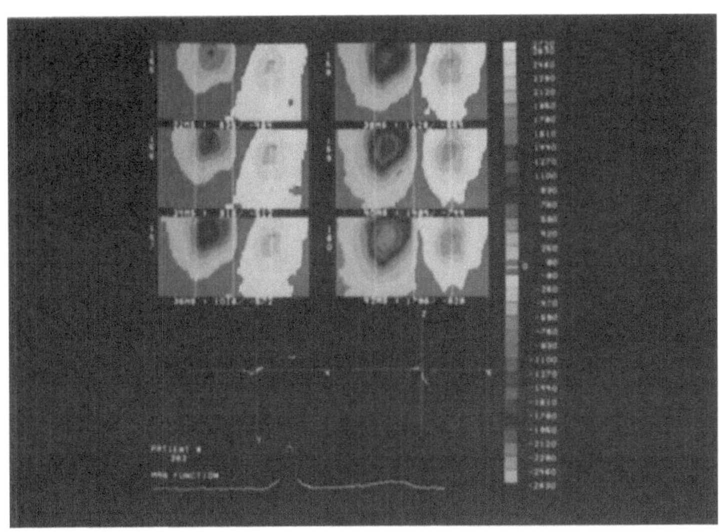

FIGURE 2. The BSPM frames (from 32 to 42 ms) are past the delta wave, and the minimum and maximum remain in the same position (as they were from 20 to 30 ms). They have expanded in area and increased greatly in magnitude. This very slow conduction is typical of muscle cell to muscle cell conduction, with no Purkinje spread.

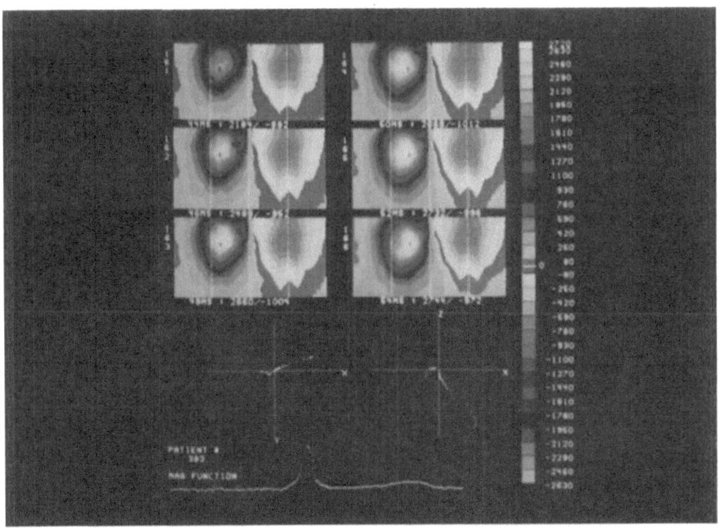

FIGURE 3. The BSPM frames (from 44 to 52 ms) continue to be in the same general position,increasing in magnitude and (with the maximum) in area as well. However, in frame 166 at 54 ms there is a notch in the maximum (in the right upper quadrant of the central area).

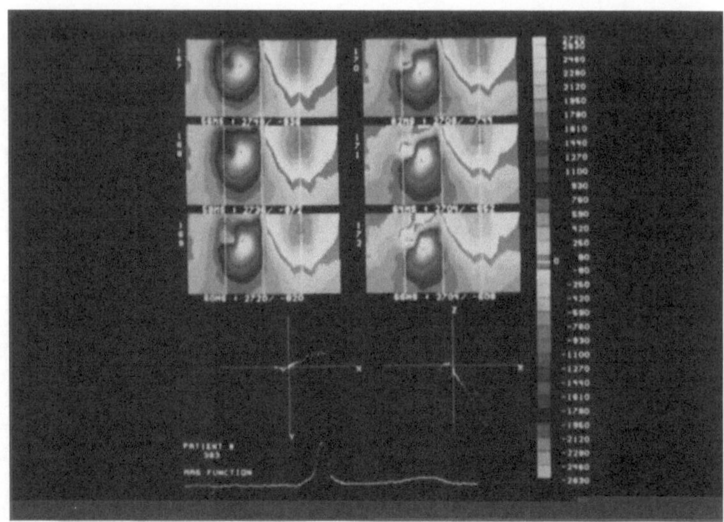

FIGURE 4. BSPM frames (from 56 to 66 ms). The minimum is beginning to recede in area and magnitude. The notch in the continuing intense maximum is dramatically expanding and a new minimum develops with that notch. This new minimum takes the shape of a typical saddle; classical right ventricular breakthrough has taken place although the pseudopod extends from the superior instead of right superior. A new maximum is developing above the area of the original notch.

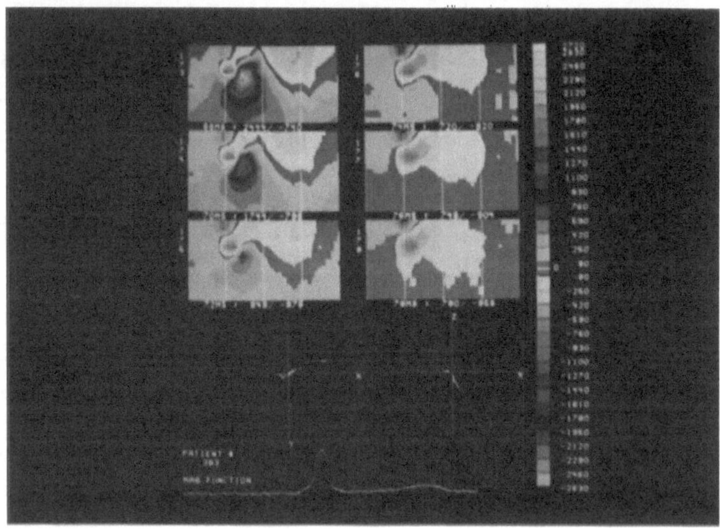

FIGURE 5. BSPM frames (from 68 to 78 ms). The pseudopod has developed into the major minimum. The original maximum is receding and the new maximum is expanding into the right anterior superior. This latter is

the typically accepted area for the right ventricular outflow tract. (It is clear that a fusion has taken place. Most of activation of the right ventricle has been from the left ventricle via the bypass tract. The remainder of the right ventricle is presumed to have been activated via the Purkinje system after normal AV conduction.

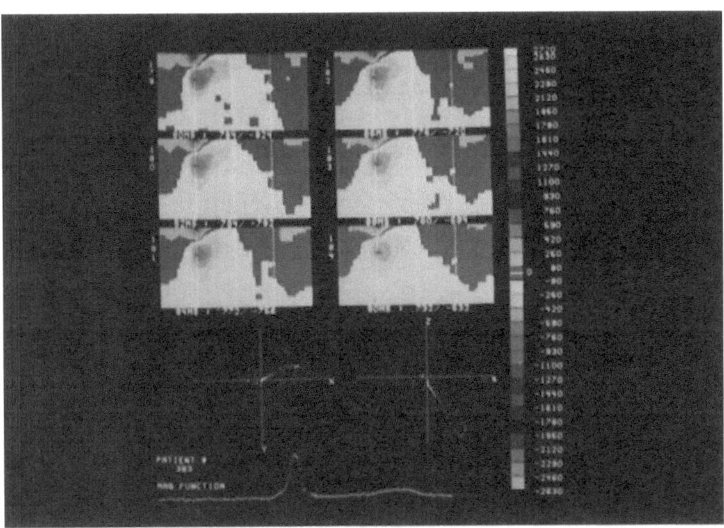

FIGURE 6. BSPM frames (from 80 to 90 ms). There is some terminal right conduction delay as manifested in the VCG and magnitude function. It is evident from the BSPM that the right anterior superior magnitude is decreasing in area and magnitude very slowly.

SUMMARY

This brief paper on ventricular conduction abnormalities has demonstrated many aspects of conduction abnormalities which could not possibly be elucidated in any other manner noninvasively. The spectrum of both partial and advanced RBBB, when surgically induced, has been delineated, and insights into the types of conduction have been delineated. That there should be clinical application is clear, one example being the ready differentiation of partial RBBB from right ventricular hypertrophy with terminal right conduction delay. Only the beginning of knowledge of mechanisms in LBBB and in the abnormally superior vector is evident, but in LBBB there is so much emerging data that there is promise of important knowledge and important diagnostic information particularly related to concurrent myocardial infarction. In the WPW syndrome with antegrade conduction across the bypass tract, the BSPM allows accurate anatomic location of the position where the tract enters the ventricle. In addition, there is the clear demonstration by the BSPM of the fusion of activation, conduction of the ventricle also occurring vis the AV conduction system, including Purkinje.

A proviso, of course, is that only so much can be presumed with the necessary concurrent basic science investigations, so as to continually confirm deductions. But, in many cases, the guide to these basic science investigations is indeed in the BSPM itself.

REFERENCES

1. Rosenbaum MB, Elizari MV, Lazzara JO, Nau NG, Levi RG, Halpern MS: Intraventricular trifascicular blocks: Review of the literature and classification. Am. Heart J. 78:450, 1969.
2. Rosenbaum MB: The hemiblocks: Diagnostic criteria and clinical significance. Mod. Concepts Cardiovasc. Disease 39:141, 1970.
3. Rosenbaum MB, Elizari MV, Lazzara JO: The hemiblocks. Tampa Tracings, Oldsmar, Florida, 1970.
4. Liebman J: Interpretation of conduction abnormalities. In Pediatric Electrocardiography, ed. Liebman, J., Plonsey, R., Gillette, P.C., Williams and Wilkins, Baltimore, Md., 1982, Chapter 2, 1972.
5. Liebman J, Rudy Y, Diaz P, Thomas CW, Plonsey R: The spectrum of right bundle branch block as manifested in electrocardiographic body surface potential maps. J. Electrocardiol. 17:329, 1984.
6. Liebman J, Thomas CW, Rudy Y, Plonsey R: Electrocardiographic body surface potential maps of the QRS of normal children. J. Electrocardiol. 14:249, 1981.
7. Liebman J, Rudy Y, Diaz P, Thomas CW, Plonsey R: Electrocardiographic body surface potential maps in advanced right bundle branch block. In Advances in Body Surface Potential Mapping, ed. Yamada, K, Musha, T., Harumi,K., Univ. Nagoya Press, Nagoya, 1983, p. 217.
8. van Dam R Th: Ventricular activation in human and canine bundle branch block. In The Conduction System of the Heart, ed. Wellens,H.J.J. Lie, K.I. and Janse, M. J., Lea and Febiger, Philadelphia, 1976, p. 377.
9. Wennemark JR, Blake DF, Kazdi P, Lev M: Extensive intraventricular conduction defect. Experimental production with destruction of total Purkinje-net system of the canine right ventricle. Circ. Res. 11:904, 1962.
10. Erickson RV, Scher AM, Becker RA: Ventricular excitation in experimental bundle branch block. Circ. Res. 5:5, 1957.
11. Walston A, Boineau JP, Spach MS, Ayers CR, Estes EH Jr: Relationship between ventricular depolarization and QRS in right and left bundle branch block. J. Electrocardiology1:155, 1968.
12. Myerburg RF, Gelband H, Nilsson K, Castellanos A, Mirales AR, Bassett AL: The role of canine superficial ventricular muscle fibers in endocardial impulse distribution. Circ. Res. 42:27, 1978.
13. Myerburg RF, Nilsson K, Gelband H: Physiology of the canine intraventricular conduction and endocardial excitation. Circ. Res. 30:217, 1972.
14. Plonsey R: A contemporary view of the ventricular gradient of Wilson. J. Electrocardiol. 12:337, 1979.
15. Plonsey R: Recovery of cardiac activity. The T wave and ventricular gradient. In New Directions in Pediatric and Fundamental Electrocardiography, ed. Liebman, J, Plonsey, R., Rudy, Y. , Martinus Nijhoff, the Hague, Holland. Chapter 2. In press.
16. Burgess MJ, Green LS: Ventricular repolarization properties and their relation to the body surface electrocardiogram. In New Directions in Pediatric and Fundamental Electrocardiography, ed. Liebman, J., Plonsey, R., Rudy, Y., Martinus Nijhoff, The Hague, Holland, 1986. Chapter 3. In press.
17. Taccardi B, De Ambrozzi L, Riva D: Chest maps of heart potentials in right bundle branch block. J. Electrocardiol. 2:109, 1969.
18. Sugenoya J: Interpretation of the body surface isopotential maps of patients with right bundle branch block. Determination of the

region of the delayed activation within the right ventricle. Jap. Heart J. 19:12, 1978.

19. Flowers NC, Sohi GS: Body surface map pattern of altered depolarization and repolarization in right bundle branch block. Circulation 61:634, 1980.

20. Liebman J, Rudy Y, Thomas CW, Plonsey R: RVH with terminal right conduction delay versus partial right bundle branch block. In New Directions in Pediatric and Fundamental Electrocardiography, ed. Liebman, J., Plonsey, R., Rudy, Y., Martinus Nijhoff, The Hague, Holland, 1986. In press.

21. Liebman J, Thomas CW, Rudy Y, Diaz PJ, Plonsey R: Clinical data with a color displayed 180 electrode ECG-BSPM system. Presented September 11, 1983. Proceedings 5th Annual Conference of the IEEE/EMBS, Columbus, OH 1983.

22. Liebman J, Rudy Y, Diaz PJ, Thomas CW, Plonsey R: Body surface potential mapping - partial right bundle branch block versus right ventricular hypertrophy with terminal right conduction delay. (Abstract) JACC 3:496, 1984.

23. Liebman J, Nadas AS: An abnormally superior vector (formerly called marked left axis deviation). Am.J.Cardiol.27:577, 1971.

24. Liebman J, Nadas AS: The vectorcardiogram in the differential diagnosis of atrial septal defect in children.Circulation22:956, 1960.

25. Toscano-Barbazo E, Brandenburg RO, Burchell HB: Electrocardiographic studies of cases with intracardiac malformations of the atrioventricular canal. Proc. Staff Meet. Mayo Clinic 31:513, 1956.

26. Burchell HB, Dushane JW, Brandenburg RO: The electrocardiogram of patients with defects of the atrioventricular canal. Am. J. Cardiol. 6:575, 1960.

27. Durrer D, Roos JP, van Dam Th: The genesis of the electrocardiogram of patients with ostium primum defects (ventral atrial septal defects). Am. Heart J. 71:642, 1966.

28. Spach MS, Boineau JP, Long EC, Gallie TM, Gabor JB: Genesis of the vectorcardiogram (electrocardiogram) in endocardial cushion defects. In Vectorcardiography 1965, ed. Hoffman, I. and Taymore, R.C., North-Holland Publishing Co., Amsterdam, 1966, p. 327.

29. Scott RV: Left bundle branch block: Clinical assessment, II. American Heart J. 70:691, 1965.

30. Grant RP, Dodge HT: Mechanisms of QRS prolongation in left ventricular conduction disturbances. Am.J.Med. 20:834, 1956.

31. Becker RA, Acker AM, Erickson RV: Ventricular excitation in experimental left bundle branch block.

32. Preda I, Balozza I, Kozmann G, Shakin VV, Szekely A, Antoloczy Z: Surface potential distribution on the human thoracic surface in left bundle branch block. Jap. Heart J. 20:7, 1979.

33. Preda I, Antaloczy Z, Kozmann G: Left bundle branch block and chronic myocardial infarction: Surface mapping evidence and electrocardiological signs. Jap. Heart J. 23 (suppl) 397, 1982.

34. Preda I, Kozmann G, Rochlitz T, Mertz J, Toth K, Antaloczy Z, Szilvasi I, Balogh I: Left bundle branch block and chronic myocardial infarction: Isointegral analysis of body surface maps. In 11th International Congress on Electrocardiology, Caen, France, 1984.

35. Stilli D, Musso E, Macchi E, Taccardi B, Rulli A, Aurier E, Favaro L, Botti G: Diagnostic value of body surface maps in left bundle branch block. Adv. Cardiol. 28:36, 1981.

36. Sohi GS, Flowers NC, Horan LG, Sridharen MR, Johnson JC: Comparison of total body surface map depolarization patters of left bundle branch block and normal axis with left bundle branch block and left axis deviation. Circulation 67:660, 1983.
37. Benson DW Jr, Sterba R, Gallagher JJ, Walston A II, Spach MS: Localization of the site of ventricular pre-excitation with body surface maps in patients with Wolff-Parkinson-White syndrome. Circulation 65:1259, 1982.
38. Gallagher JJ, Gilbert M. Svenson RH, Sealy WC, Kasell J, Wallace AG: Wolff-Parkinson-White syndrome. The problem, evaluation and surgical correction.
39. DeAmbroggi L, Taccardi B, Macchi E: Body surface maps of heart potentials - tentative localization of pre-excited areas in forty-two Wolff-Parkinson-White patients. Circulation 54:251, 1976.
40. DeAmbroggi L, Taccardi B, Macchi E, Perotta GM: Criteria for localizing pre-excited areas from body surface maps in Wolff-Parkinson-White patients. Adv. Cardiol. 21:36, 1979.
41. Iwa T, Magara T: Clinical application of body surface mapping. Correlation between localization of accessory conduction pathway and body surface maps in the Wolff-Parkinson-White syndrome. Jap. Circ. J. 45:1192, 1981.
42. Spach MS, Barr RC, Lanning CF: Experimental basis for QRS and T wave potentials in the WPW syndrome. The relation of epicardial to body surface potential distributions in the intact chimpanzee. Circ. Res. 42:103, 1978.

Chapter 11

VALIDATION (TEST SET) OF A METHOD FOR DETECTING ASSOCIATED HEART CONDITIONS IN LBBB BY MEANS OF BSM

E. MUSSO, D. STILLI, C. BRAMBILLA, G. REGOLIOSI, I. PREDA, G. KOZMANN, T. ROCHLITZ, Z. ANTALOCZY, B. TACCARDI

1. INTRODUCTION

We recently reported (1) a procedure for detecting associated heart condition(s) in left bundle branch block (LBBB), based on a multivariate analysis (Fisher's discriminant analysis (2) of 10 voltage related variables contained from body surface maps (BSM). In that study (1), we correctly classified 34 of 37 patients (90% of the cases) in whom LBBB was uncomplicated (7 cases) or complicated by: myocardial infarction (MI, 8 cases), left ventricular hypertrophy or enlargement (LVH, 8 cases), myocardial ischemia (IS, 8 cases), MI+LVH (6 cases). With a view to validating the efficacy of the method by means of a test set, we applied the same procedure to a new LBBB population studied at 1) the Institute of General Physiology of Parma and 2) the Postgraduate Medical School, 2nd Medical Clinic and the Central Research Institute for Physics of Budapest.

2. MATERIALS AND METHODS

Test set patients. Three LBBB patients were investigated at the Institute of General Physiology of Parma. In two of them the conduction defect was complicated by LVH, in one by MI. In the Hungarian study BSM were recorded from 52 LBBBs. Only 16 of them were used here, due to some differences in the criteria adopted for diagnosing the complicating heart conditions, compared with the learning set. The selected patients were three uncomplicated LBBBs, one LBBB+LVH and 12 LBBBs+MI. In the last group of patients LVH might also be present in addition to MI. Thus, the test set was constituted by 19 patients, three of whom had uncomplicated LBBB, three had LBBB+LVH and 13 had LBBB+MI, regardless of the presence or absence of LVH.

Data processing. According to the procedure followed in the learning set, we plotted as functions of time the instantaneous QRST values of the highest potential on the chest (Mxi), lowest potential (Mni), highest potential difference (ΔVi), integral of the absolute value of the potential function extended to the entire chest surface ($\int_S |Vi| dS$) and positive fraction of the thoracic area explored (Ai+%). From these functions we extracted the 10 variables (Table 1) which, in the learning set, exhibited the highest ratio: sample variance between groups/sample variance within groups. The statistical homogeneity of these variables in the learning and test set was checked by means of Hotelling test. The variables were then submitted to the procedure provided by Fisher's discriminant analysis (2) for allocating new patients in one of the group taken into consideration in the learning set. As mentioned above, in LBBB+MI cases LVH might also be present. Therefore, the classification of these patients was considered correct independently of whether they were allocated to LBBB+MI or to LBBB+MI+LVH group.

TABLE 1. Variables employed for Fisher's discriminant analysis. For the symbols Mni, ΔVi and $\int_S |Vi| dS$ see text.

1) $\Sigma\int_S |Vi| dS$(mid-QRS): sum of $\int_S |Vi| dS$ extended to the middle third of QRS
2) N$\Sigma\int_S |Vi| dS$(mid-QRS): average value of $\int_S |Vi| dS$ during middle third of QRS
3) $\Sigma\Delta$Vi(mid-QRS): sum of ΔVi extended to the middle third of QRS
4) ΣMni(QRS): sum of Mni extended to the entire QRS
5) $\Sigma\int_S |Vi| dS$(QRS): sum of $\int_S |Vi| dS$ extended to the entire QRS
6) ΣMni(mid-QRS): sum of Mni extended to the middle third of QRS
7) N$\Sigma\Delta$Vi(ST-T): average value of ΔVi during the entire ST-T
8) N$\Sigma\int_S |Vi| dS$(QRS): average value of $\int_S |Vi| dS$ during the entire QRS
9) $\Sigma\Delta$Vi(QRS): sum of ΔVi extended to the entire QRS
10) Max$\int_S |Vi| dS$(QRS): peak value of $\int_S |Vi| dS$ during QRS

TABLE 2. Mean value+standard deviation of the 10 variables submitted to Fisher's discriminant analysis in the three LBBB groups of the test set. Variables n.1,2,5,8,10 are expressed in mV.cm2, variables n.3,7,9 in mV, variables n.4,6 in -mV. The number of patients in every group is given by figures in brackets.

Variables	Pure LBBB (3)	LBBB+MI (13)	LBBB+LVH (3)
1) $\Sigma\int_S |Vi| dS$(mid-QRS)	6204.7±898.4	4115.2±926.0	8319.0±1602.4
2) N$\Sigma\int_S |Vi| dS$(mid-QRS)	246.0±43.8	174.0±41.6	295.4±36.2
3) $\Sigma\Delta$Vi(mid-QRS)	103.7±9.2	50.8±25.5	147.0±21.2
4) ΣMni(QRS)	130.0±12.4	78.8±23.3	197.8±41.4
5) $\Sigma\int_S |Vi| dS$(QRS)	10403.7±879.8	7679.5±1634.7	15623.7±2416.5
6) ΣMni(mid-QRS)	81.2±10.0	43.0±13.3	104.5±30.7
7) N$\Sigma\Delta$Vi(ST-T)	0.7±0.2	0.5±0.2	1.3±0.2
8) N$\Sigma\int_S |Vi| dS$(QRS)	142.6±18.4	105.4±23.4	183.8±18.6
9) $\Sigma\Delta$Vi(QRS)	173.3±15.4	113.8±25.4	284.7±26.8
10) Max$\int_S |Vi| dS$(QRS)	269.0±50.8	200.2±46.3	310.4±42.5

3. RESULTS

The average values of the 10 variables in the three groups of patients of the test set (Table 2) were similar to those of the corresponding groups of the learning set. In both sets, LBBBs+MI had lower values than uncomplicated cases. LBBBs+LVH had higher values. The statistical treatment of the variables by means of Fisher's discriminant analysis made it possible to properly allocate 15 of 19 patients (Fig. 1). Therefore, the percentage of correct allocation was about 80%. Of the 4 patients uncorrectly classified one had uncomplicated LBBB and 3 LBBBs+MI. The latter patients were allocated to the uncomplicated group (2 cases) and to the ischemic group (1 case). The uncomplicated patient was allocated to the ischemic group.

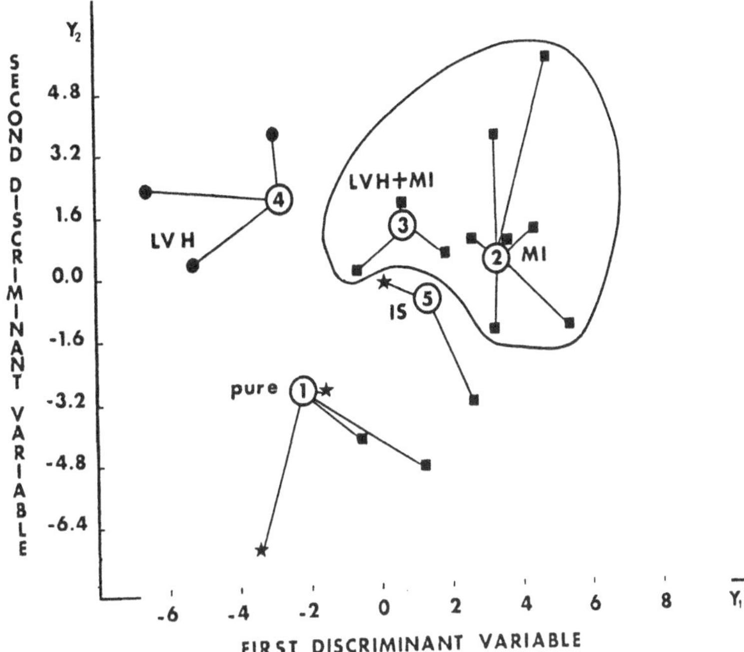

FIGURE 1. Location of the test set patients in the space of the discriminant variables provided by Fisher's discriminant analysis (Y1 and Y2 on the horizontal and vertical axis, respectively). Uncomplicated LBBBs are indicated by stars, LBBB+MI by squares, LBBB+LVH by circles. The central points of the clusters relating to LBBB groups studied in the learning set and the complicating heart condition(s) for each group are respectively indicated by the numbers 1 to 5 and by the appropriate abbreviations. The term pure specifies the uncomplicated LBBBs. The test set patients were allocated to the various groups on the basis of the minimal euclidean distance from the central point of the group (lines connecting patients with numbers). All patients with LBBB+MI surrounded by the black line were considered as correctly classified despite three of them were allocated to LVH+MI group, for the reasons indicated in the Methods. Other explanations in the text.

4. DISCUSSION

We confirmed our previous findings (1) that heart conditions complicating LBBB markedly affect the quantitative aspects of the cardiac potential field at the body surface. Specifically, chest potentials are lowered by MI and augmented by LVH presumably due to a loss or increase of active myocardial tissue, respectively. Since there is not much cancellation in LBBB, the above conditions must decrease or increase the total amount of current flowing in the chest and result in lower or higher potential values at the thoracic surface. The correct allocation of about 80% of the patients of the test set (versus 90% in the learning set) indicates that linear combination of a number of voltage related variables obtained from BSM do provide useful information for detecting complicating heart conditions in LBBB. It should be noted that a high percentage of correct allocation was achieved in the test set despite the fact that maps of most patients (Hungarian group) were obtained with recording equipment and number and location of electrodes on the chest different from those of the learning set. So far, the validation of the efficacy of the method was satisfactory for LBBB+MI. Conversely, the data relating to uncomplicated LBBB and LBBB+LVH should be considered only preliminary because of the small size of these groups in the test set. At present only 16 of 52 available patients of the Hungarian study were used. Efforts are now being made to eliminate differences between these patients and those of the learning set as regards the criteria for clinical classification of cases. This would allow to extend the size of the groups considered in the test set and to include in it other LBBB groups so far disregarded, as LBBB+IS and LBBB+MI+LVH.

REFERENCES

1. Musso E, Stilli D, Brambilla C, Regoliosi G, Rolli A, Botti G, Taccardi B: Discrimination among different groups of LBBB patients, by means of body surface maps (BSM). In: 11th International Congress on Electrocardiology. July 17-20, 1984, Caen. Abstract Book: 108.
2. Johnson RA, Wichern DW: Applied multivariate statistical analysis. Englewood Cliffs (New Jersey): Prentice Hall, 1982: 594.

Chapter 12

LOCALIZATION OF PRE-EXCITATION SITES IN THE WOLFF-PARKINSON-WHITE SYNDROME BY BODY SURFACE POTENTIAL MAPPING AND A SINGLE MOVING DIPOLE REPRESENTATION

R.A. NADEAU, P. SAVARD, G. FAUGèRE, M. SHENASA, P. PAGé, R.M. GULRAJANI, R.A. GUARDO, R. CARDINAL

1. INTRODUCTION

In the Wolf-Parkinson-White (WPW) syndrome, the Kent bundle may insert around the periphery of the A-V ring as well as in the I.V. septal region. The anomalous pathway can be localizes by intracavitary catheters during electrophysiological studies (EPS), either by stimulating the atria at multiple sites and finding the ventricular area with the greatest degree of pre-excitation, or by mapping retrograde atrial activation especially during reentrant tachycardia. Direct epicardial recordings during surgery provide a more precise localization.

The pre-excitation site can also be estimated from the electrocardiographic characteristics of the relatively slowly inscribed delta wave that corresponds to ventricular depolarization near the anomalous pathway. Various ECG, VCG, and body surface potential maps (BSPM) classification schemes have been proposed for the localization of the pre-excitation site according to the morphology of the delta wave (1-5).

In this study, BSPM were recorded in WPW patients undergoing EPS. The BSPM were analyzed by a single moving dipole (SMD) representation. The SMD location, magnitude, and angle were computed so as to reproduce on the surface of a computer torso model the measured potentials. The SMD computation techniques have been thoroughly developed in our laboratories by a series of animal experiments, computer simulations, and clinical studies (6-8). The SMD trajectories were compared to the results gathered during the course of EPS by catheter mapping, or by epicardial mapping for the patients undergoing surgery.

2. MATERIAL AND METHODS

2.1 Patients and electrophysiological investigation

The BSPM were recorded during EPS in 29 WPW patients. Different interventions were performed during EPS such as atrial pacing to modify the degree of pre-excitation, the induction of orthodromic supraventricular tachycardia and the injection of procainamide to abolish pre-excitation. The electrocardiogram and vectocardiogram were also obtained. In addition, epicardial mapping of the ventricular pre-excitation and of the retrograde atrial activation was performed during surgery in 11 of these patients.

2.2 Data acquisition and processing

The BSPM were obtained from 63 leads with 43 electrodes uniformly distributed on the front and sides of the torso, and 20 electrodes on the back. A simulation study has shown that SMD computations carried out with this array had about the same accuracy as with a 120 lead array (7). Data acquisition and processing was performed on site, with a dedicated system developed at the Institut de génie biomédical (CORDIC). With this system, the ECGs are digitized at 500 Hz with a resolution of 10 bits, and stored on disk. The ECG signals are then calibrated and displayed on a video terminal. A typical heartbeat is visually selected by the operator and baseline shift corrected.

For each sampling instant, the SMD is computed using a least-squares technique with 15 multipoles and a torso model including regions of lower electrical conductivity representing the lungs. This computation technique was found optimal when compared to other techniques in computer simulations (7) and in clinical studies with patients having implanted pacemakers (8). The SMD trajectories thus obtained were then projected onto the A-V ring plane. This new coordinate system corresponds to three rotational transformations of -70 , -40 and -45 about the standard Z, X and Y axes (9).

3. RESULTS

The SMD trajectory during the delta wave adequately depicted the ventricular pre-excitation. The SMD orientation and location projected on the A-V ring plane were oriented from the site of pre-excitation toward the center of the heart. This can be seen on Figure 1 which shows the SMD results obtained for four patients whose pre-excitation site was later localized by epicardial mapping performed before cryoablation of the accessory A-V pathway.

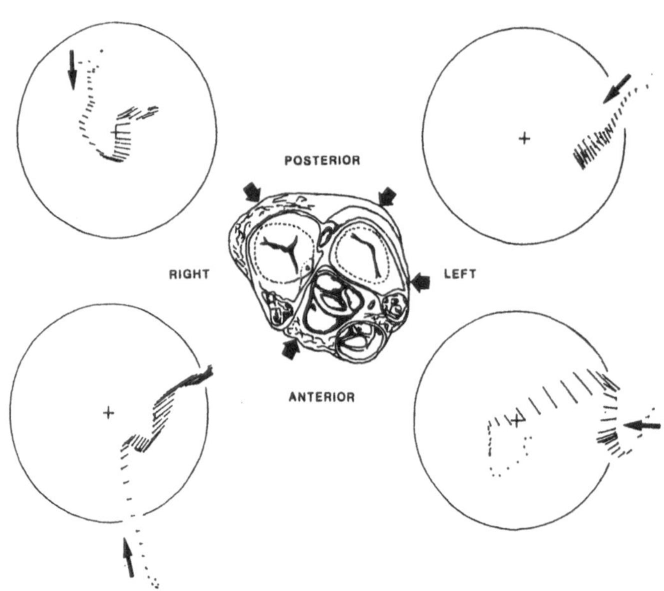

FIGURE 1: SMD trajectories during the delta wave and QRS complex of four WPW patients. The arrows around the diagram identify the location of the accessory pathway determined during surgery. The successive SMD locations projected onto the A-V ring plane at 2 msec intervals are joined by a dotted line and arrows show the direction of the trajectory. At each point, the corresponding SMD vector is projected in the same plane.

Results from other patients showed that the initial SMD trajectory depicted even moderate pre-excitation, and that its location was not significantly affected by atrial pacing. The A-V ring plane projection used for the display of these SMD trajectories provided a clearer representation of the cardiac electrical activity around the base, than frontal, sagittal or transverse plane projections.

The BSPM of the four patients presented in Figure 1 are also shown in Figure 2 and identified by asterisks. For these patients and the others who underwent surgery, the BSPM recorded at 40 ms during delta wave had a maximum which was always located in the left precordial area, whereas the minimum was located anteriorly on the right for right-sided pre-excitation, and posteriorly for left-sided pre-excitation. The lower torso was positive for anterior pre-excitation, and negative for posterior pre-excitation. The zero lines were nearly vertical for lateral pre-excitation (right or left). These findings were consistent with those of De Ambroggi et al. (2), Benson et al.(5), and Lorange et al. (10).

As shown in Figure 2, progressive changes were noted in the morphology of the BSPM recorded during the delta wave for different patients, thus reflecting the continuous distribution of pre-excitation sites around the A-V ring. We thus found a continuum of BSPM patterns instead of a small set of fixed patterns. These BSPM patterns can be attributed to dipole sources pointing from the accessory pathway site toward the apex, as illustrated in the simple heart model shown in the center of the figure.

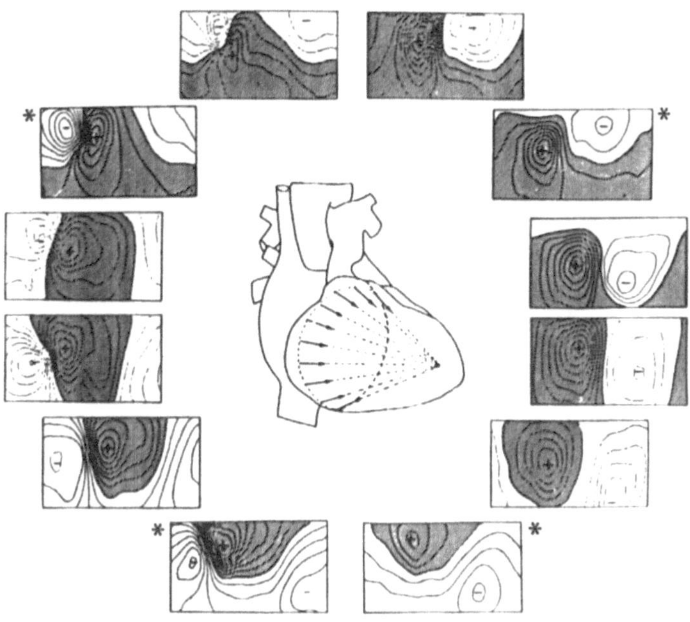

FIGURE 2: BSPM recorded during the delta wave at 40 msec after QRS onset. The left part of the maps correspond to the anterior torso, and the right part to the back. The shaded areas identify the positive regions. The location of the maps around the heart correspond to the location of the pre-excitation site determined by surgery or EPS.

4. DISCUSSION

Both BSPM and SMD could accurately localize pre-excitation sites determined by epicardial mapping (Table 1). The interpretation of the SMD trajectory was based on the orientation and location of the SMD which were oriented from the pre-excitation site, toward the center of the heart when projected on the A-V ring plane. The SMD was also able to depict the progression of activation even during moderate pre-excitation. These results suggest that the SMD might possibly be used to localize other cardiac sources such as ectopic foci.

The interpretation of the BSPM was based on the location of the negative regions on the torso surface. Since the minimum was located posteriorly for left-sided pre-excitation, this suggests that posterior recording sites can improve the accuracy of the pre-excitation localization.

TABLE 1: PRE-EXCITATION LOCALIZATION

PT	SURGERY	BSPM-SMD	EPS
LT	R ANT	R ANT	R POST SEPT
CD	R POST	R POST	L POST SEPT
PT	R POST-S	R POST	R POST
ND	L POST	L POST	L POST
DT	L LAT	L LAT	L POST
SL	L LAT	L LAT	L LAT
GJ	L LAT	L ANT	L LAT
ML	L ANT	L LAT	L LAT
CC	L ANT	L ANT	L POST SEPT
NC	L ANT	L ANT	L POST SEPT
JR	L ANT	L ANT	LAT

4. REFERENCES

1. Yamada K, Toyama J, Wada M, Sugiyama S, Sugenoya J, Toyoshima H, Mizuno Y, Sotohata I, Kobayashi T, Okajima M. Am Heart J 90:721, 1975.
2. de Ambroggi L, Taccardi B, Macchi E. Circ 54:251, 1976.
3. Frank R, Fontaine G, Guiraudon G, Archiv. Mal. du Coeur, 71:1000-1013, 1978
4. Medvedowsky JL, Nicolai P, Barnay C, Delage M, Agelou JC, Arch. Mal. du Coeur, 70:441-450, 1977.
5. Benson DW, Sterba R, Gallagher JJ, Walston A, Spach MS. Circ 65:1259, 1982.
6. Savard P, Roberge FA,Perry JB, Nadeau RA, Circ. Res., 46:415-425, 1980.
7. Savard P, Mailloux GE, Roberge FA, Gulrajani RM, Guardo R, IEEE Trans. BME, 29:700-707, 1982.
8. Savard P, Ackaoui A, Gulrajani RM, Nadeau RA, Roberge RA, Guardo R, J of Electrocardiol, 18(3), 1985.
9. Gulrajani RM, Pham-Huy H, Nadeau RA, Savard P, de Guise J, Primeau RE, Roberge FA. J Electrocardiology, 17:271-288, 1984.
10. Lorange M, Gulrajani RM, Proc. 10th CMBES, pp:49-50, 1984.

Chapter 13

COMPARISON OF BODY SURFACE MAPPING AND PHASE DISPLAY METHODS TO LOCALIZE BYPASS PATHWAYS IN WOLFF-PARKINSON-WHITE SYNDROME

I. PRÉDA, J. MÉSZÁROS, Z. ANTALÓCZY, GY. KOZMANN, J. MERTZ, L. REGŐS, E. MÁTÉ, GY. MAROSI, L. CSERNAY

1. INTRODUCTION

The advent of surgical techniques to interrupt accessory conduction pathways (ACPs) as a treatment method for Wolff-Parkinson-White (WPW) syndrome has made more apparent than ever the need to preoperatively localize the site of ACPs. With such information one can select optimal candidates for surgical intervention (lateral ACPs vs. septal ACPs), and one can choose the appropriate operative approach (thoracotomy vs. sternotomy) while intraoperative electrophysiological investigations are often hampered by limitation of time, poor patient tolerance as well as a number of technical problems (1) that may arise. The present study was designed to investigate the clinical value of both body surface mapping and phase display methods in the correct localization of ACPs in patients with WPW syndrome.

2. PATIENTS AND METHODS

2.1 Patients: 21 patients (6 female, 15 male, aged 26-60 years) with WPW syndrome were investigated. The diagnosis of WPW syndrome had been established by 12-lead ECG and Frank leads (6). The control group consisted of 10 patients (8 female, 2 male, aged 28-69 years) with Lown-Ganong-Levine (LGL) syndrome. The absence of preexcitation was proven by 12-lead and Frank-lead ECG.

2.2 Body surface mapping: For the construction of body surface insopotential maps 120 unipolar ECG leads were used. The electrodes were attached in a nonequidistant distribution to the anterior and posterior thoracic surfaces, and recordings were made on recumbent patients. After amplification of the chest leads and visual control of the quality of the signals, recordings were taken in subgroups of 12 unipolar leads and one reference tracing. The quasi-simultaneous potential field of the heart was estimated off-line from the sequentially measured analog records with a TPA/I (PDP-8 equivalent) computer (7).

2.3 Radionuclide study: Erythrocytes were labelled in vivo with 600 MBq of Tc-99m. After labelling, a list mode data acquisition was made with the detector positioned in the modified left anterior oblique view. 16 frames per cardiac cycle were collected in a 64x64 matrix. Approximately 240 K counts were acquired in each frame. Frame sequences were smoothed three-dimensionally and cyclically twice. To analyse ventricular contractions a phase display with a 13 msec time resolution was used for a heart rate of 72/min. For the presentation of ventricular parts already contracted, continuous white colour was used with the corresponding amplitude image background.

Ventricular preexcitation was localized in accordance with the Gallagher scheme (1) with all three methods applied.

3. RESULTS

3.1 Localization of ACPs using body surface mapping

By analysing the body surface isopotential maps, ACPs coult be localized in 19 of our 21 patients (Table 1). The electrocardiological analysis of

No.	Name	Age and sex	Location of Bypass Pathway		
			ECG	Mapping	Phase Display
1.	T.Z.	45 F	LT Post.	LT Post.	LT Post.
2.	F.S.	52 F	RT Lat.	RT Ant parasept.	Not detected
3.	Z.I.	58 M	LT Lat.	LT Post.	LT Post.
4.	H.D.	33 M	LT Lat.	LT Ant or Lat.	Not detected
5.	S.I.	52 M	RT Post.parasept.	RT Lat.	RT Lat.
6.	L.I.	27 M	Not detected	Not detected	RT Post.parasept.
7.	B.L.	29 M	LT Post.parasept.	LT Ant.parasept.	LT Ant.parasept.
8.	C.I.	27 F	RT Post.parasept.	RT Lat.	RT Lat.
9.	L.I.	58 M	RT Post.	RT Lat.	RT Lat.
10.	B.L.	30 M	RT Lat.	RT Ant.parasept. RT Lat.	RT Ant.parasept. RT Lat.
11.	S.A.	32 M	LT Lat.	LT Ant.	LT Ant.
12.	K.V.	32 M	RT Post.	RT Lat.or Post.	RT Lat.
13.	L.A.	56 M	LT Post.	LT Post.	LT Post.
14.	B.P.	41 M	LT Post.	LT Post.	LT Post.
15.	M.I.	21 M	LT Post.parasept.	LT Post.parasept.	LT Post.parasept.
16.	C.I.	54 F	RT Lat.	RT Lat.	RT Lat.
17.	H.T.	54 M	LT Lat.	LT Ant.	LT Ant.
18.	S.K.	31 F	LT Lat.	LT Lat.	LT Lat.
19.	A.L.	27 M	LT Ant.	LT Ant.parasept. or Ant.	Not detected
20.	V.I.	33 M	Not detected	Not detected	RT Ant.
21.	B.I.	60 M	LT Post.	LT Post.	RT Post.

TABLE 1. Locations of bypass pathways by the conventional ECG, body surface mapping and phase display methods on the 21 WPW patients.

2 patients did not show WPW syndrome at the time of examination: they probably had an intermittent form of the disease. In 7 of the 19 patients with ACP, right ventricular preexcitation was found; the remaining 12 patients displayed left ventricular preexcitation. With the Gallagher scheme (Fig.1), 5 patients exhibited lateral right ventricular ACPs, and one patient an anterior-paraseptal right ventricular ACP. The precise locations of the ACPs in the left venricle were as follows: anterior paraseptal, one case; anterior, 2 cases; lateral, one case; posterior, 5 cases; posterior paraseptal, one cases. In 3 patients (Nos. 6,19 and 20) the ACPs could not be localized precisely. A double right ventricular ACP was detected in patient No. 10.

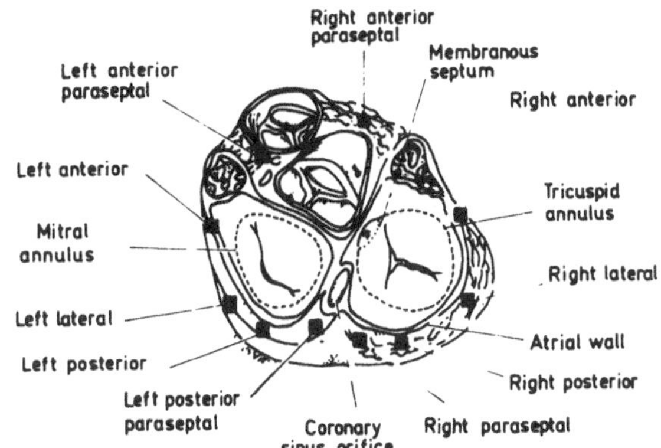

FIGURE 1. Gallagher scheme for localization of possible sites of accessory pathway around the right and left A-V rings.

3.2 Comparison of conventional ECG and body surface mapping

In 2 patients with WPW syndrome the ACP could not be detected by surface ECG methods. In 8 of the 19 patients both methods localized the ventricular preexcitations in the same position (Fig.2 and 3). In 7 cases, differences of one segment were observed whereas in two additional cases the difference in location by the two methods was two segments or more. In one case (No. 10), body surface mapping showed a double bypass tract but this was not detected by conventional ECG.

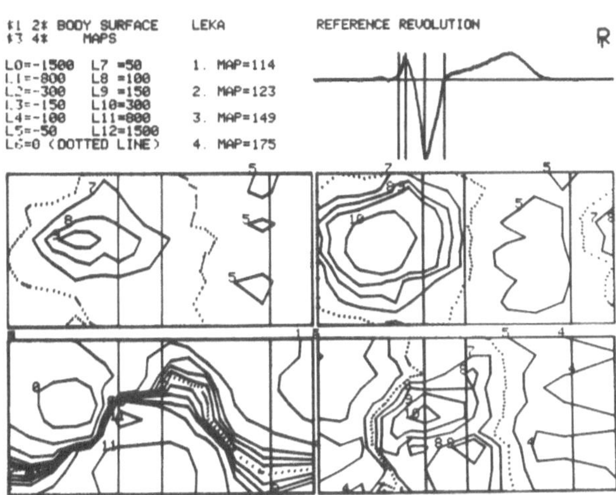

FIGURE 2. Subsequent body surface maps of patient No. 9 with right lateral accessory pathway.

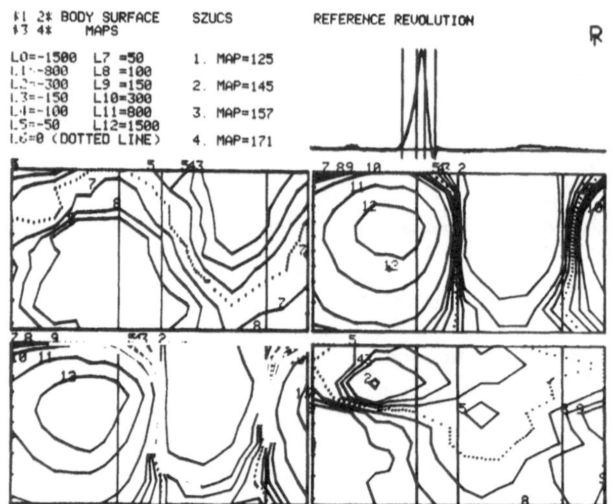

FIGURE 3. Subsequent bod surface maps of patient No. 11 with left anterio accessory pathway.

3.3 Comparison of phase display and body surface mapping

In 18 of the patients with WPW syndrome ventricular preexcitation was found on phase display. The two methods gave precisely the same locations of preexcitation within the ventricles in 15 patients. In one patient the phase display finding was right ventricular ACP; however, this was detected on the posterior wall of the left ventricle with 12-lead ECG and body surface mapping. A double bypass tract of the right ventricle (No.10) could also be detected on phase display.

3.4 Control group

The patients in the control group (LGL syndrome) did not exhibit ventricular preexcitation on ECG and body surface maps. Phase display eximination showed false-positive ACPs in two of these cases, i.e. an 80 per cent specificity for the radioisotope method.

4. DISCUSSION

Since the first reports on the clinical investigation of the WPW syndrome by body surface mapping (2,3) it is evident that various surface potential patterns occur in this disease entity, but these patterns are difficult to interpret because the distribution of heart potentials on the body surface depends not only on the site of the excitation waves, but also on the geometry of the chest and on the conductivity of body tissues. However, the interpretation of surface potential distribution is generally accepted (8), thus a potential maximum in a given area on the chest surface indicates tha an intracardiac excitation wavefront is pointing towards that area whereas a potential minimum indicates that the negative aspect of a wavefront is seen from the area on the chest surface where the minimum appears, or that a whole (breakthrough or infraction) is present in an advancing wavefront. Nevertheless, for correct interpretation, the whole depolarization pattern - indicating not only the initiation but also the course of the anomalous ventricular excitation - has to be taken into account (3). Development of intracardiac electrophysiology and intraoperative mapping studies (1,9) correlated fairly well with the ACPs localized tentatively by body surface mapping and strongly suggest the clinical value of this noninvasive method. Radionuclide high-resolution time analysis of contraction patterns of cardiac ventricles with cine format display was recently described (10) anc was proved to be a useful method for investigating conduction disturbances (4,5). The clinical significance of this method has been pointed out by several authors (11,12,13,14) and almost the same methodology was used in these studies. Points have identical phase values on the phase display images which are displayed in most groups. Our modification includes continuous plotting of points with phase values lower than the actual ones (13) with a time resolution of 5.6 grade. The results are consistent from the aspect of the applicability of this method in ventricular preexcitation, however, its capacity remains uncertain.

As is also evident from our study, body surface potential mapping is a useful procedure in localizing preexcitation waves and the accuracy of the method is better than that of 12-lead ECG (2,3,6). The method is non-invasive, complex and time-consuming, but probably if it is combined with the applied phase display method offers higher accuracy in localizing ACPs. In our present series the sensitivity of both methods was 79 per cent whereas the specificity was 100 per cent for body surface mapping and 80 per cent for the phase imaging method. In one case a double right ventricular ACP was detected using both body surface mapping and phase display methods, however, its confirmation by direct electrophysiological methods is lacking.

In conclusions, body surface potential mapping and phase display methods are both suitable for the detection of ventricular preexcitation in patients with WPW syndrome, but the invasive validition of these methods is still lacking. Ventricular localization of ACPs using body surface mapping has led to results similar to those obtained by the radionuclide method. The simultaneous application of both procedures might the useful for non-invasive screening prior to electrophysiological investigations, and also for monitoring the effectiveness of surgical intervention and of drug prevention of paroxysmal tachycardias in WPW syndrome.

REFERENCES

1. Gallagher JJ, Sealy WC, Wallace AG and Kassel J: Correlation between catheter electrophysiological studies and findings on mapping of ventricular excitation in the W.P.W. syndrome, in: The Conductions System of the Heart, eds: HJJ Wellens, KI Lie and MJ Janse, p: 588, Stenfert Kroese, Leiden (1976)
2. Yamada K, Toyama J, Wada M, Sugiyama S, Sugenoya J, Toyoshima H, Mizuno Y, Sotohata I, Kobayashi T and Okajima M: Body surface isopential mapping in Wolff-Parkinson-White syndrome: Noninvasive method to determine the localization of the accessory atrioventricular pathway. Amer. Heart J. 90: 721 (1975)
3. De Ambroggi L, Taccardi B and Macchi E: Body-surface maps of heart potentials. Tentative localization of pre-excited areas in forty-two Wolff-Parkinson-White patients. Circulation, 54: 251 (1976)
4. Botvinick E, Frais M, O'Connel W, Faulkner D, Scheinmann M, Morady F, Sung R, Shosa D and Dae M: Phase image evaluation of patients with ventricular pre-excitation syndromes. J.Am.Col. Cariol. 3: 799 (1984)
5. Underwood SR, Walton S, Laming PJ, Ell PJ, Emanuel RW, Swanton RH: Patterns of ventricular contraction in patients with conduction abnormality studied by radionuclide angiocardiography. Br. Heart J. 51: 568 (1984)
6. Antalóczy Z, Regős L and Strommer M: Vektorkardiographische Untersuchungen beim WPW-Syndrome. Z. Kardiol. 66: 150 (1977)
7. Kozmann GY, Préda I, Shakin VV, Szlávik F and Antalóczy Z: Computer-aided method for the comparison of surface potential and accelaration maps, in: Computer in Cardiology, Washington University, St. Luis, 29 (1976)

8. Taccardi B, De Ambroggi L and Viganotti C: Body surface mapping of heart potentials, in: The Theoretical Basis of Electrocardiology eds.: CV Nelson and DB Gaselowitz, Clanderon Press, Oxford, p: 436 (1976)
9. Wallace AG, Sealy WC, Gallagher JJ and Kasell J: Ventricular excitation in the Wolff-Parkinson-White syndrome, in: The Conduction System of the Heart, eds: HJJ Wellens, KI Lie and MJ Janse, p: 613, Stenfert Kroese, Leiden (1976)
10. Adam WE, Tarkowska A, Bitter F, Stauch M and Geffers H: Equilibrium (gated) radionuclide ventriculography. Cardiovasc. Radiol. 2: 161 (1979)
11. Swiryn S, Pavel D, Byrom E et al.: Sequential regional phase mapping of radionuclide gated biventriculograms in patients with left bundle branch block. Am. Heart. J. 102: 1000 (1981)
12. Rakovec P, Kranjec I, Fettich J et al.: Localization of accessory pathways in Wolff-Parkinson-White syndrome by phase imaging. Cardiology 70: 138 (1983)
13. Mester I, Préda I, Kozmann GY, Máté E, Regős L, Havasi GY, Antalóczy Z and Csernay L: Localization of accessory conduction pathways in Wolff-Parkinson-White syndrome through phase display and body surface mapping: A comparative study (in preparation)
14. Nakajima K, Bunko H, Tada A et al.: Phase analysis of Wolff-Parkinson-White syndrome with surgically proven accessory pathways: Concise communication. J. Nucl. Med. 25: 7 (1984)

Chapter 14

BODY SURFACE MAP AND LOCATION OF ORIGIN OF VENTRICULAR TACHYCARDIA. COMPARISON WITH EPICARDIAL MAP

C. KLERSY, M. VIGANO', L. MARTINELLI, M. CHIMIENTI, J.A. SALERNO

Ventricular tachycardia (VT) following a myocardial infarction may require surgical correction, when resistant to medical treatment. For precise and less damaging surgery, a careful preoperative and intraoperative mapping is mandatory, as the morphology of VT on standard ecg has been demonstrated not to be indicative of its origin (1).

The purpose of our study was to evaluate the correspondence between the location of the potential minimum at 50 ms on chest maps and the epicardial break-through during VT, in order to improve the preoperative electrophysiologic characterization of VT.

Chest mapping was formerly used by some authors to localize the site of ventricular preexcitation in Wolff-Parkinson-White syndrome (2,3,4), but at present time no attempt is reported in the literature of the identification of the epicardial breakthrough during VT by means of body surface maps in analogy with ventricular preexcitation.

1. MATERIALD AND METHODS

Nine patients (8 male and 1 female), aged 47-70 years (mean age 50 yrs), undergoing surgery for VT, were selected for chest mapping. In 7 patients VT followed a myocardial infarction, whether 2 patients had a cardiomyopathy. All were referred to our CCU for intractable ventricular arrhythmias.

Heart potentials were recorded from 140 electrodes, fixed on rubber straps and distributed over the anterior and posterior chest in 4 groups of 35 electrodes each: 3 groups explored the anterior part of the torso, with a particularly high density of electrodes on the precordial area, and 1 group explored the back. The blocks of informations thus obtained were related to 4 different cardiac beats, due to the acquisition system provided for 35 electrodes, but could be processed in unitary form after time-alignment using the II Einthoven lead as reference.

Data recorded from those 140 exploring sites were amplified, sent to a conversion unit, that contains the multiplexer and the anolog-to-digital converter and which makes the physical and logical connection to computer and to a monitor on line that allows a quality control of the acquired signals on line, group by group. The computer was a Data General Nova 4C (central memory of 64 Kbytes); software and patients' files are contained on floppy disks; data were elaborated by computer and isopotential maps were visualized on a video-terminal or transferred onto paper by means of a hard-copy unit.

On surgery, 35 unipolar electrodes were distributed on an elastic net, which was placed over the heart by the surgeon. Two columns of 5 electrodes each explored the right ventricle, while 5 columns of 5 electrodes collected potentials from the left ventricle. The acquisition and processing system was the same as that used for chest mapping. Activation times were determined by an algorithm that identified the maximal negative derivative of the ecg curve and the final results appeared on video-terminal in the form of an isochronic map.

In all patients standard ecg was performed during preoperative study as well as intraoperatively to ensure that VT morphology was comparable.

RESULTS

During surface mapping all patients had a VT, which was spontaneous in 8 patients and electrically induced in one. The arrhythmias were fairly tolerated from the hemodynamic point of view in all cases. VT showed a pattern of right bundle branch block in all patients but 2; left axis deviation was present in 4 patients, while 5 patients had a vertical or a right axis (table 1).

TABLE 1.

PATIENT	VT MORPHOLOGY	EPICARDIAL BREAKTHROUGH	CHEST MINIMUM
1	RBBB pattern right axis	left anterior paraseptal	upper right anterior quadrant
2	RBBB pattern right axis	left anterior	upper left anterior quadrant
3	RBBB pattern inferior axis	left anterior	upper left anterior quadrant
4	RBBB pattern left axis	left anterior	upper left anterior quadrant
5	RBBB pattern left axis	left posterior paraseptal	lower anterior quadrants
6	RBBB pattern left axis	left posterior paraseptal	lower anterior quadrants
7	LBBB pattern inferior axis	left anterior	lower anterior quadrants
8	RBBB pattern inferior axis	left posterior paraseptal	lower anterior quadrants
9	LBBB pattern left axis	left posterior paraseptal	posterior

Abbreviations: RBBB=right bundle branch block; LBBB=left bundle branch block.

The minimum of potential at 50 ms was localized in the upper anterior quadrants in 4 pts: in 3 patients the minimum was located in the left upper anterior quadrant (pts 2, 3, 4) and in 1 patient in the right upper anterior quadrant (pt 1), whereas the minimum appeared on the lower anterior quadrants in 4 patients (pts 5, 6, 7, 8) and on the back in 1 patient (pt 9) (figure 1).

At surgery epicardial maps were performed during electrically induced VT in all cases; standard ecg allowed to ensure that VT were comparable with the preoperative arrhythmia.

Epicardial breakthrough was on the anterior wall of the left ventricle in 4 patients (pts 2, 3, 4, 7) and in the paraseptal region in 1 (pt 1): we could observe a good spatial correspondence between the location of minimum in the upper anterior quadrants and the breakthrough on the anterior epicardium. On the other hand, all but one minima located in the inferior quadrants and the dorsal minimum were related to an epicardial breakthrough near the posterior interventricular groove, with a poor spatial correlation between the two maps.

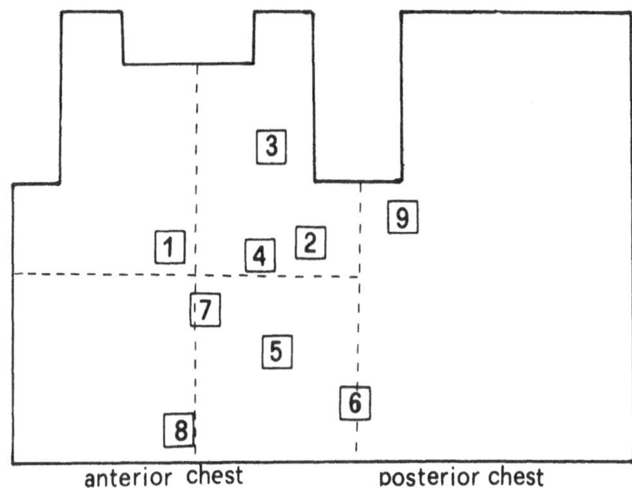

FIGURE 1. Representation of anterior and posterior torso and location of potential minima at 50 ms of patients 1-9, indicated by squares with numbers.

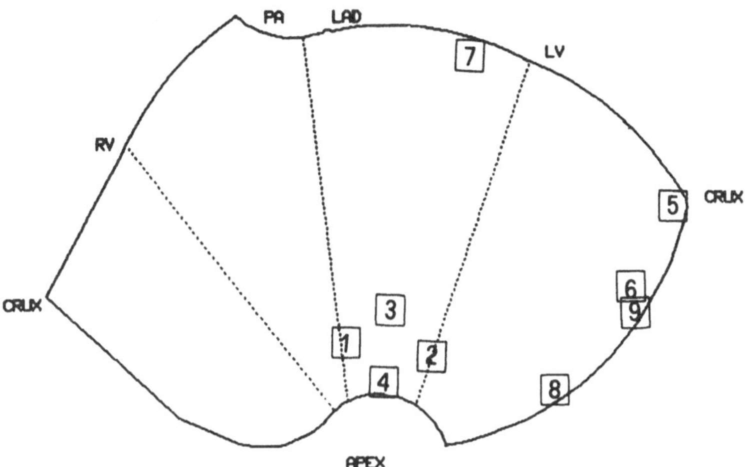

FIGURE 2. Representation of the epicardium, opened like a book after a cut along the posterior interventricular groove; squares with numbers indicate the location of epicardial breakthrough in patients 1-9. RV=right ventricle; PA=pulmonary artery; LV=left ventricle.

DISCUSSION

Other authors (2,3,4) have previously demonstrated that the pattern of surface potential distribution during QRS and ST-T wave and the location of potential minimum and maximum during delta wave may be important in predicting the location of a single preexcited site; they used body surface maps which were compared to catheter or surgical location of the pathway; this non invasive location of preexcited area may help the surgeon to choose the most appropriate access and limit epicardial mapping to a small area.

The preoperative diagnostic approach for identifying the site of origin of VT is at present focused on the measurement of local activation times at multiple sites in the right and the left ventricle with catheters; our data show that chest maps may give further informations concerning the initial activation of the heart during VT, which do not immediately emerge from the examination of standard ecg. Moreover it appears in table 1 and in figures 1 and 2 that in our patients same morphologies of VT did not correspond to similar epicardial breakthrough; similarly other Authors demonstrated that there was poor correspondence between standard ecg and endocardial origin of VT (1).

These data on chest maps in man seem partially in accordance with experimental results of Spach and al. (5), which showed that ectopic ventricular stimulation in chimpanzee was closely related to potential distribution on the torso.

The discrepancy that we found between the good correlation of anterior epicardial breakthrough and minimum on the upper anterior chest and the poor predictive value of an inferior and posterior minimum may account for the distance of the epicardial event to the recording site on the body surface; this hypothesis is in accordance with the experimental results of Spach (5) that demonstrated the role of volume conductor.

However an effort should be made to verify on a larger number of patients the value of chest maps in predicting the origin of VT, in order to add a reliable computerized and non invasive information to the preoperative evaluation of VT, that may better the surgical approach to these highly compromized patients.

REFERENCES

1. Josephson M.E., Horowitz L.N., Waxman H.L., Cain M.E., Spielman S.R., Greenspan A.M., Marchlinski F.E., Ezri M.D.: Sustained ventricular tachycardia: role of the 12-lead electrocardiogram in localizing site of origin. Circulation 64: 257, 1981.
2. Yamada K., Toyama J., Wada M., Sugiyama S., Sugenoya J., Toyoshima H., Mizuro Y., Sotohata I., Kobayashi T., Okajima M.: Body surface isopotential mapping in Wolff-Parkinson-White syndrome. Non invasive method to determine the location of accessory atrio-ventricular pathway. Am Heart J 90: 721, 1975.
3. De Ambroggi L., Taccardi B., Macchi E.: Body surface maps of heart potentials. Tentative localization of preexcited areas in 42 Wolff-Parkinson-White patients. Circulation 54: 251, 1976.
4. Benson D.W., Sterba K., Gallagher J.J., Walston II A., Spach M.S.: Localization of the site of ventricular preexcitation with body surface maps in patients with Wolff-Parkinson-White syndrome. Circulation 65: 1259, 1982.
5. Spach M.S., Barr R.C., Lanning C.F.: Experimental basis for QRS and T wave potentials in the WPW syndrome. The relation of epicardial to body surface potential distributions in the intact chimpanzee. Circ Res 42: 103, 1978.

Chapter 15

LOCALIZATION OF CARDIAC ELECTRICAL ACTIVITY BY A SINGLE MOVING DIPOLE FOR VENTRICULAR TACHYCARDIA IN DOG: VALIDATION BY EPICARDIAL ACTIVATION MAPPING

P. SAVARD, S. BOUCHER, R. CARDINAL, R. GIASSON

1. INTRODUCTION

The localization of the site of origin of ventricular tachycardia (VT) is an important pre-requisite for an effective surgical treatment of VT (1). Various techniques have been proposed for this purpose. Pre-operatively, the site of origin can be estimated according to ECG morphology during VT (2), or during pacing with an endocardial catheter at a location which best reproduces the ECG morphology observed during VT (3). The site of earliest activation during VT can also be determined with endocardial catheters (4), and intraoperatively, the VT origin can be determined with greater accuracy by epicardial and endocardial mapping (5).

The objective of this study was to evaluate a non-invasive electrocardiographic technique for the localization of arrhythmogenic activity. This technique is based on a representation of the cardiac electrical activity by a single moving dipole (SMD) which is computed from the potentials measured over the entire torso surface. This technique has been developed through a series of animal experiments, computer simulations and clinical studies (6-8), and it is well suited to represent the relatively simple activation sequences of ectopic beats with a single focus.

We thus recorded body surface potentials during VT induced by programmed electrical stimulation (PES) in dogs with a chronic infarct. To validate the results, epicardial isochronal maps recorded with a sock electrode array were used to localize the site of origin and the rest of the activation sequence of VT episodes with uniform ECG morphology.

2. MATERIAL AND METHODS

2.1 Experimental protocol

The experiments were carried out on 17 dogs with chronic infarcts produced by a permanent occlusion of the left anterior descending coronary artery after methylprednisolone administration (9). Three days later, the animals were subjected to PES through epicardial electrodes implanted during the occlusion. The body surface potentials were recorded on digital magnetic tape during VT episodes and pacing at known sites. The electrode array consisted of 43 needle electrodes on the front and sides of the torso, and 20 electrodes on the back. In addition, ECG leads I and AVF were continuously recorded on analog magnetic tape and a chart recorder during the experiment.

After recording VT episodes with different ECG morphologies, a sternotomy was performed and a sock electrode array with 64 unipolar contacts was placed over the ventricles. The animals were again subjected to PES, and during VT, the 64 electrograms were recorded instead of the 63 ECGs.

2.2 Data acquisition and processing

A data acquisition system capable of simultaneously recording 64 ECGs or electrograms was used. The signals were amplified, filtered, multiplexed, digitized at 500 Hz with a resolution of 10 bits, and stored on magnetic tape for subsequent processing on a PDP 11/34.

The initial phase of this processing consisted in selecting a heart beat, correcting the time skew between channels introduced by the multiplexing, calibrating the signals from a known waveform, and correcting the baseline shift by selecting a baseline between two successive isoelectric segments. The determination of a baseline was approximated for tachycardias with high heart rates because of the absence of any isoelectric interval.

For each sampling instant, the location, magnitude and orientation of the SMD were computed from the 63 ECGs. The SMD computations were performed using a least-squares technique with 15 multipoles and a finite and homogeneous torso model having a surface made of 780 discrete triangles (6-7).

Each electrogram from a selected time window was displayed on a video terminal. Activation times were automatically detected by the program and indicated by vertical cursors. Local activation time was detected as the point of most rapid decrease of potential with a slope in excess of -1 mV/msec. The operator edited these activation times to eliminate artifacts and finally, the isochronal map of the selected beat was displayed on the terminal.

Since the epicardial electrograms were recorded after the body surface potentials, the ECG morphologies (leads I and AVF) of VT episodes occuring before sternotomy were compared to those occuring after sternotomy. Thus, thoracic and epicardial recordings for the same type of VT were obtained. Epicardial activation sequences of different VT episodes with the same ECG morphologies in the same dog were reproducible and showed the validity of this procedure. A common time reference was obtained by determining the QRS onset on the RMS signals of the thoracic potentials and of the epicardial potentials. Also, a spatial reference was taken as the location of the initial SMD location following pacing at a known site, and was used to center the heart silhouette at the corresponding site.

3. RESULTS

We were able to induce VT with uniform ECG morphology in 10 of the 17 dogs. We found 5 VT episodes which had uniform ECG morphology and similar ECG morphologies before and after sternotomy. The period was superior to 270 msec in 3 cases, and shorter in 2 cases.

An example of a VT episode with a 400 msec period is illustrated in Figure 1. The epicardial isochronal map shows that activation started on the anterior part of the left ventricle, then progressed away from the focus in a concentric fashion, and finally ended near the base of the right ventricle. The SMD trajectory adequately depicted this activation sequence: it also started anteriorly in region of the left ventricle, moved away and ended near the base of the right ventricle. Between 0 and 20 msec, the SMD trajectory showed large, erratic movements because of the low signal-to-noise ratio. After about 20 msec, it became slower and coherent. The depolarized epicardial region then had a diameter of about 4 cm, and the cardiac body surface potentials were larger than the noise on the body surface.

Similar features can be found in Figure 2, but with an opposite VT origin. The activation started anteriorly on the right ventricle near the base, moved away toward the apex, and ended over the left ventricle. The SMD trajectory also started anteriorly near the base, on the right, then moved toward the left and the apex. Figure 3 shows a very different type of VT: instead of a focal origin, there is continuous propagation around two regions of functional block over the infarct, with the activation sequence showing a figure-of-eight reentry circuit. The SMD trajectory does not show a straightforward displacement accross the entire heart. It moves from the base toward the apex, then moves back toward the base, thus depicting the activation sequence but with one exception: the SMD is located posteriorly instead of anteriorly at 0 msec, which is probably due to the overlap of anterior depolarization and posterior repolarization.

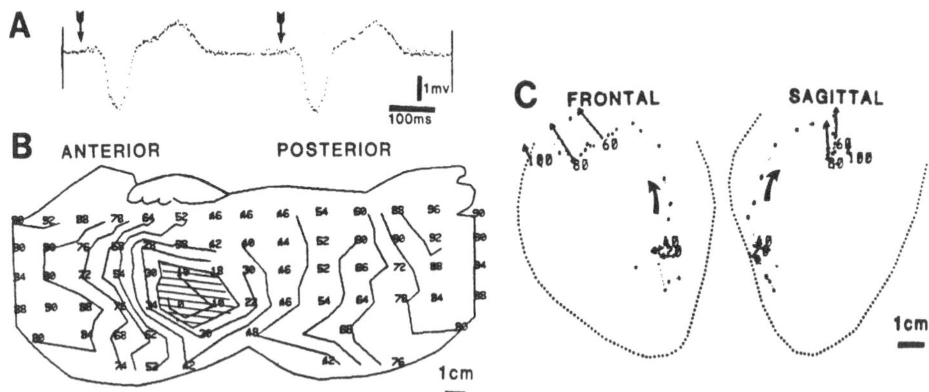

FIGURE 1: Epicardial activation sequence and SMD trajectory during VT. A) ECG lead AVF, arrows indicate the zero time reference. B) Isochronal map, numbers indicate the activation time in msec, isochronal lines are drawn at each 10 msec, the hatched area represents the region that was depolarized after 20 msec. C) SMD trajectory during QRS, successive SMD locations at 2 msec intervals are joined by dotted lines and curved arrows show the direction of the trajectory, the corresponding SMD vectors are projected at every 20 msec.

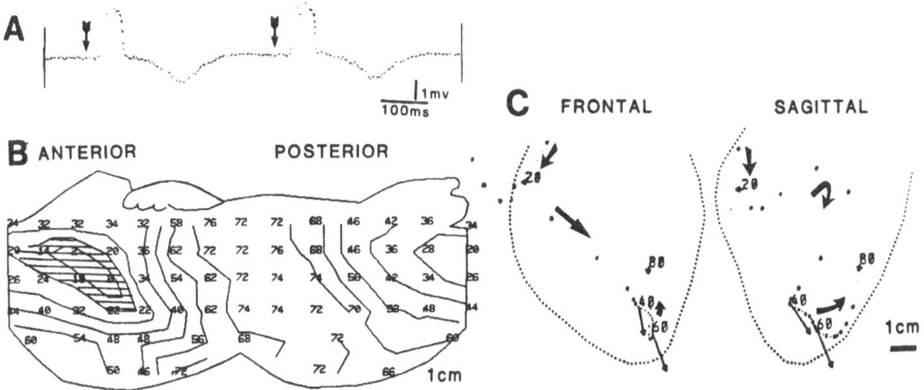

FIGURE 2: Epicardial activation sequence and SMD trajectory for a VT episode with a 380 msec period.

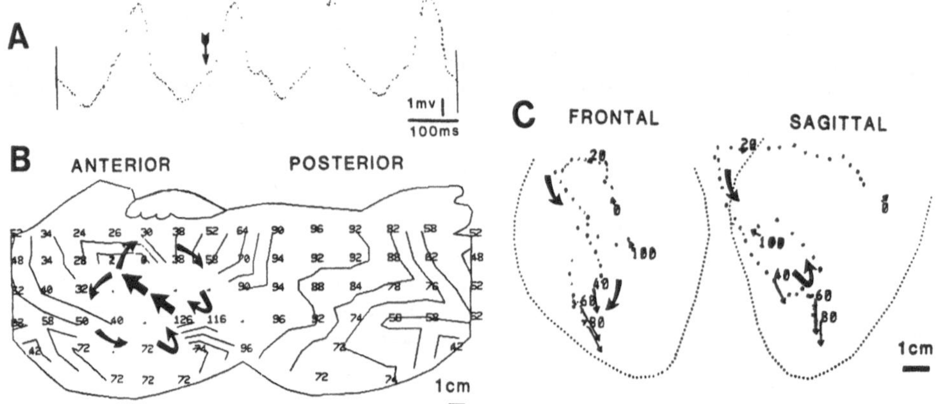

FIGURE 3: Epicardial activation sequence and SMD trajectory for a VT episode with a 190 msec period. The dots on the map indicate electrode sites where no local activation was detected, and around which no isochronal lines were drawn.

4. DISCUSSION

We found that the SMD locations at QRS onset and offset corresponded to the the initial and terminal wavefronts seen on the isochronal maps, and that the SMD trajectory depicted the main features of the activation sequence. The SMD trajectory became slow and coherent when the signal-to-noise ratio was sufficiently high, which was at about 20 to 40 msec after QRS onset when an epicardial region with a diameter of about 4 cm was depolarized. This diameter represents the limit of the SMD localization accuracy of the VT origin. In some cases when the VT rate was high, an accurate measurement of the body surface potentials with respect to an isoelectric baseline was not possible because of the absence of T-P segment, however, acceptable SMD trajectories were obtained by using approximate baselines. We thus consider that the SMD is a promising technique for the electrocardiographic localization of VT foci.

5. REFERENCES

1. Mason JW, Stinson EB, Winkle RA, Oyer PE, Griffin JC, Ross DL. Am J Cardiol, 49:241-248, 1982.
2. Josephson ME, Horowitz LN, Waxman HL, Circ., 64:257-272, 1981.
3. Josephson ME, Waxman HL, Cain ME, Gardner MJ, Buxton AE. Am J Cardiol, 50:11-22, 1982.
4. Josephson ME, Horowitz LN, Farshidi A, Spear JF, Kastor JA, Moore EN. Circ., 57:440-447, 1978.
5. Horowitz LN, Josephson ME, Harken AH. Circ., 61:1227-1238, 1980.
6. Savard P, Roberge FA,Perry JB, Nadeau RA. Circ. Res., 46:415-425, 1980.
7. Savard P, Mailloux GE, Roberge FA, Gulrajani RM, Guardo R. IEEE Trans. BME, 29:700-707, 1982.
8. Savard P, Ackaoui A, Gulrajani RM, Nadeau RA, Roberge RA, Guardo R. J of Electrocardiol., 18(3), 1985.
9. Cardinal R, Savard P, Carson DL, Perry JB, Pagé P. Circ, 70:136-148, 1984.

Chapter 16

ISOINTEGRAL ANALYSIS OF BODY SURFACE MAPS OF VENTRICULAR PREMATURE BEATS

H. HAYASHI, K. MIYACHI, T. ISHIKAWA, K. TAKAMI, S. YABE, S. OHSUGI, T. OHTA

1. INTRODUCTION

Ventricular gradient or QRST area is theoretically independent of the ventricular activation sequence provided that the repolarization property is constant (1,2). The QRST isointegral map obtained from body surface maps has been proven to be independent of the activation sequence but dependent of the recovery property by animal experiments (3,6).

There are, however, some conflicting evidences regarding the consistency of QRST area under various conduction patterns of the ventricle and clinical studies on this matter have not been precisely performed yet.

The present study was carried out to examine the consistency of the isointegral map between normal sinus conduction and ventricular premature beat (VPB).

The study was also focused on the difference, if ever, of the isointegral map by the site of origin of VPB.

2. SUBJECTS AND METHODS

The subjects were 131 patients with VPBs and they were divided into two groups. Group N consisted of 60 patients who were without obvious underlying cardiovascular disease as detected by standard 12-lead ECG or other diagnostic procedures. Group D consisted of 71 patients who had various cardiovascular diseases. Group N consisted of 30 men and 30 women with the mean age of 34.4 $\pm$ 18.8 (SD) years old and group D consisted of 58 men and 13 women with mean age of 56.8 $\pm$ 14.9 years old.

Group D was subdivided into two groups; D_1 and D_2. Group D_1 included the patients whose QRST isointegral map pattern in sinus conduction, as described below, was similar (correlation coefficient > 0.90) to the mean QRST isointegral map which was obtained based on 60 patients in group N. Group D_2 included the patients whose QRST isointegral map pattern in sinus conduction was largely different from the mean QRST isointegral map with correlation coefficient of less than 0.90, and this group was excluded from the study analysis. The mean age of group D_1 was 48.7 $\pm$ 14.8 years old. Those VPBs with premature index less than 1.0 were excluded from the study.

Unipolar lead ECGs of VPB were recorded from 87 lead points over the precordium (59 points) and the back (28 points) with Wilson's central terminal as the reference point. These data were fed into the mapper, HPM-6500 (Chunichi-Denshi Electric Company) (7) and isopotential maps were drawn for every 1-2 ms.

The artificial pacemaker stimulus was applied at various sites of both ventricles and pacemaker maps were recorded to compare the similarity with VPB maps and these findings were taken into consideration to presume the site of origin of VPB.

Isointegral maps were made for QRS, ST-T and QRST of sinus conduction and VPB. Correlation coefficients were obtained to examine the similarity of map pattern.

3. RESULTS

Based on the pacemaker maps, VPB maps were divided into nine types: A, B, C, D, E, F, G, H and I and the site of origin of each VPB was presumed as shown in table 1.

TABLE 1. Types of VPB and their presumed sites of origin

Type	Presumed site of origin	
A	RV outflow tract*	
B	RV inflow tract*	RV origin
C	RV apex*	
D	IVS base*	IVS origin
E	LV posterior base*	
F	LV anterolateral base*	
G	Posterior division of LBB	LV origin
H	Anterior division of LBB	
I	LV apex*	

RV: right ventricle; LV: left ventricle; IVS: interventricular septum; LBB: left bundle branch.
(* Site of origin of VPB was presumed by the comparison with pacemaker maps.)

The locations of the minimum and the maximum at 10, 20, 30 and 40 ms in normal sinus conduction and in each type of VPB in group N were studied and those at 30 ms are shown in Fig. 1. In normal sinus conduction they were at the right shoulder region and near V_4 position.

In VPB types A, D, G and H, the minimum was located in the upper sternum region and the maximum was at slightly below V_4.

In types B, the minimum was at V_1 area and the maximum was at slightly above V_4.

In type C, the minimum was at the mid-lower aspect of the chest and the maximum at the upper back.

In type E, the minimum was at the middle of the back and the maximum at the middle of the chest.

In type F, the minimum was at the left upper precordium and the maximum was at V_3.

Fig. 2 is an example of QRS, ST-T and QRST isointegral map in normal sinus conduction. In QRS map the minimum is located near V_2 position and the maximum is near V_5. In QRST map the minimum is right upper sternal region and the maximum is at V_4.

QRS isointegral maps in VPBs of various origin are shown in Fig. 3. In each VPB, the map pattern is quite different and the position of the minimum indicated the relationship with the site of origin of VPB.
For example, in type A VPB, the focus of which is presumed to be at the right ventricular outflow tract, the minimum was at the upper sternal re-

gion and in type E VPB, the focus of which is presumed to be the posterior base of left ventricle, the minimum was at the middle of the back.

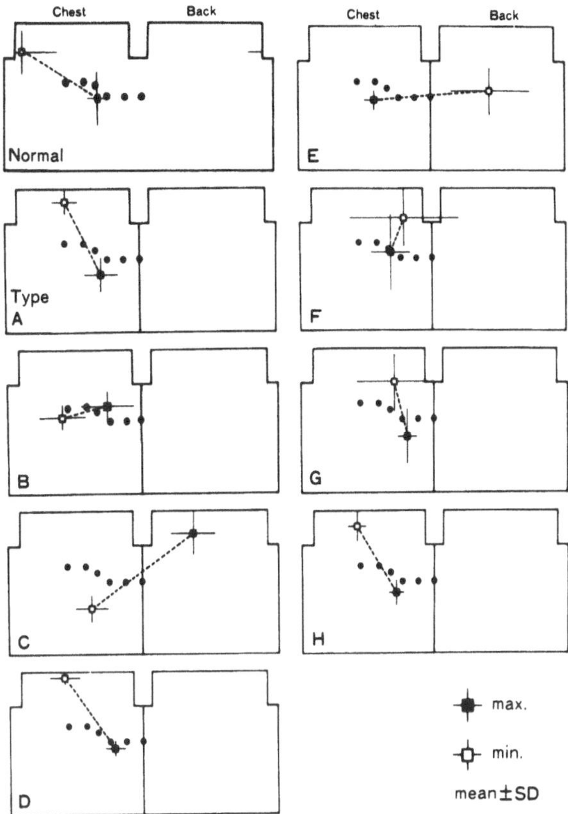

FIGURE 1. Positions of the maximum and the minimum at 30 ms in normals and VPBs of different site of origin. For the site of origin of VPB, refer to table 1.

Fig. 4 summarizes the mean position of the minimum in the QRS isointegral map for each VPB with different focus in relation to V_1 to V_6 in the standard 12-lead ECG. The minima of VPBs of right ventricular origin (Types A, B and C) were in the region of V_2 and slightly below V_3. On the other hand, those of VPBs of left ventricular origin (Types E, G and H) were located further to the left of the anterior axillary line or V_5. The minima of types D and F were in the region above V_{2-3}. The minimum of type H was below the region of V_4.

Fig. 5 shows QRST isointegral maps in normal sinus conduction and in VPB for each group studied.

In group N, isointegral map patterns of sinus conduction and VPB (type B) were very similar to each other and the correlation coefficient was 0.97. The isointegral map of sinus conduction in group D-1 resembled that of group N and it was also very similar to that of VPB (type A) with the correlation coefficient of 0.96. In group D-2, on the other hand, QRST isointegral map in sinus conduction was quite different from that of group N, but it resembled that of VPB (type C) with a correlation coefficient of 0.97.

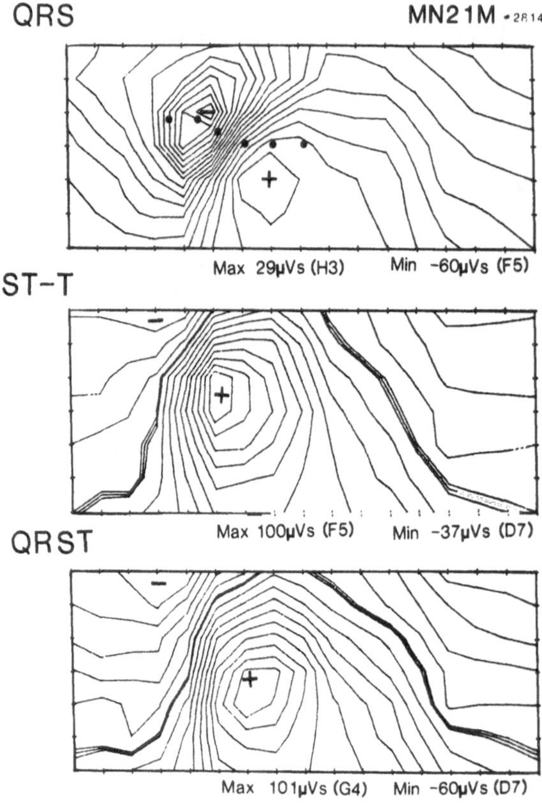

FIGURE 2. QRS, ST-T and QRST isointegral maps in normal sinus conduction.

Fig. 6 shows the mean position of the maximum of QRST isointegral map of sinus conduction and VPB in groups N and D-1. All maxima were located very close to each other in the region of V_4 and no significant difference was observed.

The positions of the maximum of QRST isointegral map of VPBs are shown by the site of origin (Fig. 7). When the VPB focus was divided into three groups; right ventricle (RV), left ventricle (LV) and interventricular septum (IVS), the position of the maximum for each group of VPB indicated the anatomical relationship of both ventricles; the maximum of RV was located more to the right as compared with that of LV and vice versa and that of IVS was in between these two maxima. When the VPB focus was divided into two groups; cardiac base and apex, the maximum of the former was located more superiorly as compared with that of the latter and vice versa. The mean position of the maximum of QRST isointegral map of VPB are shown by the site of origin (Fig. 8). They are located close to each other and

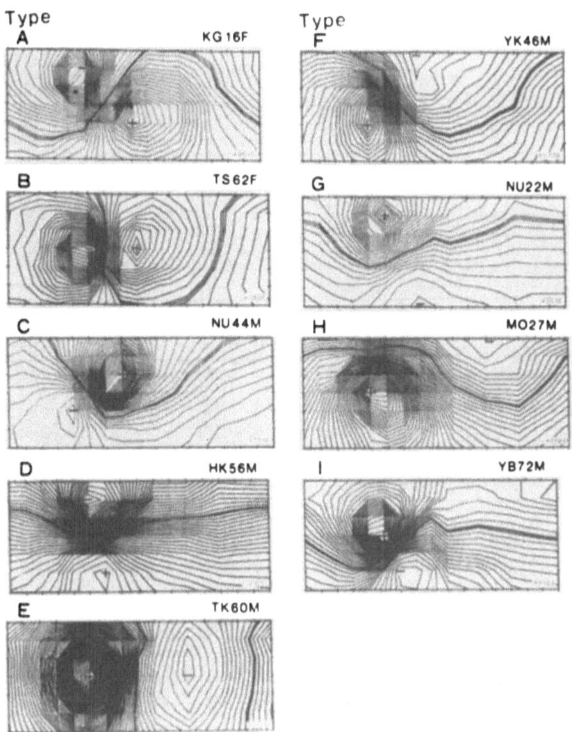

FIGURE 3. QRS isointegral maps in VPB of different site of origin.

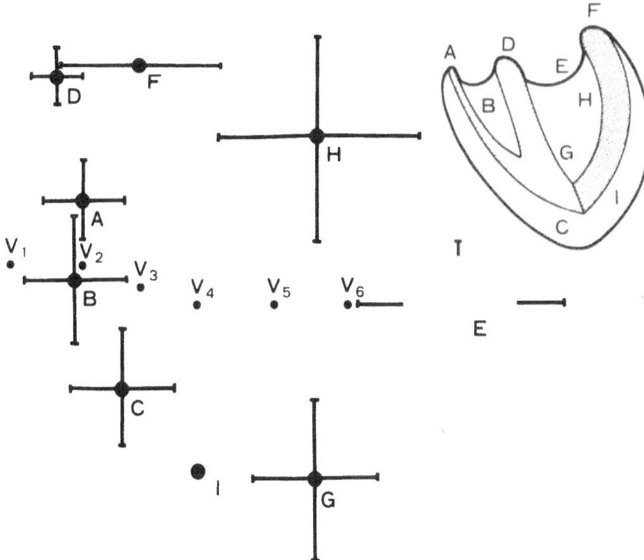

FIGURE 4. The position of the minimum of QRS isointegral maps in VPBs having different sites of origin.

However, they indicated the relative anatomical relationship; the position of the maximum was to the right of V_4 in VPBs of right ventricular origin (types A, B and C). It was superiorly to V_4 region in VPB of interventricular origin (type D) and to the left of V_4 in VPBs of left ventricular origin (types E, F, G, H and I).

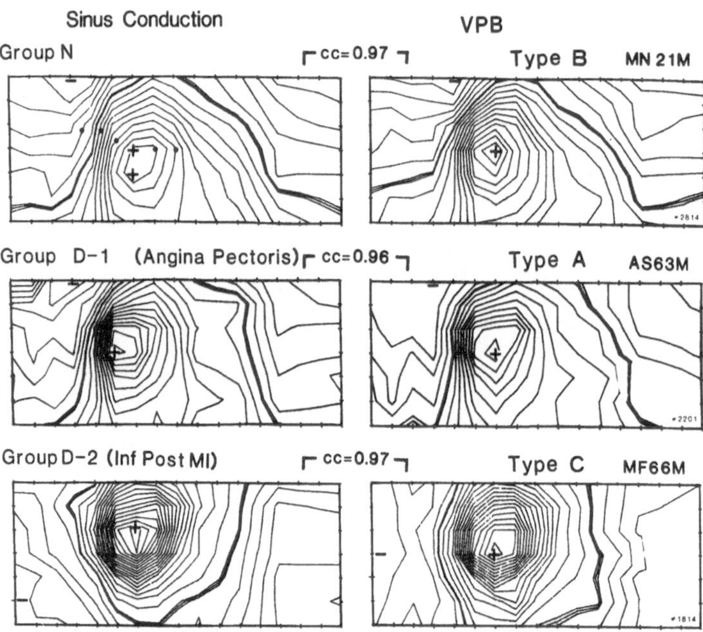

FIGURE 5. QRST isointegral maps of sinus conduction and VPB in groups N, D-1 and D-2.

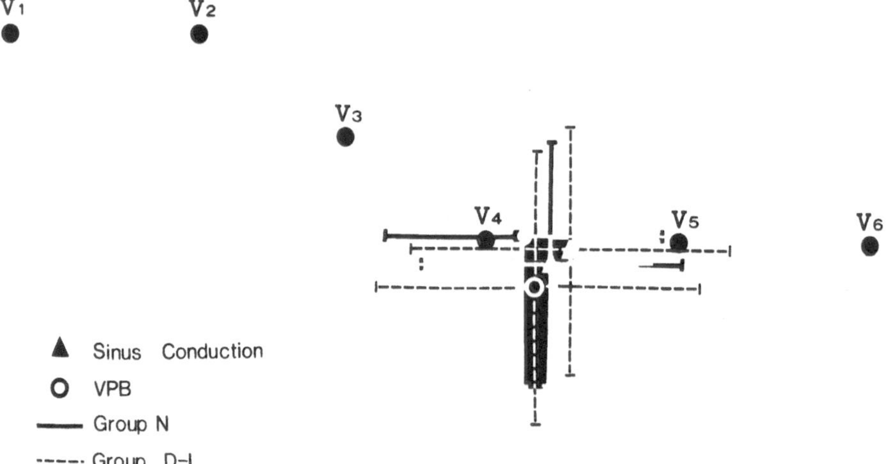

FIGURE 6. The position of the maximum in QRST isointegral maps of sinus conduction and VPB.

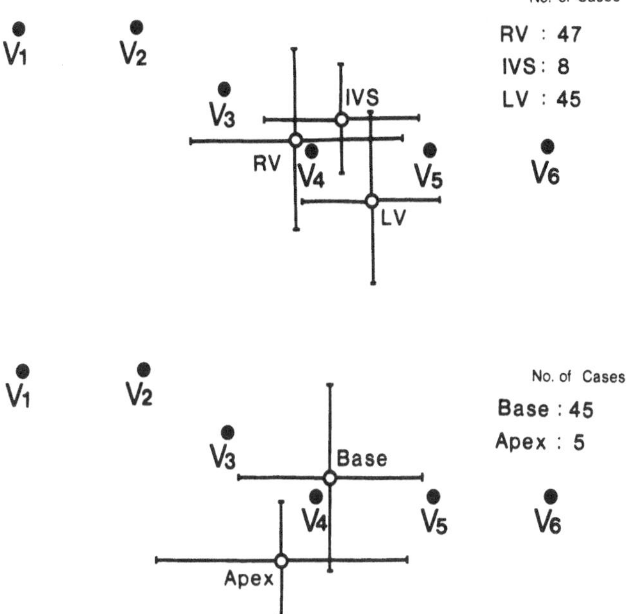

FIGURE 7. The position of the maximum in QRST isointegral maps in VPBs.

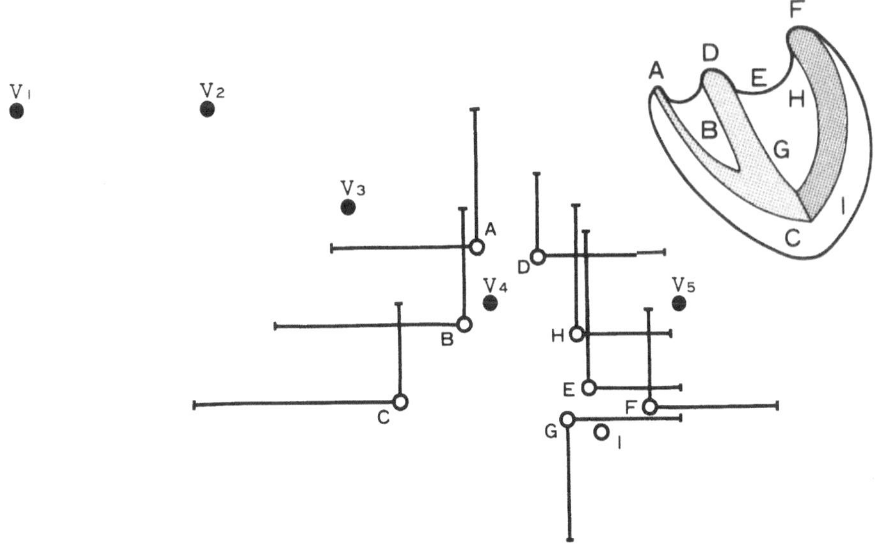

FIGURE 8. The position of the maximum in QRST isointegral maps in VPBs of different site of origin.

4. DISCUSSION

The QRST area is theoretically independent of the ventricular activation sequence provided the ventricular recovery property is uniform. However, it has been shown in animal experiments that the ventricular recovery process is influenced to some extent by ventricular ectopic stimulation and this causes the slight change in QRST area (1,6,8,-13). The mechanism to explain the difference is not clear but this corresponds to the change of recovery properties due to the difference in electronic interaction in the various activation patterns (9,12,-18). Abildskov et al. (16) also suggested the possibility of inconsistency of ventricular gradient due to the significant difference of refractory period according to the change in the ventricular activation order. The clinical observation also supported the change in the ventricular gradient of VPB as compared with that of normal sinus conduction (11,12,19). Despite the theoretical importance of ventricular gradient, physiological or clinical validity has not been fully elucidated at the present time.

In group N of the present study, QRST isointegral map of sinus conduction was quite similar to that of VPB irrespective of its focus with a very high correlation coefficient with a mean of 0.95. The same applied to groups D_1 and D_2 and it was verified that the QRST area was not influenced by the difference of the activation order of the ventricle irrespective of the presence or absence of underlying heart diseases despite that QRST isointegral map of sinus conduction in group D-2 was largely different from group N. Since the QRST isointegral map of sinus conduction in group D-1 was very similar to that in group N (mean correlation coefficient 0.94), only the former was included into the study group and patients of group D_2 were excluded from the study because the correlation coefficient of sinus conduction was less than 0.90 and the recovery property in these patients might be different from normal. The site of origin of VPB was presumed to be 9 regions of the ventricle on the basis of the similarity of the isopotential map during the electrical pacing at various sites of both ventricles (20). The direction of the vector pointing from the minimum to the maximum at 30 ms in each type of VPB indicated the major direction of activation and the position of the minimum was related closely to the focus of VPBs. This relationship was easily understood in those cases in which the activation was primarily through the muscle conduction but in types G and H in which the activation was presumed to be through the specialized conduction system, the position of the minimum at 30 ms did not necessarily indicate directly the site of origin of VPB.

The position of the minimum in QRS isointegral map was another useful indicator to presume VPB focus. Its position was very similar to that in isopotential map at 30 ms as shown in Fig. 2 except types G and H. For the latter two cases, the position of the minimum in QRS isointegral map indicated more likely anatomical position for VPB focus than that of the minimum at 30 ms in isopotential map. The position of the minimum QRS isointegral map was shown to indicate the position of bypass tract in WPW syndrome and VPB focus in animal experiments (21).

The present study revealed the significant difference in the position of the minimum by the site of origin of VPB.

It also revealed that the QRST isointegral map pattern and the position of the potential maximum in sinus conduction were very similar to those in VPB when all VPBs were taken into consideration. However, when the position of the maximum was analyzed by the site of origin of VPB, it was found that the maximum shifted slightly to the body surface region which is considered to correspond to each VPB focus.

Han et al. (22) noted in animal experiment the significant reduction of repolarization time as measured by functional refractory period at the ventricular region where the ectopic stimuli were applied.

If this fact could be extrapolated in clinical situation, the ventricular gradient ($\hat{VG}$) is expected to be influenced by the change in recovery property associated with the difference in ventricular activation sequence.

This brings about the result that VG vector loses its consistency and it directs to the site of origin of VPB. Abildskov et al. (8) proved this hypothesis in their animal experiment, however, clinical study on this matter has not been performed very precisely yet (19).

Although the present study did not deal with $\hat{VG}$ itself directly, the direction pointing from the minimum to the maximum in QRST isointegral map or the position of the maximum is comparable to $\hat{VG}$ in a vectorial sense. The close relationship is understood in this respect between the VPB focus and the position of the maximum of QRST area.

The QRST area depends on differences in duration of repolarization properties (3). In muscle conduction where the conduction speed is slow, the disparity of recovery property is considered to increase resulting in increase in QRST area (3). In VPBs with the focus at the ordinary ventricular muscle (i.e. types A,C,D,E,F and I), the QRST area was large in the present study which has been pointed out by Abildskov et al. (3). The shift of $\hat{VG}$ has also been explained by the change in the morphology and the direction of the alignment of the myocardial cells due to the difference in contractile pattern of the ventricles accompanied by the change of the ventricular activation sequence (11,12,23,24). In order to prove very precisely that $\hat{VG}$ is not kept constant in VPB, it is crucial to examine this using body surface leads sensitive enough to the electrical phenomenon of both depolarization and repolarization of the ventricle in the same manner (8). This was carefully examined and its importance was stressed by Fruehan et al. (23) in intermittent left bundle branch block. In this regard the study using body surface map is considered to be of value as lead points are distributed over the entire thorax but the methodology for this specific purpose needs to be examined more carefully in future.

As heart rate does not seem to influence the direction of $\hat{VG}$ (25,26) the shift of the maximum in QRST isointegral map will not be due to the prematurity of VPB. The magnitude of the maximum and the minimum in QRST isointegral map of VPB was not analyzed in the present study, as it is expected to be influenced stronger by the time factor, heart rate (3) and probably the coupling interval, rather than the difference in VPB focus. To avoid the influence by the change in recovery property of VPB and also to obtain as much as possible the correct QRST area, those VPBs with prematurity index less than 1.0 were excluded from the study.

The important thing is that this clinical observation does not deny the concept of $\hat{VG}$ by Wilson (1), but it implies that the changes of recovery property associated with the occurrence of VPB did influence $\hat{VG}$ if it is examined by the site of origin of VPB and this was reflected on body surface as the slight shift of the maximum in QRST isointegral map.

5. CONCLUSION

The site of origin of ventricular premature beat (VPB) was deducted from body surface isopotential maps and QRST isointegral maps of 131 VPB with different sites of origin were studied to find out whether it would be influenced the ventricular activation order. The study revealed the following results.

1. The site of origin of VPB was presumed to be located at 9 regions.
2. The position of the minimum in QRS isointegral map of VPB indicated VPB focus.
3. The QRST isointegral maps of sinus conduction and VPB were very similar to each other irrespective of the presence or absence of the underlying heart diseases.
4. The position of the maximum in QRST isointegral map of VPB shifted slightly to the direction of the presumed site of origin of VPB.
5. The position of the maximum of QRST isointegral map shifted probably due to slight changes in the ventricular recovery properties associated with VPB occurrence. Therefore $V\hat{G}$ was presumed to lose its consistency to some degree and its directional change was suggested clinically to be related to the site of origin of VPB.

REFERENCES

1. Wilson FN, Macleod AG, Barker PS and Johnston FD: The determination
AG and the significance of the areas of the ventricular deflections of the electrocardiogram. Am Heart J 10: 46, 1934
2. Plonsey R: A contemporary View of the Ventricular Gradient of Wilson. J Electrocardiology 12: 337, 1979
3. Abildskov JA, Green LS, Evans AK and Lux RL: The QRST Deflection Area of Electrograms during Global Alterations of Ventricular Repolarization. J Electrocardiology 15: 103, 1982
4. Lux RL, Urie PM, Brugess MJ and Abildskov JA: Variability of the body surface distributions of QRS, ST-T and QRST deflection areas with varied activation sequence in dogs. Cardiovasc Res 14: 607, 1980
5. Abildskov JA, Burgess MJ, Urie PM, Lux RL and Wyatt RF: The unidentified information content of the electrocardiogram. Circ Res 40: 3, 1977
6. Burgess MJ, Lux RL, Wyatt RF and Abildskov JA: The relation of localized myocardial warming to changes in cardiac surface electrograms in dogs. Circ Res 43: 889, 1978
7. Toyama J, Ohta K and Yamada K: Newly developed body surface mapping systems for clinical use. Advances in Body Surface Potencial Mapping, eds Yamada K et al. The University of Nagoya Press, Nagoya, 1983
8. Abildskov JA, Burgess MJ, Millar K and Wyatt R: New Data and Concepts Concerning the Ventricular Gradient Chest 58: 244, 1970
9. Abildskov JA, Evans AK, Lux RL and Burgess MJ: Ventricular recovery properties and QRST deflection area in cardiac electrograms. Am J Physiol 239: H227, 1980
10. Abildskov JA and Klein RM: Cancellation of electrocardiographic effects during ventricular excitation. Circ Res 11: 247, 1962
11. Cosma J, Levy B and Pipberger H: The spatial ventricular gradient during alterations in the ventricular activation pathway. Am Heart J 71: 84, 1966
12. Simonson E, Schmitt OH, Dahl J, Fry D and Bakken EE: The theoretical and experimental basis of the frontal plane ventricular gradient and its spatial counterpart. Am Heart J 47: 122, 1954
13. Urie PM, Burgess MJ, Lux RL, Wyatt RL and Abildskov JA: The electrocardiographic recognition of cardiac states at high risk of ventricular arrhythmias. Circ Res 42: 350, 1978
14. Cranefield PF and Hoffman BF: Propagated repolarization in heart muscle. J Gen Physiol 41: 633, 1958

15. Mendez C, Mueller WJ, Merideth J and Moe GK: Interaction of transmembrane potentials in canine Purkinje fibers and at Purkinje fiber-muscle junctions. Circ Res 24: 361, 1969
16. Abildskov JA: Effects of activation sequence on the local recovery of ventricular excitability in the dog. Circ Res 38: 240, 1976
17. Toyoshima H and Burgess MJ: Electronic interaction during canine ventricular repolarization. Circ Res 43: 348, 1978
18. Weidman S: The electrical constants of Purkinje fibers. J Physiol London 118: 348, 1952
19. Berkun MA, Kesselman RH, Donoso E and Grishman A: The White syndrome, intermittent left bundle branch block and ventricular premature contractions. Circulation 13: 562, 1956
20. Uematsu H, Hayashi H, Ishikawa T, Wada M, Ishikawa S, Sotobata I and Yasui S: Ventricular activation sequence in patients with pacemaker implanted at different site determined by body surface isopotential maps. Proceedings of the VIth World Symposium on Cardiac Pacing, Montreal, 1979. Chapter 2
21. Oguri H, Lux RL, Burgess MJ, Wyatt RF and Abildskov JA: Body Surface Distribution of QRS Deflection Areas in Experimental Ventricular Preexcitation. J Electrocardiology 13: 237, 1980
22. Han J, Garcia de Jalon P and Moe GK: Fibrillation threshold of premature ventricular responses. Circ Res 18: 18, 1966
23. Fruehan CT, Crain B, Burgess MJ, Millar K and Abildskov JA: Observations concerning the validity of the ventricular gradient concepts. Am Heart J 78: 796, 1969
24. Angle WD: The ventricular gradient vector and related vectors. Am Heart J 59: 749, 1960
25. Mashima S, Fu L and Fukushima K: The normal ventricular gradient determined with Frank's lead system and its relation to the heart rate change induced by various procedures: Studies on the ventricular gradient (I). Jpn Heart J 5: 337, 1964
26. Brambilla I: Correlation between the spatial ventricular gradient, its vectorial component, and the duration of the different phases of the cardiac cycle. Acta Cardiol 19: 71, 1964

Chapter 17

CHEST MAPPING IN THE EVALUATION OF PSEUDOISCHEMIC T WAVES RELATED TO INTERMITTENT LEFT BUNDLE BRANCH BLOCK

E. MARANGONI, L. GUASTI, M. PREVITALI, M. CHIMIENTI, J.A. SALERNO

T-wave changes can be observed in many clinical situations and they are classically divided into primary and secondary T-wave changes. Secondary T-wave changes occur during anomalous ventricular activation while primary changes occur when the activation sequence is normal, thus appearing independent from the pattern of ventricular activation. However, at the resumption of normal intraventricular conduction, after a certain period of anomalous activation, a peculiar type of T-wave changes occurs, which mimics ischemic-type modifications. Such a change needs some time to appear and to reach the maximum level, till anomalous activation is present, and a longer time to disappear, after the disappearance of the abnormal QRS pattern. This phenomenon is suggestive of modulation of repolarization related to the entity and duration of the anomalous activation (1-3).

In order to evaluate the relation between ventricular activation and T-wave modulation, we studied repolarization changes occurring in intermittent left bundle branch block (LBBB). LBBB is usually associated with a clinical evidence of heart disease but less frequently it is idiopathic (4). In our study we considered only the latter condition excluding patients whose repolarization abnormalities could be related to myocardial ischemia or other causes of primary T-wave changes.

1. MATERIALS AND METHODS

Three patients showing intermittent LBBB and negative T waves in antero-septal leads in the normally conducted beats, were studied with 24-h Holter monitoring and chest mapping. These examinations were repeated after 20, 23 and 60 days, and 12, 24 and 25 months respectively. All patients, 1M and 2F aged 57$\pm$3 years, were asymptomatic. Intermittent LBBB was tachycardia-dependent (phase 3 block) in all cases. At the time of the first study and during the following controls, clinical, radiological and laboratory examinations were carried out. During continuous electrocardiographic monitoring, changes in cycle length were obtained by means of hyperventilation and carotid sinus compression in order to determine temporal zones of LBBB and normal conduction. These observations were repeated at the time of Holter monitoring and chest mapping. Holter monitoring was performed by means of an Oxford Medilog II tape recorder using a two-lead system (modified lead II and V5); then the recordings were analysed using a high speed computerized system (Reynolds Medical Pathfinder II) which provided information on the number of normally conducted beats and beats with LBBB. At the end of Holter monitoring, each patient underwent automatic chest mapping by means of Battaglia-Rangoni Cardimap II. Chest electrodes were grouped in 7 rubber straps containing 5 electrodes each, at an interelectrode distance of 4 cm. The first strap was applied to the patient's chest along the right hemiclavicular line with the first lead in the second intercostal space; the other straps were positioned along the following lines: right parasternal, left parasternal, mid line between left parasternal and hemiclavicular left hemiclavear, anterior and mid axillary, so that lowest lead of strap 7 was placed in the sixth intercostal space along mid axillary line. Recording of electrograms was always made at the end of a normal expiration. The electrograms recorded from the 35 chest electrodes and one standard lead (II) were conveyed by the automatic device to 36 amplifiers and, after an analog-to-digital conversion, they were processed by a computer Data General Nova 4/C. The beginning of QRS was determined by visual examination of the reference lead or by the root mean square of potential values in order to detect the beginning of ventricular activation. After instantaneous elaboration of all recorded signals, chest maps or other processed data were displayed on a Tektronix 4025/A video terminal. The following parameters were examined: <u>ΣT</u>, sum of T-wave maximum potential in the 35 chest leads, expressed in mV; <u>T area</u>, sum of the values of T-wave area integral, expressed in mV.msec; <u>T-area map</u>, display of T-area values and of lines joining points at the same value of T-wave area (isoarea lines).

RESULTS

At the time of the first study, all patients were asymptomatic and presented tachycardia-dependent block (phase 3 block). At the second and third observation, no change in clinical condition was observed; intermittent LBBB was still present in 2/3 patients; in patient 3, since the second observation, LBBB was no longer present in basal condition nor it appeared after changing heart rate by hyperventilation or carotid sinus compression. The relationship between intraventricular conduction pattern and cardiac cycle length was evaluated in each case. A modification of the temporal zone of block occurred in each patient: patient 1 and 2 showed a shift of the block zone towards shorter values of the cardiac cycle (shortening of effective refractory period of left bundle branch) while in patient 3, after 60 days, LBBB was neither present nor inducible. Table I shows data from Holter monitoring and chest mapping in each patient at the time of 1st, 2nd and 3rd study. It can be observed that T-wave area and T-wave sum get more negative values if the majority of beats is conducted with LBBB; on the contrary, in absence of anomalous ventricular activation, chest mapping parameters reach positive values. Moreover, comparing changes in the temporal zone of block with chest mapping data, a correlation between repolarization changes and left bundle branch refractoriness may be observed.In each patient T-area map shows a similar pattern in anterior chest leads, both for negative and for positive values and the location of the maximum value occurred where QRS area of beats with LBBB presented the maximum value. Figures 1 and 2 show chest electrograms and isoarea maps, in patient 1, at first and second observation, respectively.

TABLE 1

	I			II			III		
	N%	T area	ΣT	N%	T area	ΣT	N%	T area	ΣT
case 1	100	-1678	-16	90.8	-1048	-10	13.7	+45	+1
case 2	93.9	-587	-6	37.5	-383	-5	29.2	+330	+9
case 3	95.7	-630	-7	0	+1127	+10	0	+1127	+10

Abbreviations: N%=percentage of sinus beats with LBBB at 1st, 2nd and 3rd study; T area=sum of the values of T-wave areas; ΣT=sum of T-wave maximum potentials.

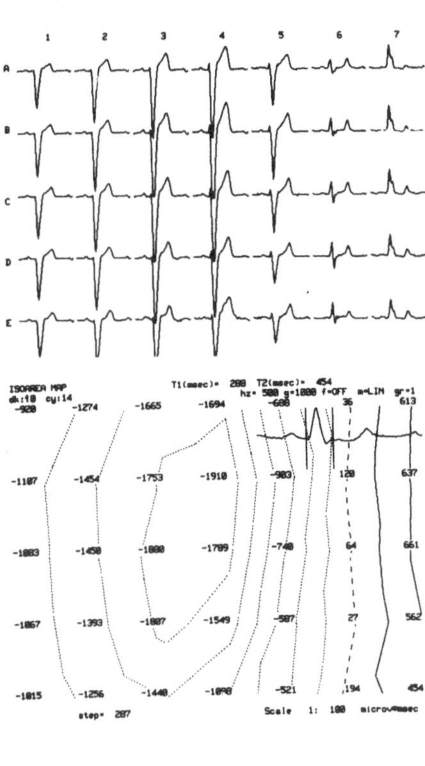

a

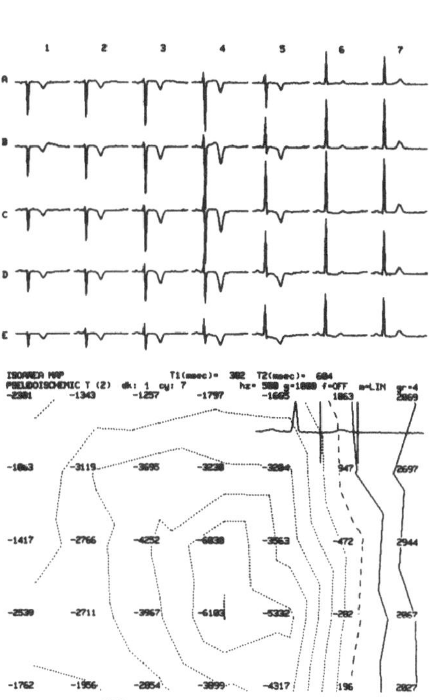

b

FIGURE 1: a. Chest electrograms and QRS isoarea map of a beat with LBBB, at first observation.
b. Chest electrograms and T area map at resumption of normal conduction.
It can be observed that the negativity of T and QRS isoarea show approximatively the same distribution on the anterior chest surface.

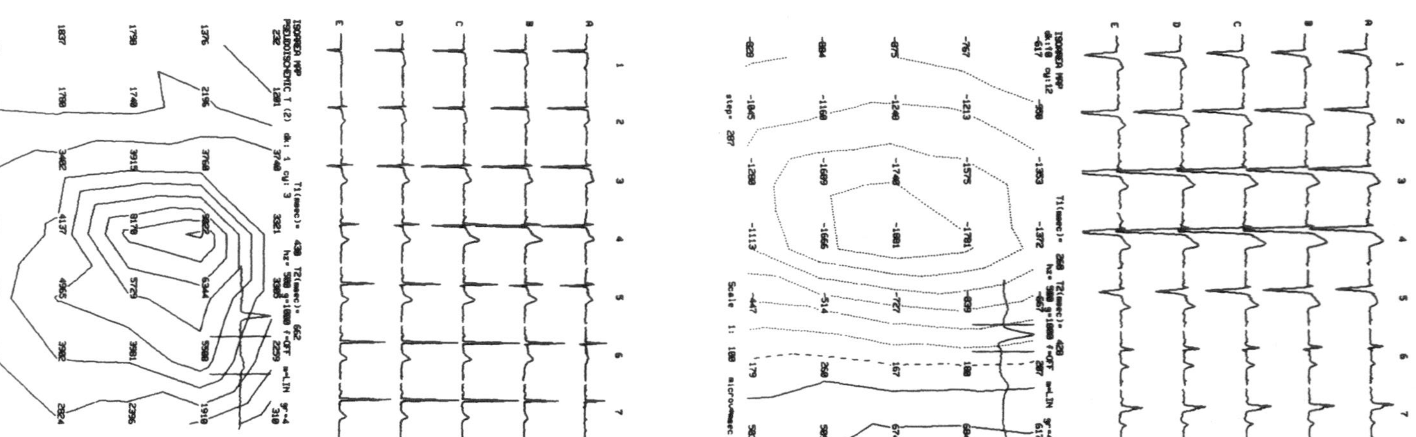

FIGURE 2: a. Chest electrograms and QRS isoarea map of a beat with LBBB, at second observation.
b. Chest electrograms and T area map at resumption of normal conduction.
At the time of the second observation, in spite of a QRS potential distribution nearby identical to that observed in figure 1, T-wave polarity during normal conduction was completely different.

DISCUSSION

Negative T-waves,like those observed in the cases described here, are not to be referred to myocardial ischemia (3,4). The relation between the abnormal polarity of T wave and the previous anomalous ventricular activation observed in our patients is in accordance with other reported findings (1-3). It must be pointed out that, in each lead, these pseudo-primary T-wave changes exhibit the same polarity as the QRS of beats with LBBB. Moreover, the possible direct relation between the duration of anomalous activation and the degree of T-wave changes in normally conducted beats suggests that this phenomenon could be related to a sort of "accumulation" (3). In order to examine better the latter aspect, we used these two techniques, Holter and mapping, to have quantitative informations about duration of anomalous activation and entity of repolarization changes. From our preliminary data, it appears that a direct relationship exixts between the number of anomalous beats and the negativity of repolarization parameters and between the reduction of anomalous beats and the resumption of positive values of T area.

REFERENCES

1. Chatterjee K, Harris A, Davies G, Leatham A: Electrocardiographic changes subsequent to artificial ventricular depolarization. Br Heart J 31: 770, 1969.
2. Nicolai P, Medvedowsky JL, Delaage M, Barnay C, Blache E, Pisapia A: Wolff-Parkinson-White syndrome: T-wave abnormalities during normal pathway conduction. J Electrocardiol 14: 295, 1981.
3. Rosenbaum MB, Blanco HH, Elizari MV, Lazzari JO, Vetulli HM: Electrotonic modulation of ventricular repolarization and cardiac memory. In: Rosenbaum MB, Elizari MV (eds). Frontiers of cardiac electrophysiology. Boston, The Hague, Dordrecht, Lancaster: Martinus Nijhoff pb, 1983, p 67.
4. Salerno JA, Costantini M, Bressan MA, Chimienti M, Previtali M, Medici A: Significato clinico ed evoluzione del blocco di branca sinistra. In: De Ponti CF, Rovelli F (eds). Aggiornamenti in Cardiologia. Roma: Luigi Pozzi pb, 1980, p 161.

PART 4

RECORDING AND DISPLAY TECHNIQUES

Chapter 18

CONTINUOUS DIGITAL RECORDING OF 240 ECG LEADS FOR BODY SURFACE POTENTIAL MAPPING

E. MACCHI, P. BARONE, P. CIARLINI, D. DOTTI, B.M. HORACEK, P. MACINNIS, B. TACCARDI, G. VESCOVINI

INTRODUCTION

The three-dimensional cardiac electric field is subject to changes relating to respiration, heart rate, diastolic and systolic volume, nervous activity, pathologic processes, etc. To study these changes it is necessary 1) to record as many leads as possible from the entire body surface for long periods of time, 2) to display results on-line for quality control and for interacting with the experimental conditions.

To this end we developed a hardware-software system for continuous digital recording of 240 simultaneous electrocardiographic signals at the overall sampling rate of 120 Kbyte/s.

The signals are amplified, multiplexed and digitized by an already existing instrument (1,2). Through ping-pong buffers (3) a PDP 11/40 minicomputer receives direct memory access (DMA) data and transfers them at a higher rate to a large storage disk while updating its device directory. The capacity of our disks (two RM03 disk drives) limits continuous data recording to a maximum of 20 minutes.

The RT-11 single-job monitor runs on-line data collection, while the TSX-Plus time-sharing operating system efficiently supports data processing and displaying. The recorded signals are displayed on-line for quality control and any selected sequence of body surface potential maps (BSPM) can also be displayed within minutes by means of isocontour lines on an electrostatic plotter.

Permanent data storage is performed on magnetic tape. Each data file contains all information relevant to the recording conditions according to the Halifax BSPM tape format for easy data exchange among different laboratories.

The acquisition software can run on any other smaller DIGITAL computer with an RT-11 system whose bus can handle simultaneous DMA and disk data transfers for an assigned number of input signals at a given sampling rate. If a different operating system is used only minor changes are needed. The processing and displaying software is designed to handle different input signal sampling rates, different numbers of input signals and variable electrode grid formats.

ANALOG INSTRUMENT

The general features of an analog instrument for BSPM are here reported. Almost all of these features are implemented in our analog instrument (1,2).

The measuring chain for BSPM can be designed according to the characteristics of the signal source and the desired performace. A set of environmental conditions for the signal source might be as follows:

1) source impedance not greater than 100 KΩ;
2) offset voltage not higher than 100 mV (absolute value);
3) low frequency noise picked up by connections lower than 10 mV.

The desired performance may be specified by an input signal range of ± 8 mV with overall resolution of 1 μV or 0.2% whichever the higher. Fig. 1 illustrates an analog acquisition system, conceived to meet that specification, so configured:

- ECG probes;
- twisted pairs, connected to probes and a reference signal;
- pre-amplifiers with:
    a) galvanic insulation for the subject safety;
    b) input impedance: 50 MΩ;
    c) input noise within the considered frequency band: 1 μV;
    d) gain: 20 or 40 dB;
    e) common mode rejection ration: 80 dB;
- offset subtractor, with capacitive memory, featuring at least 10^5 s discharge time constant;
- main amplifier with variable gain: 20, 30 or 40 dB;
- anti aliasing filter, with proper cut off frequency: e.g. a 4 pole Bessel device, which offers the best phase constancy;

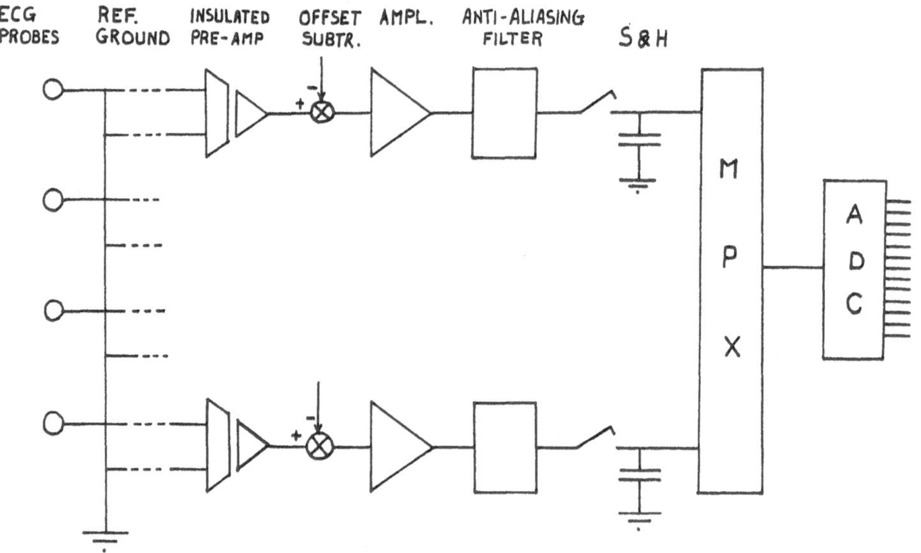

FIGURE 1. Analog acquisition system.

- sample and hold stage, to give instantaneous measures for the same map, if needed: discharge time constant should be not less than 1 s;
- signal selector, for multiplexing the ECG probes;
- analog to digital converter (ADC) with 14 bits resolution and 5 μs conversion time.

Some of these features cannot be easily met, although many of the present day mapping systems are based on the described scheme. However a new design is today made possible by the impressive advances in digital device technology. An example of a new signal conditioner partially based on digital electronics is represented in Fig. 2.

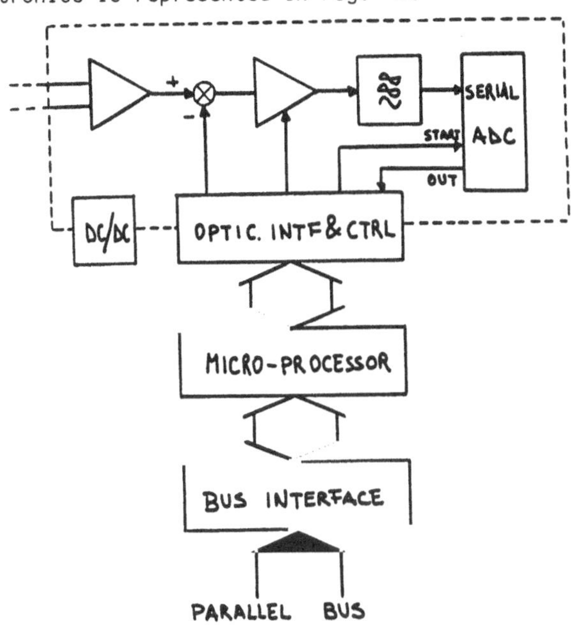

FIGURE 2. New signal conditioner.

The analog part of the measuring chain consists of an insulated board which gets power supply from a DC/DC converter; it also houses a serial ADC so that communication with grounded digital circuitry can take place through optoelectronic devices. A small microprocessor system provides control for regulating offset subtraction, amplifier gain, system calibration, etc. In addition it can operate variable system filtering and sample decimation by software means, whilst the analog signal is passed through a filter with constant cutoff frequency and converted to digital form at a constant rate. Signal multiplexing can be digitally obtained through bus connection between the different acquisition modules and the processing unit, not shown here.

The advantages of this acquisition system can be summarized as follows:
- the input pre-amplifier does not require internal insulation: this allows improved noise figure and better frequency response at the same cost;
- digital offset subtraction eliminates problems due to discharge time constant;

- analog to digital conversion can be simultaneously achieved in each individual acquisition module, eliminating sample and hold devices, since data can be temporarily stored in the microprocessor memory;
- analog to digital conversion can be obtained at a lower rate thus providing improved resolution.

The cost for producing such modules (a few tens) has been evaluated to be about 500 $.

Insofar two extreme solutions have been considered: the former uses one ADC for the whole acquisition system, while the latter uses one ADC for each module. However intermediate solutions can represent an advantageous and practical compromise such as, for instance, the system being developed at the Politecnico of Milano, which provides complex modules comprising 16 analog data channels and a very precise 16 bit ADC.

PING-PONG BUFFERS

The data from the ADC are fed to computer core memory and simultaneously transferred to magnetic disk. To handle these functions the PDP 11/40 computer uses a single communication path called UNIBUS that allows easy data transfer and control. All computer system components and peripherals connect to and communicate with each other on the UNIBUS. With bidirectional and asynchronous lines, peripheral devices can send, receive and exchange data independently by means of "non processor request" (NPR) operation.

Core memory functions as a buffer between the acquisition system (user device) and the disk drive. Two memory buffers of equal size are used (Fig. 3):

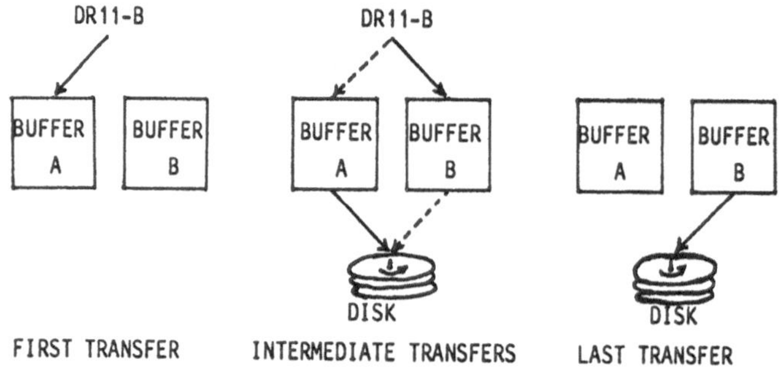

FIGURE 3. Ping-pong buffers.

when buffer A is being filled, buffer B is simultaneously deplenished, and viceversa. In two occasions the operation takes place in one direction only: the first transfer is from user device to buffer A, while the last transfer is from buffer to disk. It is necessary that data transfer from a buffer to disk be finished before the other buffer is full. The largest time interval of recorded data is limited by the total disk capacity, while the shortest time interval is fixed by the memory buffer size.

The following PDP 11/40 peripherals are used:
1) DR11-B DMA interface,
2) two RM03 disk drives.

The block diagram of the data collection system is displayed in Fig. 4.

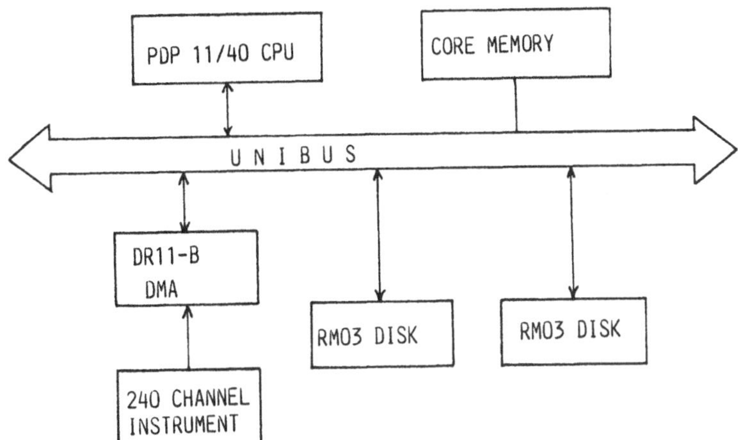

FIGURE 4. Block diagram of data collection system.

DIRECT MEMORY ACCESS INTERFACE

The DR11-B DMA interface is identified on the UNIBUS by a set of registers. The relevant registers are: Word Count (DRWC), Bus Address (DRBA) and Status and Command (DRST). In addition, user output signals are provided by the DR11-B to the user device, and user input signals are provided to the DR11-B by the user device. Some of these signal lines are derived from bits of the DR11-B registers.

The user input signals comprise 8 lines for ADC 8-bit bytes which compress analog data in a quasi-logarithmic scale. The ADC conversion rate is 120 KHz. A user made circuitry is merged into the DR11-B to interface user input and user output signals. This additional interface accomplishes input data demultiplexing by loading two bytes into one word and by forcing sequential word addressing. The cycle request pulse is thus shaped every two bytes halving the input frequency to 60 KHz. It also performs initial resetting and it checks for the reference input channel which primes data acquisition.

Transfer operation is initiated under program control by:
a) loading DRWC with the 2's complement of the number of transfers;
b) specifying the initial address of the core memory buffer;
c) loading DRST register with DMA operation function bits.

The user device recognizes these function bits (user output signals) requesting the first transfer (bus cycle) when the reference input channel is being multiplexed. This feature ensures input channel and data identification. Successive transfers take place under external clock control, thereby eliminating processing time. The processor is notified by an interrupt on DRWC overflow when all the data of one buffer have been transferred. The program may then request a new transfer by loading DRWC,

DRBA and DRST: the content of DRBA register is now the address of the other memory buffer. The buffer is dimensioned by 0.512 s of input data, equal to 61,440 bytes. The number of transfers relative to a single buffer is then 30,720. This same number is loaded into DRWC register to prior any transfer operation. The user interface times a fixed number of cycles during interrupts to keep input data in phase and it halts cycle requests when a DMA transfer error occurs.

MAGNETIC DISK STORAGE

The memory to disk transfer rate must be higher than the DMA transfer rate in order to avoid memory overwriting. The high speed RM03 disk drive fills this demand. To operate this disk a high speed controller is needed to interface to the computer memory bus. This provides a high-speed path for direct memory transfer to take place. All data transfers use the NPR facility for DMA.

The formatted RM03 disk drive is specified by:

disks/pack	3 (top and bottom disks are for protection only)
data surfaces	5
tracks/surface	823
sectors/track	32
bytes/sector	512
data capacity	67,420,160 bytes
spindle speed	3600 rpm

The time for one revolution is 16.66 ms. The number of bytes transferred during one revolution is (512 x 32) = 16,384 (bytes/track) equal to a transfer rate of 983,040 byte/s or to a cycle time of 1.017 μs/byte. A single memory buffer (61,440 bytes) may entirely fit into one cylinder (81,920 bytes). The transfer time of one buffer from memory to disk is (1.017 μs x 61,440) = 62.5 ms. If the transfer from memory to disk takes place in between two successive cylinders, an additional 6 ms seek time interval has to be added for a total amount of 68.5 ms. The time required to transfer the same amount of DMA data is 512 ms. Thus the RM03 disk drive can transfer data about 7 times faster than DMA.

SOFTWARE INTERFACE

Data transfers between user device and memory and between memory and disk drive take place simultaneously and at a high speed on the UNIBUS. For this reason the computer governs data acquisition by means of the RT-11 single job monitor and no other interrupt can take place on the UNIBUS during real time data collection. A user made handler takes over RM03 disk drive which is not supported by the RT-11 system. Such disk handler supports 4 virtual drives for each physical disk drive.

Prior to data collection relevant parameters have to be defined. Then data transfer can take place. The entire sequence of operations is the following:

1) get number of input channels;
2) check for RT-11 system;

3) check for valid date and time;
4) check for calibration table;
5) determine disk drive(s) to be used;
6) claim all unused disk areas of reasonable size (fragments);
7) identify each fragment with a 'filespec' (ddhhmm.fgn):
   filename = ddhhmm (6 characters), dd day, hh hour, mm minute
   file type = fgn (3 characters), fragment number;
8) enter number of seconds to record;
9) perform data acquisition;
10) delete unused fragments;
11) write fragment header.

The data acquisition routine is the kernel of the software interface and it runs as a stand alone program, taking over the data transfers instead of the operating system. A block diagram describing data acquisition logic follows:

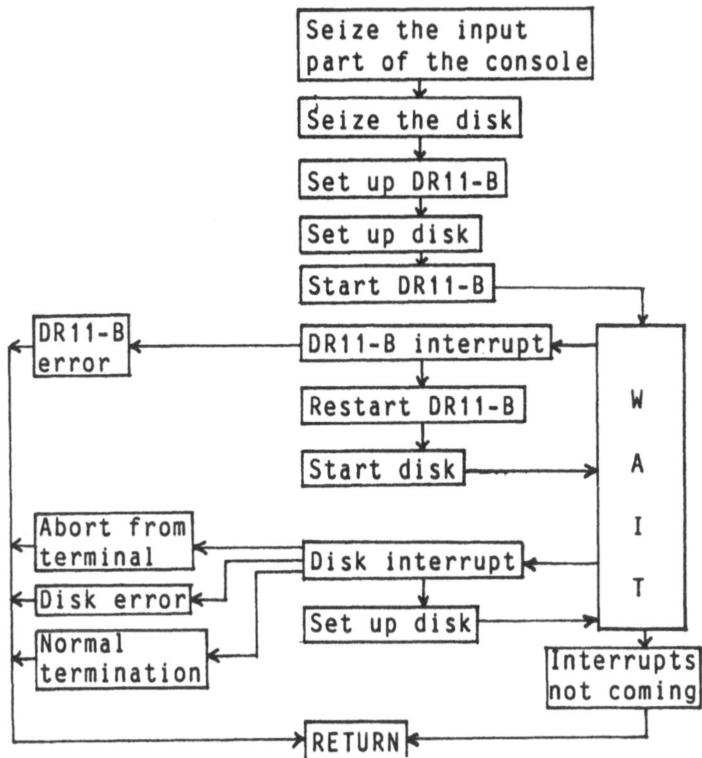

The computer falls through the WAIT on each interrupt (DR11-B, disk, terminal and 50 Hz clock). A flag is reset to 150 (3 seconds) on each disk interrupt and it is counted down at least 50 times a second because of the line frequency clock that is bumping the control out of the above WAIT. Data acquisition ceases when the requested number of transfers is completed, an early termination command is typed in at the terminal, a disk or DR11-B error occurs.

A file is terminated and it is continued by a new file with the same filename whose fragment number is stepped up due to bad blocks on disk or when moving to the next virtual drive. A device directory can list all the files obtained during data acquisition. As regards file length, 240 disk blocks are allocated for each second of input data, in addition to 32 blocks for the file header. The maximum time interval duration for input data is only limited by the available space on disk. One second is the shortest interval, while little less than 20 minutes is the maximum interval when utilizing two physical disk drives.

The header contains all information regarding the hardware parameters set for the input channels, the calibration table, the electrode grid format. Thus each file contains all the parameters needed for processing its data. Permanent storage of the files is obtained by means of a magnetic tape data library. The maximum transfer speed between disk and tape is obtained by means of data transfer functions of the RT-11 system subroutine library.

The main advantage feature of this acquisition software is that the data are stored on disk as any other system or user file, thus avoiding the need for a disk dedicated to the data (4).

DATA PROCESSING AND DISPLAYING

To fully exploit computer memory and CPU time the TSX-Plus time-sharing operating system runs data processing. Multiple users and programs can work simultaneously, utilizing the different graphic peripheral devices. Quality control of any signal relating to the entire recorded time interval, or part of it, is obtained interactively within seconds on a graphic display (Fig. 5).

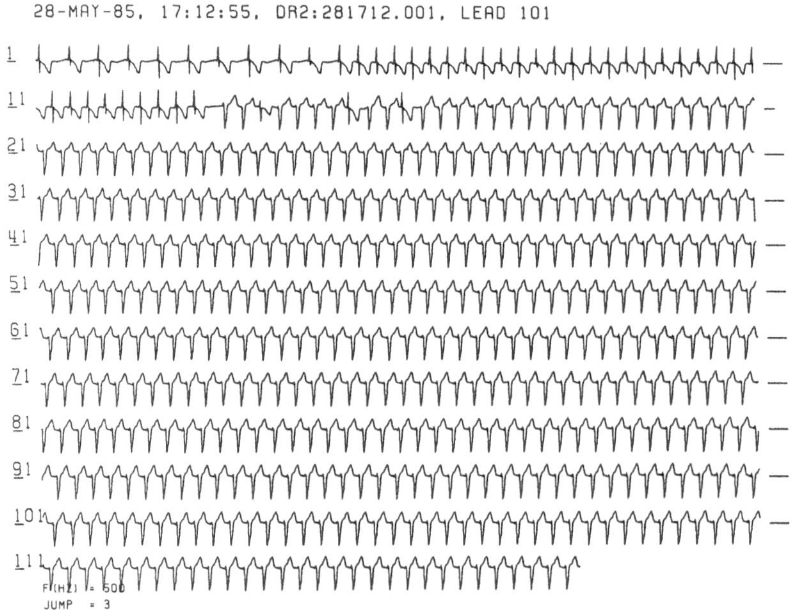

FIGURE 6. On-line display of one of 240 epicardial leads in dog (10 s/row).

It is also possible to select subintervals of 1,024 ms duration, or less, for further processing. Successive beats relating to a long time interval can be time aligned for averaging in order to improve the signal-to-noise ratio during time intervals and in body regions of low potentials (5).

The signals relating to a selected interval are displayed on-line on an electrostatic plotter in the electrode grid format. The interactive programs account for different grid formats, different number of input signals and different signal sampling rates as defined in the file header. The display of maps by means of isopotential lines and/or the printing of maps in tabular form relating to a given sequence within the selected interval can also be obtained in a few minutes on the electrostatic plotter (Fig. 6).

Long interval recordings make it possible to remove low frequency baseline drifts of the signals due to instrumental noise and physiological artifacts. To this end a new method is proposed (6) which works in the time domain instead of the frequency domain as most filters do. The non linear trend, defined as a smoothing cubic spline $f(t_j)$ j=1,N to the data r_j j=1,N is the solution of the following optimization problem:

$$s = \min_{f \in H} \left\{ \int_a^b (f'')^2 + \sum_{j=1}^{N} q^{-1} \cdot \left[r_j - f(t_j) \right]^2 \right\}$$

where q is the smoothing parameter of given value, N is the number of data samples in the time interval examined, H is the Hilbert space of absolute continuous functions and s measures the compromise between accuracy to the data and smoothness of the spline function, controlled by the norm of the second derivative of the spline function weighted by the smoothing parameter q (0 q). The Kalman filter (7) is used to compute the values $f(t_j)$ j=1,N. The value of the weighting parameter q can be chosen interactively by displaying the computed trend for a signal for values of q in a given range. The optimal value of q is the one which corresponds to a smooth trend containing frequencies lower than the ones due to cardiac activity. In fig. 7 the computed non linear trend for a given signal is displayed for different values of q. For given values of q (Fig. 7 A,B) the oscillations in the computed trend correspond to periodic cardiac activity. In fig. 7 C,D for higher values of q, the oscillations are in phase with the respiratory activity which was recorded separately through one of the input channels. For a higher value of q the computed non linear drift may relate to long term physiological changes (Fig. 7 E).

While this system is designed for laboratory research, the functions it performs may be conveniently implemented in a smaller machine of low cost for acquisition, processing and displaying of BSPM in clinical practice. Such a system is open to upgrades, changes and to the addition of new software for more elaborate data processing.

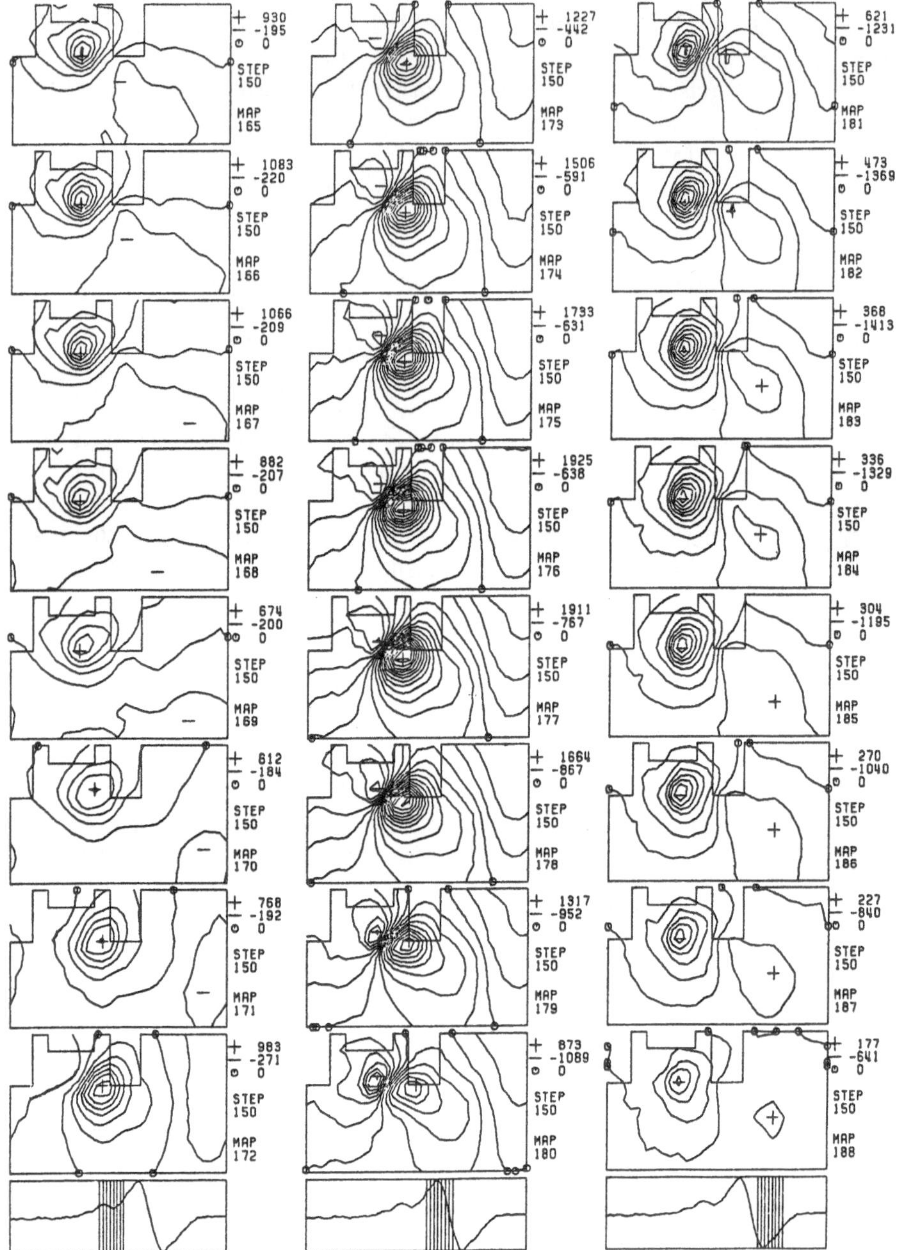

FIGURE 6. Display of body surface isopotential maps during ventricular activation in a patient suffering from anterior myocardial infarction. In each map numerals by the + and - signs indicate the maximum and minimum potentials in μV; the MAP number refers to the time sequence in 2 ms steps from a time reference; STEP is the increment in μV between two isopotential lines; the small circles indicate the zero potential line. The vertical bars on the reference electrocardiogram refer to the sequence of maps displayed in the column above.

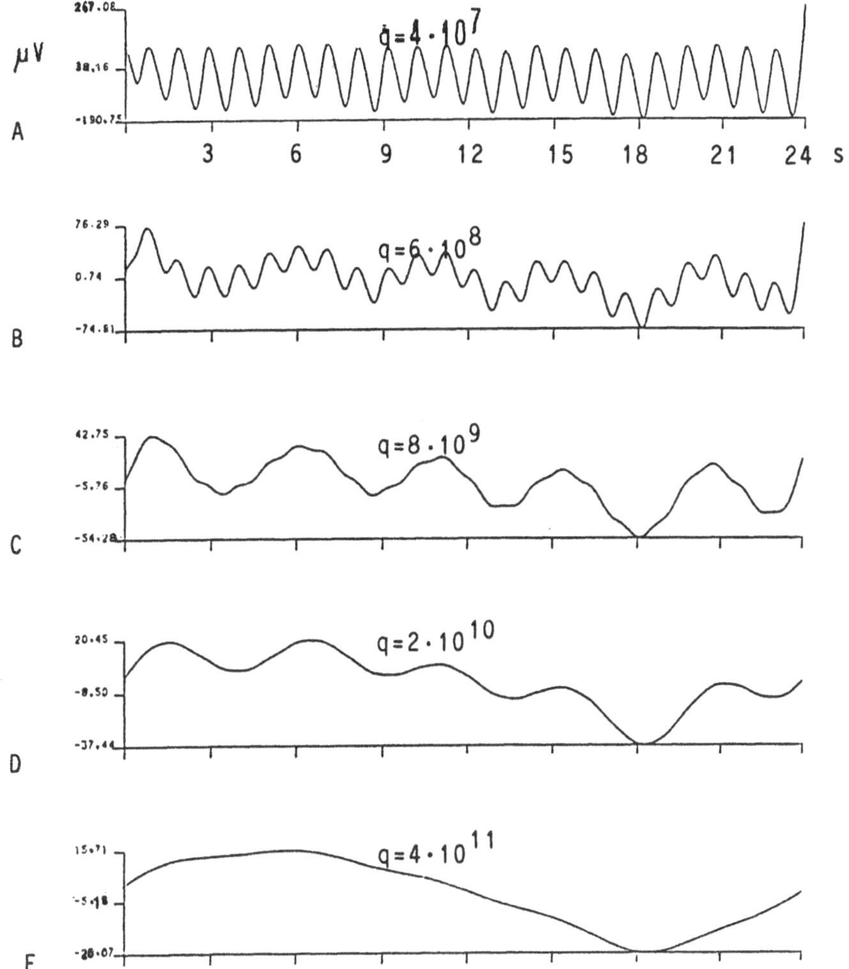

FIGURE 7. Non linear drift computed for one surface lead in a 24 s time interval for different values of the weighting parameter q. Amplitude units are microvolts.

REFERENCES

1. Cottini C, Dotti D, Gatti E, Taccardi B: Uno strumento a 240 sonde per la mappatura del potenziale cardiaco. Alta Frequenza, 41: 988, 1972.
2. Cottini C, Dotti D, Gatti E, Taccardi B: A 240 instrument for mapping cardiac potentials. Proceedings of the Satellite Symposium of the XXVth International Congress of Physiological Sciences, The Electrical Field of the Heart, Rijlant P ed., Presses Academiques Europeennes, Bruxelles, 1972, p. 99-102.
3. Soucek B: Minicomputers in data processing and simulation. Wiley-Interscience, J Wiley and Sons, New York, 1972.

4. Macchi E, Dotti D: Real-time high speed digital data acquisition: a small computer facility. Istituto per le Applicazioni del Calcolo "Mauro Picone", Consiglio Nazionale delle Ricerche, Quaderni, Serie III, n. 98, Roma, 1979.
5. Regoliosi G, Barone P, Ciarlini P, Guspini A, Macchi E, Musso E, Stilli D, Taccardi B: Interactive procedure for automated averaging of body surface maps. In 'Advances in Body Surface Potential Mapping', Yamada K, Harumi K, Musha T ed.s, The University of Nagoya Press, Nagoya, 1984, p. 85-91.
6. Barone P, Ciarlini P, Guspini A: Recursive computation of low-frequency baseline drifts in body surface potential mapping. In Computers in Cardiology, Linkoping, Sweden, Sep. 8-11, 1985.
7. Weinert HL, Byrd RH, Sidhu GS: A stochastic framework for recursive computation of spline functions: Part II, Smoothing splines. Journal of Optimization Theory and Applications, vol. 30, 2, 1980.

Chapter 19

GRID OF ELECTRODES USED AT THE INSTITUTE OF GENERAL PHYSIOLOGY, PARMA, ITALY

E. MUSSO

Two hundred and nineteen silver silver-chloride electrodes, 8 mm in diameter, are mounted on 22 rubber straps. The distances between electrodes on the straps are 3 to 6 cm. The straps are 3 cm width and are vertically attached to the anterior, posterior and lateral chest walls by means of 3M double coated Medical tape. The location of the electrodes on the chest is schematically illustrated in Figure 1. The straps n 1 and 2 are respectively located behind and before the right midaxillary line. Straps n 3 to 13 are attached to the chest surface by placing them side by side starting from strap n 8 which lies on the sternal midline. Straps 14 to 16 are approximately located on the anterior, mid and posterior axillary line, respectively. Straps n 17 to 22 are equally spaced on the back starting from straps n 19 and 20 located on the paravertebral lines. Thus, the vertical distances between electrodes are fixed in every patient, 3 or 6 cm, while the horizontal distances may slightly depart from these values in the various patients, depending on chest geometry.

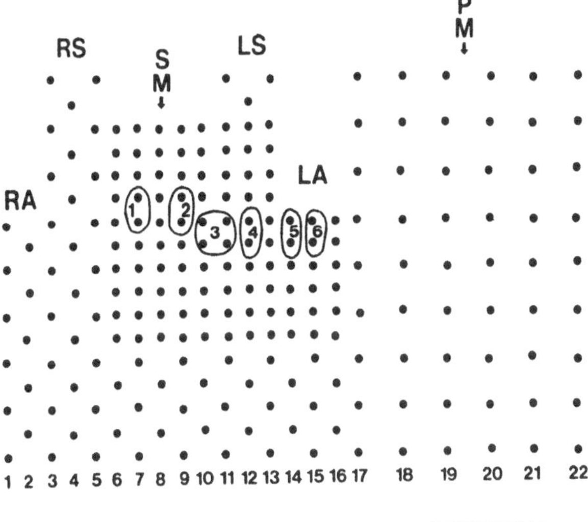

Fig. 1: Schematic drawing illustrating the location of the electrodes on the anterior and posterior chest surface. The thoracic areas surrounded by the black lines roughly correspond to those occupied by the standard precordial leads (1 to 6) in the various patients. The figures 1 to 22 at the bottom of each column of electrodes indicate the numbers of the rubber straps. RA = right axilla, RS = right shoulder, SM = sternal midline, LS = left shoulder, LA = left axilla PM = posterior midline.

Chapter 20

TOWARDS A COMMON DATA-FORMAT IN CARDIAC POTENTIAL MAPPING

B.M. HORACEK, R.K. HELPPI, P. MACINNIS, J.D. SHERWOOD

1. INTRODUCTION

Data bases with adequately sized groups will be needed to positively identify the diagnostic information in cardiac mapping data. Assembling such groups may be too difficult and expensive a task for any single research group; thus pooling of data from different laboratories seems to be an inevitability. Such cooperation is hindered by a paucity of standards, the prevailing opinion being that it is premature to get tied up with standards that would fix, among other things, the number of recording electrodes and their location. One way to overcome this stalemate is to adopt a data-format convention that would accommodate all existing recording protocols as well as all existing data-acquisition-hardware features. This would permit easy conversion of data originating in different places to whatever standard form may be negotiated in the future. The present paper is a proposal for such a common data-format, for both "raw" and processed data. The proposed format bears many similarities to the one used in Japan (2), and thus we hope that the formulation of generally acceptable definitive standards is not too far away.

2. FORMATS OF CARDIAC POTENTIAL MAPPING DATA

2.1. Background

Our first data-acquisition system (1) was designed to record continuously, for up to four minutes, 128 simultaneous electrocardiograms on 9-track digital magnetic tape. Channel amplifiers had a fixed gain, their filters were set for a fixed bandwidth, and an analog multiplexer with an A/D converter produced 10-bit samples at 500 samples/sec/channel. All these parameters were chosen for the recording of electrocardiograms at the body surface; however, it soon became obvious that the acquisition system should be versatile enough to satisfy the requirements of cardiac mapping techniques used in the clinical electrophysiological laboratory or in the operating room. Therefore, our second-generation acquisition system for cardiac potential mapping (which has been in use since 1983) was designed to allow flexibility in choosing the number of recorded channels, the array of recording electrodes, the gain of amplifiers, the sampling rate, the A/D converter resolution, etc. This system can record simultaneously up to 256 unipolar/bipolar cardiac electrograms or body-surface electrocardiograms. Data acquisition can be performed at up to 2000 samples/second/channel with the total data throughput being up to 192 kbytes per second. The amplitude resolution is up to 0.5 μV per bit with a maximal dynamic range of up to 100 mV. Data are continuously recorded on digital magnetic tape. This modified design concept required also new software to provide flexibility conveniently and to produce data files that store all the particulars of a recording protocol as well as hardware parameters of an acquisition system. Our present data-formats are described in sections 2.2 and 2.3.

----

*From the Department of Physiology & Biophysics, Dalhousie University, Halifax, Nova Scotia, Canada

2.2. Acquisition tape format

2.2.1. Basic concepts. We are using Digital Equipment Corporation's PDP-11/24 computer as a basis of the data acquisition system, and Digital's VAX-11/780 computer running the VMS operating system to process data. Our acquisition system (with a Kennedy 9300 tape drive) produces "recording tapes" that can have a density of either 800 bpi or 1600 bpi. The VAX-11 can read those "recording tapes" and subsequently store processed data using 800, 1600, or 6250 bpi density. The interrecord gap decreases the actual density of data on the magnetic tape. To allow higher throughput of the acquisition system, we allow record sizes of up to 30,000 bytes. With the tape drive's capstan speed of 120 ips and a recording density of 1600 bpi, we capture nearly 192,000 bytes per second; thus we can record 256 channels at 500 12-bit samples/sec/channel or 128-channels at 1000 12-bit samples/sec/channel. Data on magnetic tape are organized into files. Because the magnetic tape file-system which normally provides header-records for each file is computer-dependent, we created our own header-records with the idea of portability, and we designed them specifically for cardiac mapping applications.

2.2.2. General description. Our mapping data are preceded by two header-records, and provision is made for an optional third header-record. The first header-record contains information about the installation, the subject, the recording protocol, and the acquired data, and the second is of variable length and contains specifications for all channels. The third header-record can be specified by the user; its length and description are given in the first header-record. The first and second header-records are composed entirely of ASCII characters; the same should apply to the third header-record. Variable-width pure numeric fields are right justified with either zero or blank fill; variable-width alphanumeric fields are left justified with blank fill. The fields marked with an asterisk ('*') are required; all other fields are optional.

2.2.3. First header-record.

Field Description	Position (bytes)	Length (bytes)	Example/Remarks
Header identification	*1-2	2	'H1' identifies the first header-record. No other characters accepted.
Installation	*3-8	6	'YHZ001' - a unique identifier for the particular hardware installation. It defines the geographic location by a three-character airport code, and the computer/front-end configuration of the system.
Version	9-12	4	'001A' - minor revisions of the software increment the letter; major revisions (including changes to the tape format) increment the numeric field.
Date and Time (YYYYMMDDHHMMSS)	13-26	14	'19850117211007' - year, month, day, hour, minute, second of the recording.

Session number	27-32	6	'001234' - free-form fielden-tered at the start of each re-cording session; used as a cross-reference to the paper file for the recording.
Protocol code	*33-40	8	'100/XYZ' - free-form alphanumer-ic field describing the record-ing protocol; electrode posi-tions, etc.
Patient number	41-56	16	'111-222-333-10'- free-form alphanumeric field; Social Insur-ance Number (SIN) in Canada.
Patient name	57-88	32	'JONES,JOHN P.' - alphabetic field for name; surname first, followed by a comma (',').
Hospital file #	89-98	10	'123456-02' - patient hospital-record identifier; free form.
Birthdate	99-106	8	'YYYYMMDD'
Sex	107	1	'M' or 'F'
Pacemaker	108	1	'Y' or 'N'
Patient status	109-112	4	'RSUP' - a four-character stan-dardized mnemonic descriptor for the patient state; RSUP = resting supine, etc.
Diagnostic information	113-208	96	An array of four-character strings (each 24 characters in length)giving up to four differ-ent diagnostic descriptions. This field is free format; we use the New York Heart Association nomenclature (4).
Cardiologist	209-218	10	Name of the referring cardio-logist; free form.
Technician	219-228	10	Name of the recording technician; free form.
Remarks	229-338	110	Optional; free form.
Reserved for future use	339-402	64	-
Number of channels (NCH)	*403-406	4	'0128' - number of multiplexed channels.

Number of samples per channel per record	*407-410	4	'0156' - redundant information for convenience.
Sample size in bits	*411-412	2	'12'
Sample-to-sample interval in usec	*413-418	6	'002000' - this example corresponds to 500 samples per second per channel.
High-pass filters	419-482	64	'.2500E-1' - an array of up to 8 character strings, each 8 bytes long, defining the -3 db point (Hz) of high-pass filters in the acquisition system; E8.4 format. The channel specifications include a pointer into this array.
Low-pass filters	483-546	64	'.1250E3' - similar to the high-pass filter array above. Defines the -3 db point in Hz for the low-pass filters.
Coordinate system	547-550	4	'CYLI' - standardized 4-character mnemonic code for the electrode coordinate system; CYLI = cylindrical; GRID = grid system defining an electrode location on the map-display rectangle (cf. grid described in (2)).
Data type	*551-554	4	'IBM2' - 4-character standardized mnemonic code defining the type of binary data in the data records. 'IBM2' - 2's complement IBM tape format; 'DEC2' - 2's complement PDP-11 tape format; 'IBMF' - offset binary IBM tape format, etc.
Data record size in bytes	*555-560	6	'030000' adjusted such that each record begins with the same channel (e.g. channel #1). This count does not include the 32-byte preamble. The maximal permissible data-record size is 30,000 bytes; records shorter than 4 kbytes are recommended if the throughput is not critical.
Size of the second header-record; in bytes	561-566	6	'004096' - this count does not include the 32-byte preamble; it must be equal to CHD*NCH where CHD is the size of channel descriptor in the second header and NCH is the number of channels.

Size of the channel descriptor (CHD) in the 2nd header-record; in bytes	567-568	2	'32' - normally, CHD size is 32 bytes.
Size of the optional 3rd header-record; in bytes	569-574	6	the user defined 3rd header-record is provided to accommodate the specific features of the given installation; '0' indicates there is no third header-record.
Description of the 3rd header-record contents	575-699	125	Optional, free form.
Reserved for future use	700-1024	325	

2.2.4. <u>Second header-record.</u> The second header-record must have 'H2' in the first 2 bytes. This record contains--in addition to the 32-byte preamble--the channel specifications. Each channel has its own channel descriptor, which is CHD bytes long (see the first header-record); CHD = 32 is recommended. Thus for NCH channels (see the first header-record), the second header-record must be (32 + NCH * CHD) bytes long.

Field Description	Position (bytes)	Length (bytes)	Example/Remarks
Header identification	*1-2	2	'H2' - identifies the 2nd header-record.
Installation	*3-8	6	'YHZ001' - as in 1st header-record.
Version	9-12	4	'001A' - as in 1st header-record.
Reserved for future use	13-32	20	-
Electrode coordinates	33-44	12	An array of three elements, each four numeric characters long. The values are in integer format; the coordinate system and its units can be inferred from the coordinate system code in the first header-record.
Resolution	*45-52	8	'.2500E-5' - the resolution of the least significant bit of the sample values for this channel; units specified in the following field; E8.4 format.
Resolution unit	*53	1	'V' - standardized one-character code specifying MKS units of the measured signal.

Time skew from first channel	54-61	8	'.1000E-4' - if sample & hold circuit not used on every channel, this parameter defines the skew in seconds; E8.4 format.
High-pass filter index	62	1	'0' - index into the high-pass filter array in the first header-record; (0/1/2/3/4/5/6/7).
Low-pass filter index	63	1	'0' - index into the low-pass filter array in the first header-record; (0/1/2/3/4/5/6/7).
Channel attribute	64	1	'N' - standardized one-character numeric code; e.g. 'N' - not sampled, 'R' - rejected, etc.

Specifications for channels #2 to #NCH follow in blocks of CHD bytes (usually 32 bytes) in the format identical to that for channel #1.

2.2.5. Third header-record. The third header-record is optional; it is defined by the user to accommodate his specific needs (e.g., as in (3), storing calibration constants of the logarithmic A/D converter in this header-record). The length and format of the record should be specified in the first header; 'H3' must appear in the first 2 bytes and the record must be composed entirely of ASCII characters.

Field Description	Position (bytes)	Length (bytes)	Example/Remarks
Header identification	1-2	2	'H3' - identifies the optional 3rd header-record.
User defined field	3-	-	It is suggested that this field is composed entirely of ASCII characters.

2.2.6. Data records. Data records are in packed binary, i.e., there are no empty bits between samples regardless of their size. IBM or DEC formats are permitted as defined by the 'data type' variable in the first header-record.

Field Description	Position (bytes)	Length (bytes)	Example/Remarks
Sequence count	1-4	4	'0001' - starts at 1 and increments for each data record.
Date and time	5-18	14	this field is a copy of the same field from the header, i.e. the time field does not increment.
Reserved for future use	19-32	14	-
Data	33-	≤30000	binary data up to 30000 bytes

A tape mark follows the last data record. This may be followed by a header-record of another file, or a second consecutive tape mark (signifying end of tape).

2.3. Tape format of processed data (Version '1-85'; VAX-11/780 VMS)

2.3.1. General description. Processed data are written into files on "output tapes". None of the "output tapes" are volumes of a multivolume set, i.e. the data written on them do not continue to any other tape volume. The density is 6250 bpi.

2.3.2. Header format. The following description is an abbreviated preliminary version. The header-record is 12800 bytes long; it is composed entirely of ASCII characters, and all numerical values are integers. The first part contains subject identifiers, recording identifiers, and information pertinent to the results of the processing program (optionally modified by the over-reader's entries); the second part essentially copies header-records of the "recording tape" (these can be accommodated completely for any number of recorded channels not exceeding 256, with the channel-descriptor size not exceeding 32 bytes).

Position (bytes)	Length (bytes)	Variable name	Field Description
1-100	100	-	Installation information in free format
101-116	16	JPN	Subject number
117-120	4	JSTAT	Subject state
121-124	4	JAREA	Area code
125-128	4	JSEQ	Additional identifier (sequence etc.)
129-141	13	-	Not used
142-145	4	TAPE81	Input tape number
146-149	4	BEGIN81	Input file number
150-153	4	JSAMP	Number of samples per second per lead
154-157	4	SINT	Sampling interval in usec
158-221	64	INVPRBS	Bit array specifying the valid probes for up to 512 leads
222-229	8	-	Not used
230-235	6	SIDR	Size of data records in bytes
236-239	4	NSPR	Number of samples per lead in each data record

240-241	2	SASI	Sample size in bytes
242-245	4	IVER	Processing program version ID
246-261	16	IDT	Date of processing
262-269	8	STRTIME	Time of processing
270-273	4	ISCW	Selected lead for the QRS detection
274-275	1	NTCHED	Notch-filter indicator ("1"=.TRUE.; "0"=.FALSE.)
276-278	3	IHR	Number of QRS complexes per minute
279-282	4	NC	Number of QRS complexes found in the data
283-286	4	NCAV	Number of complexes averaged
287-292	6	MYNPL	Total number of samples in the averaged complex
293-296	4	NPL	Number of averaged samples per lead
297-300	4	JRON	QRS onset; sample number
301-304	4	JDUR	QRS duration in samples
305-312	8	PON	P-wave onset in usec from the beginning of averaged complex
313-320	8	PMAX	P-wave spatial (VCG) maximum in usec
321-328	8	POFF	P-wave offset in µsec
329-336	8	PRMIN	Time in µsec into the averaged data, where the electrical activity is minimal between P and QRS
337-344	8	RON	R-wave onset in µsec
345-352	8	RPK	Time in usec to the QRS spatial (VCG) maximum
353-360	8	ROFF	QRS offset in µsec
361-368	8	SPMAXT	Time in µsec to the T-wave

			spatial (VCG) maximum
369-376	8	TOFF	T-wave offset in µsec
377-400	24	-	Not used
401-1424	1024	-	Copy of the first input header-record
1425-1600	176	-	Not used
1601-9824	8224	-	Copy of the second input header-record
9825-10000	176	-	Not used
10001-12048	2048	-	Copy of the third input header
12049-12800	752	-	Not used

2.3.3. Data format. The averaged data are stored in parallel fashion. Since the size of the data records may vary from one application to another, information about the size of the records, the number of samples per lead in one record, and the sample size is given in the header-record (bytes 230-241). The last data record should be of the same size as other data records and thus it may have to be filled with zeroes beyond the last valid averaged sample value. Presently, we are still using the old format for our output tapes (1): each sample is 2 bytes long and there are 50 samples in one data record; for the 128-lead recordings this means that the first samples of leads 1-128 are stored in the first 256 bytes of the first record, and the record length for the 50 samples, therefore, is 12800 bytes.

3. DISCUSSION

Digital Equipment Corporation computers produce digital tapes in which the words are written starting with the least significant byte. The format used by most of the rest of the industry writes the most significant byte first. If only character data are involved this presents no problem since characters are also stored internally in swapped format. With binary data, however, care must be taken that the computers used for writing and reading the tapes allow for the possibility of a swap. To make matters worse, the swapping depends upon the word size of the computer. Thus a PDP-11 does a different swap than a VAX. Compared to the IBM format, the PDP-11 format has the odd and even bytes interchanged. To circumvent these problems the header-records of both "recording tape" and "output tape" are entirely character format in a form which may be deciphered with a formatted READ or DECODE in FORTRAN.

4. ACKNOWLEDGMENTS

We gratefuly acknowledge the contribution and criticism of Dr. Robert Guardo from the Institut de génie biomédical, Université de Montréal, who first suggested the expandable second header-record of the "recording tape" and pointed out to us several omissions in our original concept. This work was supported in part by the Medical Research Council of Canada (PG-30) and by the Nova Scotia Heart Foundation.

5. REFERENCES

1. Horacek BM, Eifler WJ, Gewirtz H, Helppi R, MacAulay PB, Sherwood JD, Smith ER, Tiberghien J, Rautaharju PM: An automated system for body-surface potential mapping. In: Ostrow HG and Ripley KL (Eds.), Computers in Cardiology, IEEE Computer Society, Long Beach, Calif. 1977, pp 399-407

2. Teramachi Y, Musha T, Harumi K: Proposal for "Standardization of the body surface potential mapping system". In this volume.

3. Macchi E, Barone P, Ciarlini P, Dotti D, Horacek BM, MacInnis P, Taccardi B, Vescovini G. Continuous digital recording of 240 ECG leads for body surface potential mapping. In this volume.

4. The Criteria Committee of the New York Heart Association. Nomenclature and criteria for diagnosis of diseases of the heart and great vessels. 8th Edition. Little, Brown and Company, Boston, 1979.

Chapter 21

PROPOSAL FOR "STANDARDIZATION OF THE BODY SURFACE POTENTIAL MAPPING SYSTEM"

Y. TERAMACHI, T. MUSHA, K. HARUMI

We propose a standardized data file format for the floppy disk to make possible mutual exchange of data files between different BSPM systems. Each BSPM system has its original arrangement of leads. This makes a universal data transformation method between all kinds of BSPM systems complicated. Therefore we propose 128 standard display points that are uniformly arranged on the BSPM. Standard display points may not be the real positions. Potentials at standard display points are calculated from data collected by an arbitrary BSPM system. In the standardized data file, these calculated data are stored instead of original data. For display, these standardized data are re-transformed to the data corresponding to the positions of another BSPM system's leads. With this method, only one pair of programs for transformation between standardized data and system data is necessary.

BSPM co-ordinates are proposed to describe the original lead positions on the BSPM. Standard vertical lines are right midaxillary line, median line, left midaxillary line and mid-spinal line. The Y-axis is aligned on the right midaxillary line. The X-axis is aligned on the top of the BSPM. Y-distances of the second intercostal space and V5 lead are described in the heading of the data file as positions of the vertical reference points.

Eight inches, double density and dual sides floppy disks are used as data media for mutual data exchange. The track and sector format is IBM type, but the file format is original.

This proposal for "STANDARDIZATION OF THE BODY SURFACE POTENTIAL MAPPING SYSTEM" had the approval of the Committee on Standardization of the Body Surface Potential Mapping in Japan.

SPECIFICATIONS OF BSPM DATA FILE FORMAT

I. Cylinder and sector map:

cylinder	side	sector		data-type
0			not used	
1	0	1	volume label	(character)
		2	directories	(integer)
		3	file table 1	(integer)
		4	file table 2	(integer)
		5	file table 3	(integer)
		6	old file table	(integer)
		7 - 8	for future use	
	1	1	total number of electrodes	(integer)
		2 - 4	coordinates of original electrodes	(integer)
		5 - 6	for future use	
		7 - 8	not used	
2 - 73			data area	
74 - 76			not used	

II. File Managing area:

II-1. Directories:

The First 960 bytes of this sector are divided into 60 directories. These directories are composed of 16 bytes. File managing parameters are stored in remaining 64 bytes.

II-1.1. Structure of each directory:

field	position	bytes	
1. Delete mark	1 - 2	2	0:available file 15:deleted file 63:used file -1:abnormal end
2. File attribute	3 - 4	2	0:read/write -1:read only
3. First cluster number in the file	4 - 6	2	(1- 144)
4.	7 -16		for future use

II-1.2. File managing parameters:

field	position	bytes	
1. Abnormal file	961-962	2	0:all normal files -1:abnormal file exists
2. Volume attribute	963-964	2	0:read/write -1:read only
3. Number of available files	965-966	2	
4. Number of remaining clusters	967-968	2	
5.	969-1024	56	for future use

II-2. File Table:

Data are either read from or recorded on a floppy disc in the unit of a cluster. One cluster consists of eight sectors in one side of one cylinder. The first cluster, the second cluster and the 144th cluster are located at side 0 in cylinder 2, side 1 in cylinder 2 and side 1 in cylinder 73, respectively. The number of the first cluster in one file is recorded in the directory of this file. The next cluster number in this file is recorded on the position of the present cluster number in the file table. In the position of the last cluster, the number of used sector is recorded. Three file tables with the same contents are prepared for safety. These three file tables are renewed when a file is deleted or a new file is added. One more file table called old file table is prepared. This old file table is renewed only when a new file is added. Thus, even deleted files can be reconstructed.

Contents of File Table:

0:available
1-144:following cluster number
193-200:this number minus 192 indicates the number of the last sector in the last cluster of one file
255:reserved for system use

II-3. Volume Label:

field	position	bytes	
1. File Format Identifier	1 - 8	8	'BSPM-STD' This character string indicates that this file is the BSPM standard file
2. Version	9 - 16	8	'V1.1'
3. Name of BSPM system	17 - 48	32	
4.	49-1024	976	for future use

III. Coordinates of electrodes in the original system:

III-1. Total number of electrodes in the original system:

field	position	bytes	
1. Total number of electrodes	1 - 2	2	
2.	3 - 1024	1022	for future use

III-2. BSPM coordinates of electrodes in the original system:

Coordinates of original electrodes in the BSPM coordinate are recorded on the third sector in sequence as X1,Y1,X2,Y2, ,Xn,Yn where n is the total number of electrodes. If n is larger than 256, data will be recorded on the fourth and fifth sectors.

IV. File structure:

IV-1. File Label:

field	position	bytes	
1. Patient name	1 - 32	32	
2. ID number	33 - 44	12	
3. Clinical diagnosis	45 - 172	128	
4. ECG diagnosis	173 - 300	128	
5. Remarks	301 - 556	256	
6. Original floppy disc number	557 - 568	12	
7.	569 -1024	456	for future use

IV-2. Parameters:

field	position	bytes	
1. Age	1 - 2	2	
2. Sex	3 - 4	2	0:Male, 1:Female
3. Birthdate, year	5 - 6	2	in A.D.
4. month	7 - 8	2	
5. day	9 - 10	2	
6. Height	11 - 12	2	in mm
7. Weight	13 - 14	2	in hectogr. 1(hg)=100(g)
8. Chest girth	15 - 16	2	in mm
9. Date of measurement, year	17 - 18	2	in A.D.
10. month	19 - 20	2	
11. day	21 - 22	2	
12. Time of measurement, hour	23 - 24	2	
13. minute	25 - 26	2	
14. second	27 - 28	2	
15. Posture of patient	29 - 30	2	0:others, 1:standing, 2:sitting, 3:lying, 4:lying at 45 degree
16. Phase of respiration	31 - 32	2	0:free, 1:expiratory, 2:inspiratory
17. Heart rate	33 - 34	2	in beats per minute
18. Y coordinate of the second intercostal space in the BSPM coordinates	35 - 36	2	c.f. a in Fig. 4
19. Y coordinate of the V4 lead in the BSPM coordinates	37 - 38	2	c.f. b in Fig. 4
20. Displacement between these two points in Y axis	39 - 40	2	in mm between a en b in Fig. 4
21. Vertical length of the BSPM	41 - 42	2	in mm Displacement between E1 and E8 in Fig. 4 on the body surface
22. Indifferent electrode	43 - 44	2	0:others, 1:Wilson's central electrode
23. Resolution of AD converter	45 - 46	2	in bits
24. Total frame number	47 - 48	2	
25. Sample-to-sample interval	49 - 50	2	in ms *1
26. Sample-to-sample interval	51 - 52	2	in ms *1
27. Channel-to-channel time skew	53 - 54	2	in ms *1
28. Channel-to-channel time skew	55 - 56	2	in ms *1
29. Input voltage range	57 - 58	2	in ms *1
30. Input voltage range	59 - 60	2	in microvolts *1

31. Total number of averaging	61 - 62	2	
32.	63 - 1024	966	for future use

IV-3. Measured BSPM data:

Data are stored in 16 bits, two's complement format. If the resolution of the AD converter is less than 16 bits then data should be justified left. Then, maximum input voltage is expressed as 32767. The words are written starting with the most significant byte. These data are stored on the floppy disc in the sequence of A1,A2, A8,B1, P8 (c.f. Fig.1).

*1 These expressions of numbers are employed to realize wide valuerange without using floating point numbers. Let values of fields 25 and 26 be IA and IB respectively, then real sample-to-sample interval is

$$IA \times 10^{-3} + IB \times 16^{-6} \text{ seconds.}$$

If the sample-to-sample interval is 1.25 ms, 1 is recorded on field 25 and 250 is recorded on field 26.

*2 Future space areas in a sector of which data-type is character should be filled with '(space)';20H. Future use area in a sector of which data-type is integer should be filled with 0;00H.

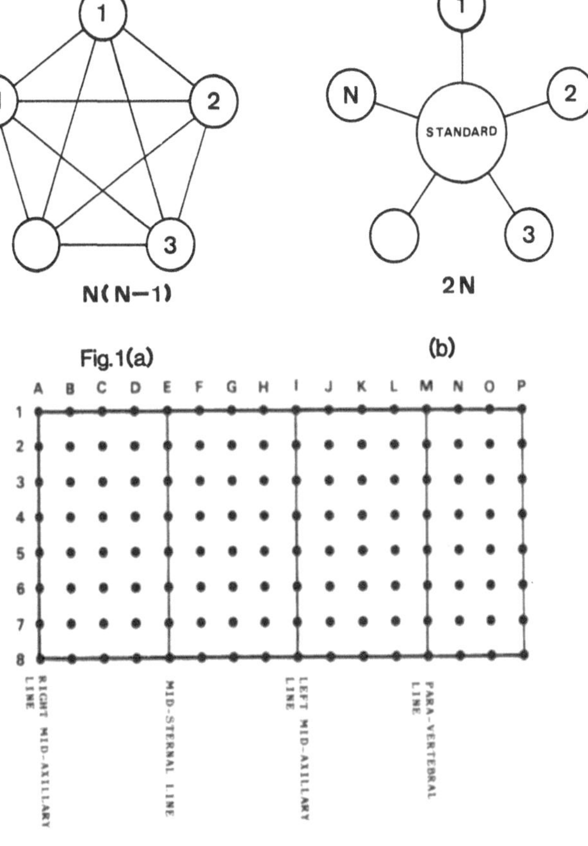

Fig.1(a) (b)

Fig.2 STANDARD DISPLAY POINTS

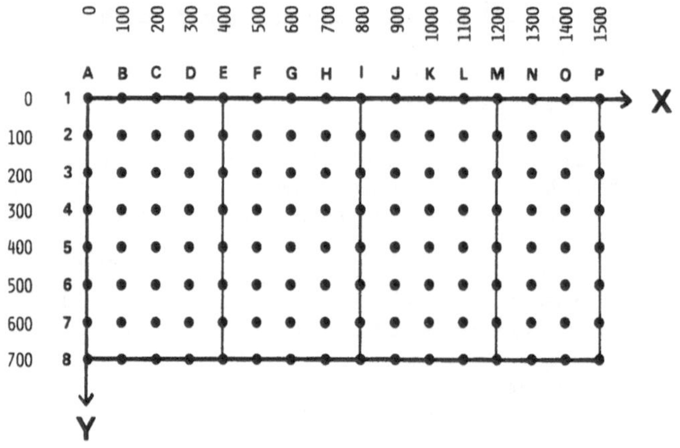

Fig.3 BSPM COORDINATES

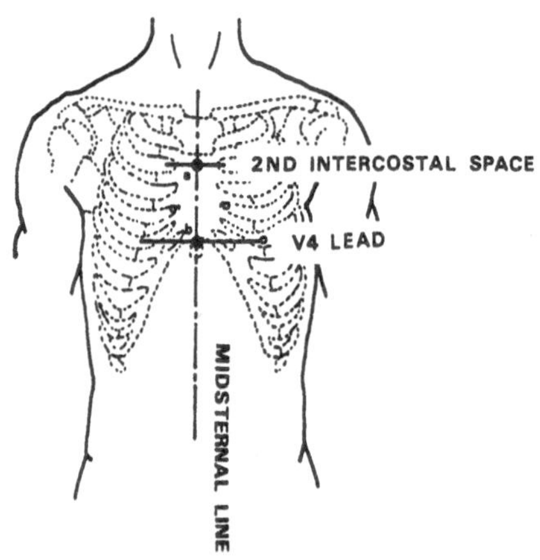

Fig.4 VERTICAL REFERENCE POINTS

Chapter 22

DATA REPRESENTATION PROBLEMS OF BODY SURFACE POTENTIAL MAPPING

GY. KOZMANN, ZS. CSERJÉS, T. ROCHLITZ, F. SZLÁVIK

1. INTRODUCTION

The representation of cardiac potential fields is fundamentally a five dimensional problem. Three dimensions are needed to define space dependence, one to determine the time coordinate and, finally, the fifth dimensions is for the potential values. In order to reduce dimensionality the torso is assumed to be a cylinder which is cut along a generating line (usually along the right axilla) and is unrolled; it thus becomes flat so only two dimensions are needed to identify a surface point. A further dimension-reducing possibility is offered by sampling in the time domain; in other words the time course of the field formation is represented by a series of instantaneous potential distributions. Thus, finally, the elementary unit to be represented is a two dimensional scalar-scalar function. The display of this is already a routine task in computer graphics.

The required accuracy of the time domain representation can be ensured by an adequate sampling rate, as is done in high speed film techniques. The quality of the space domain representation is also determined by the sampling density; in other words, by the interelectrode distance of the measuring array.

In this paper two groups of problems are briefly touched on.

In the first the influence of the space and time domain sampling rate and interpolation strategy on the expected error of field reconstruction is discussed in terms of a mean square relative error criterion.

The second problem group concerns representation methods which have proved to be useful for visualizing test results performed on an arbitrary individual and with some further methods introduced for characterizing field properties of a homogeneous group or groups of patients.

2. SAMPLING RATE REQUIREMENTS OF BODY SURFACE POTENTIAL MAPPING

2.1 Time-domain sampling rate requirements

In the last decade several papers have been published on the spectral content and on the sampling requirements of ECG signals. From the viewpoint of body surface mapping the most important paper was that of Barr and Spach (1).

In their paper the expected interpolation error as a function of sampling rate was formulated in graphic form, parametrized by the interpolation strategy used. For adults a sampling rate of 500 samples per sec ensures a time domain reconstruction of ECG curves with less than 1% mean error (defined as the squared difference between the original waveform and the reconstructed wave, divided by the mean square value of the original waveform). From the practical point of view it is advantageous that in the sampling frequnecy range considered no sophisticated interpolation (quadratic, Shannon) is needed instead of the simple linear method to reconstruct the time-course of ECG waveforms (Fig. 1).

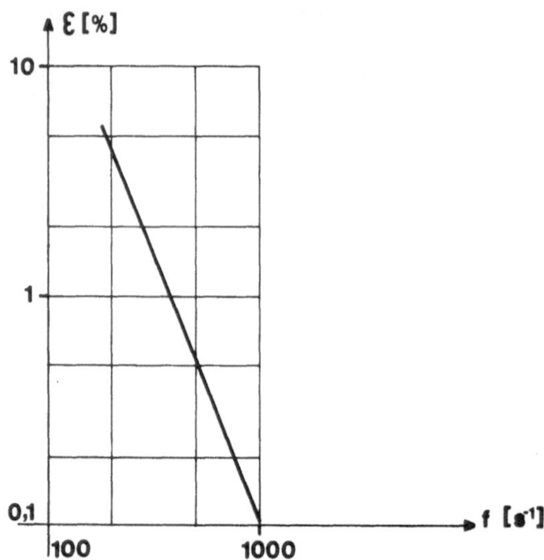

FIGURE 1. Time-domain mean error of ECG wave reconstructions as a function of sampling rate (simplified diagram after Barr and Spach)

Most body surface mapping equipment reported earlier works at a sampling rate of 500 Hz, so the requirements of accurate time characterization are fulfilled. However, in pediatrics, a minimum of twice this rate may be justified.

2.2 <u>The space-domain sampling</u>

Only a few papers have dealt with the problems of spatial sampling. Zywietz has published the average number of spatial harmonics needed in different rows and columns for a field reconstruction of 5% error at the time of QRS maximum (2). Monro and Attwood demonstrated the rapidly decreasing envelope of spatial power spectrum at the most energetic instants of the different ECG waves based on measurements perfomed in the presumably most energetic electrode row and column (3). Though their work was mainly concerned with the band-limited Fourier interpolation valuable comparisons with other schemes (Chebishev and spline interpolation) were also submitted. According to a study of Watanabe et al. a 2.5 cm or lower interelectrode distance is necessary to reliably detect the characteristic field pattern at the time of right epicardial breakthrough (4).

Based on a result obtained in our laboratory the relationship between the spatial sampling rate and the "mean error" (error power divided by signal power) of field reconstruction by linear interpolation is depicted in Fig. 2. This relationship is approximately valid during the QRS and ST-T waves for all the rows and columns delineated in Fig. 3, with the exception of right posterior columns where the actual error was significantly lower. As is demonstrated in Fig. 3, in this study the "accurate potential profile" was measured by 30 electrodes (in the case of rows) and 15 electrodes (in the case of columns), with a constant interelectrode distance of 3 cm. The lower sampling rates were simulated by systematically disregarding the signals of certain electrodes. Note that the relationship was actually calculated only for interelectrode distances of 6, 9 and 12 cm (solid line segment); the dotted line segment is the result of an extrapolation.

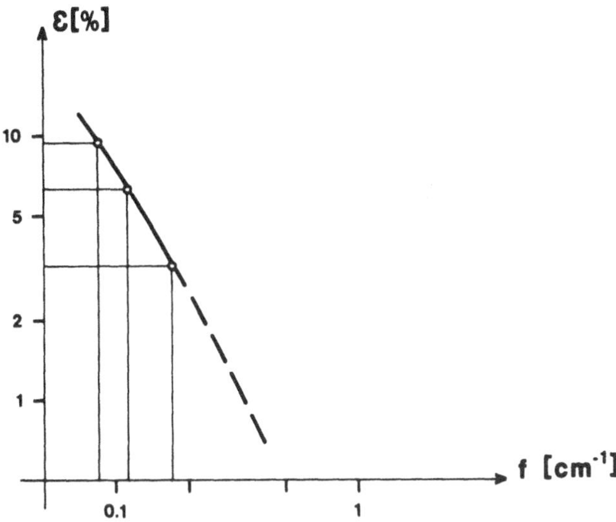

FIGURE 2. Space-domain mean error of body surface potential field reconstruction by linear interpolation as a function of spatial sampling rate ($f = \Delta^{-1}$, Δ: interelectrode distance in cm)

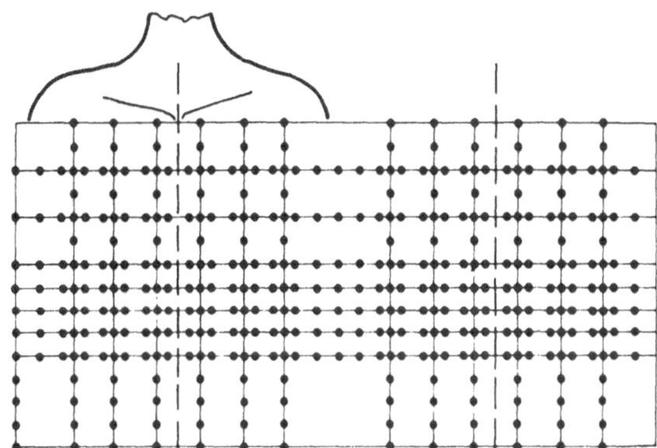

FIGURE 3. Layout of the electrode array used for the determination of space-domain sampling requirements

It is noteworthy that by the use of cubic spline interpolation instead of the linear one the accuracy of estimation increased in general, however this increase was not usually significant nor was it spatially uniform.

Taking into consideration the results in Fig. 2, it seems reasonable to suggest that for a spatial sampling comparable in error with that of a 500 samples per sec time-domain sampling an equidistant electrode matrix with 3 cm spacing is needed. The realization of this electrode density in the area usually considered informative from the medical point of view would require data acquistion equipment with some 350-500 channels. Fortunately, without serious compromise in accuracy, the use of a nonequidistant electrode arrangement enables the total number of electrodes to be reduced considerably. Nonequidistant positioning preserves, the high electrode density in the precordial area whereas in the regions outside this a sparse arrangement is used. Thus, finally one can estimate that for a spatial reconstruction error of about 1%, a system with approximately 150-200 electrodes is required.

If we apply the results of Fig. 2 to the analysis of the precordial electrode density of several existing systems we may conclude that the majority of these probably have an error of 3-5%.

3. REPRESENTATION METHODS

3.1 Representation of the instantaneous body surface potential distribution of an arbitrary individual

As has already been mentioned in the introduction, the depiction of body surface potential distribution (BSPD) is reduced to the representation of instantaneous two dimensional scalar-scalar functions. In Figs. 4 and 5 the two most frequently used methods of body surface potential distribution representations are illustrated. Some further possibilities of BSPD representations are given e.g. in reference (5). The photos of

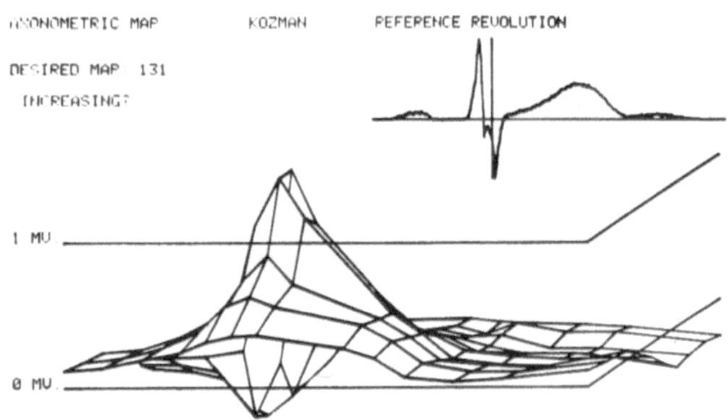

FIGURE 4. Axonometric representation of instantaneous BSPD.

Figs. 4 and 5 were taken from the display unit of the body surface potential mapping system developed at the Central Research Institute for Physics, Budapest. In line with common usage, in both cases the time instant sampled is marked on a reference ECG tracing. The geometrical landmarks in Fig. 5 are the following; the upper horizontal line is at the height of the sternal notch, the lower horizontal borderline is 42 cm below it (usually a few cm below the umbilicus). The leftmost vertical borderline coincides with the right anterior axilla, the next vertical line with the left anterior axilla, and then the left posterior axilla and finally the right posterior axilla follows.

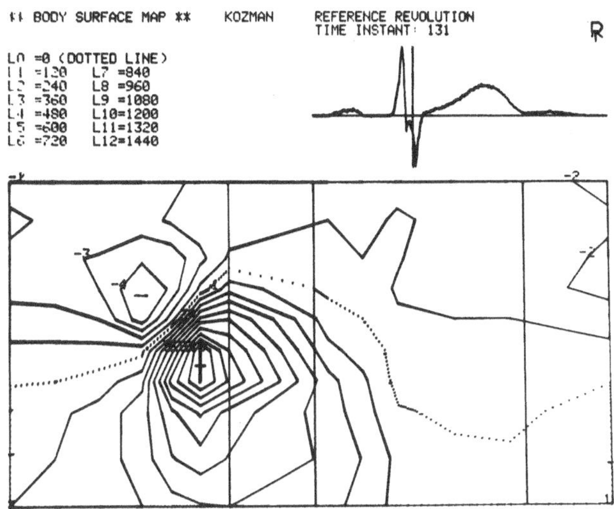

FIGURE 5. Isopotential line representation of instantaneous BSPD (the potential values corresponding to the contour lines are listed in μV units in the left upper corner)

It is necessary to note that there are significant discrepancies between the existing measuring systems in respect of the area explored by electrodes and the location of the line along which the torso is "cut". The latter can probably be arranged simply by repeating a portion of a map - as was recently suggested by Plonsey (6). The first problem cannot overcome so easily if we glance at Fig. 6 where the area explored by some systems is drawn. There is little doubt that in the future, at least a clear indication of the area considered is needed.

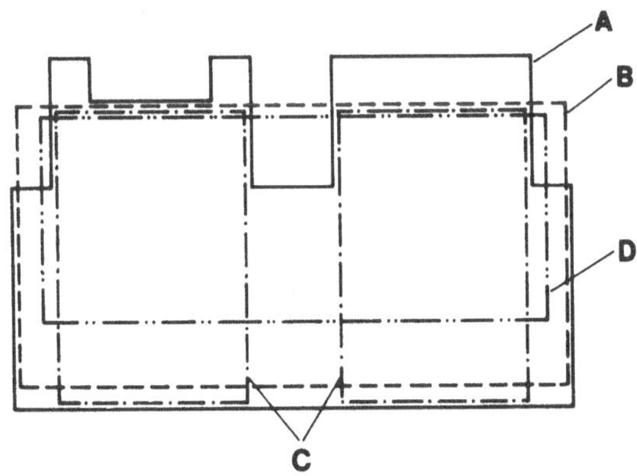

FIGURE 6. Schematic representation of the body surface area explored by electrodes by some working groups (A: Parma, B: Salt Lake City, C: Budapest, D: Halifax, Brussels).

ent n and m values in (11). The results of the lead-by-lead test are summed up either in contour maps of the D_{nm} G-K distance (see Fig. 7b) or by the significance maps.

a)

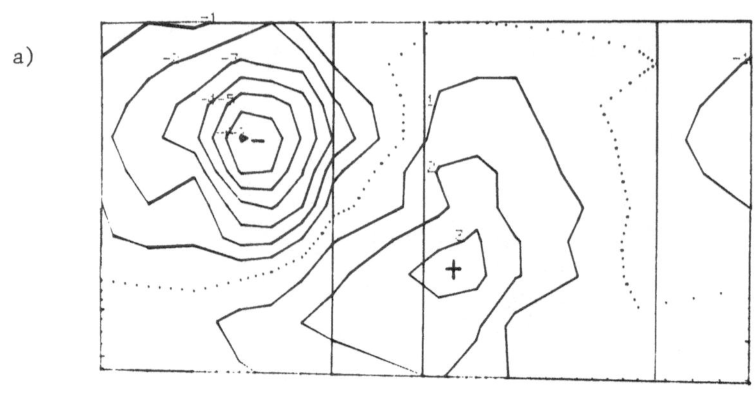

b)

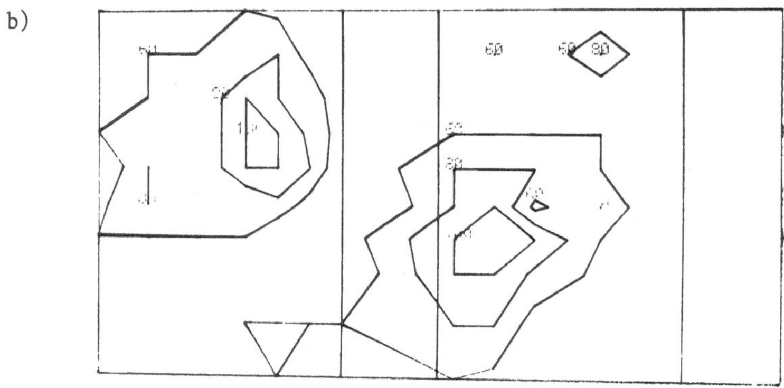

FIGURE 7. a) Difference of group mean QRS isointegral maps of pure left axis type left bundle branch block (LBBB) patients and that of patients of LBBB complicated by extensive anterior myocardial infarction. b) G-K distance map of the previous two groups of patients (G-K distance are expressed in per cent values).

Here we would draw attention to the fact that - depending on the sample size of the classes compared - already at the moderate level of D_{nm} a highly significant conclusion could be made for the homogeneity of the groups compared, but this does not mean that the distribution functions are not overlapping, i.e. they are easily separable by a threshold type decision. The lack of the overlapping property of the distributions is fulfilled only when and where $D_{nm} = 1$ (in our G-K distance maps 100 per cent). The two-class comparison of several subgroups of left bundle branch block and Wolff-Parkinson-White syndrome patients has revealed that very often the most significant discriminative areas are not explored at all

With the appearance of colour display units, the problem of colour code standardization has arisen too (6), though this kind of incompatibility between the representation methods is no great obstacle concerning the comparability of the published results.

3.2 Representation of the time dependence of the body surface potential distribution

Until recently a series of static pictures on display units and in the literature was the only means available to represent the time sequence of caridac fields. With regard to the publications, probably this type of representation will continue to be used though the dynamic display methods that have been applied recently offer attractive alternative for qualitative routine analysis (e.g. 5).

3.3 Link with conventional electrocardiology

Body surface mapping extends the conventional methods of electrocardiology. Logically its application starts where the diagnostic power of the conventional systems begins to fail. In view of this, it is clearly advisable to retain representation modes which link the two methods. Practically all of the systems available offer a possibility to represent the recorded unipolar waveforms in an arangement similar to the electrode layout. Some systems provides the representation of Frank leads, Lissajous loops and 12-lead ECG signals as well.

3.4 Representation of average within and between group properties

With regard to the representation of average within and between group properties it should be emphasized that its use is far from being a generally accepted practice nor is the method fully elaborated yet.

Average within group properties are mainly visualized by the so called group mean maps or by the set of group mean ECG curves in an arrangement similar to the measuring point layout. In the latter case around the average ECG curves usually a band of one or two standard deviation in width is depicted as well (e.g. 7,8,9).

Between groups comparison is usually done by the use of the difference maps of the group mean maps of the subpopulations compared (see Fig. 7a). Unfortunately this kind of characterization is not suitable for identifying those subregions where the difference of group means is not only large but statistically significant as well. Therefore some methods use statistical tests - rigorously valid only in case of normal distributions - to determine significantly different spatio-temporal subregions (8). To eliminate the above shortcoming, i.e. the application of parametric statistical tests, a new method was developed and tested in our laboratory (10).

3.4.1 Non-parametric method of between group comparisions of BSPDs. The method is based on the systematic use of the Gnedenko-Koroljuk (G-K) test of homogeneity. This test is a small sample variant of the well known Kolmogorov-Smirnov type non-parametric test of homogeneity. In the course of data preparation two groups of patients are always defined; n subjects are classified - on the basis of ECG independent evidences - into pathological group A, and m patients in group B. Within each group, an empirical distribution function (F_n (x_k), and G_m (x_k) respectively) is ordered; to every lead position. These epirical distributions are computed from the x_k values of the group members. If the maximum absolute difference between the two empirical distributions is D_{nm}, the null hypothesis, i.e. the homogeneity of the empirical distributions compared can be rejected at a p_{nm} level of significance. The p_{nm} probabilities are tabulated for differ-by the frequently used ECG and VCG lead systems (12). This finding supports our view concerning the potential superiority of body surface mapping methods in the solution of heart electrodiagnostic problems. In almost all cases strongly discriminative areas on the back - in some cases mainly on the back - were identified by the G-K method. The mean difference maps corresponding to the cases studied usually showed low amplitude in the very same areas. An example supporting the above statement is given in Fig. 7. These observations indicate that in several cases diagnostic features are hidden in low amplitude regions. In other words high signal energy regions and informative regions do not necessarily cover each other.

REFERENCES

1. Barr RC, Spach MS: Sampling Rates Required for Digital Recording of Intracellular and Extarcellular Cardiac Potentials. Circulation, 55: 40, 1977
2. Zywietz C: Informationsgehalt von EKG Ableitungssystemen. Biomedizinische Technik, 23: 6, 1978
3. Monro DM, Attwood DR: Sampling and Reconstruction of Electrocardiographic Surface Maps. In: Proc. of the 2nd Annual WAMI Meeting, 404, 1979
4. Watanabe T, Toyama J, Toyoshima H, Oguri H, Ohno M, Okajima M, Naito Y, Yamada K: A Practical Microcomputer-Based Mapping System for Body Surface, Precordium and Epicardium. Computersand Biomedical Res. 14: 341, 1981
5. Furukawa T, Yajima K, Tanaka H: A Body Surface Potential Mapping System Equipped with a Microprocessor for the Dynamic Observation of Potential Patterns. In: Advances in Body Surface Mapping. (Eds.: Yamada K, Harumi K, Musha T), 117, Univ. Nagoya Press, Nagoya, 1983
6. Yamada K, Harumi K, Musha T (Eds): Round Table Discussion. In: Advances in Body Surface Potential Mapping, 289, Univ. Nagoya Press, Nagoya, 1983
7. Montague TJ, Smith RE, Cameron DA, Rautaharju PM, Klassen GA, Flemington CS, Horacek BM: Isointegral Analysis of Body Surface Distribution and Temporal Variability in Normal Subjects. Circulation, 63: 1116, 1981
8. Kornreich F: Selection of Optimal ECG Leads and Map Features for the Diagnosis of Myocardial Infarction by Multivariate Analysis of Body Surface Potential Maps. In this volume.
9. Green LS, Lux RL, Haws CW, Burgess MJ, Abildskov JA: Features of Body Surface Maps from a Large Normal Population. In this volume.
10. Kozmann GY, Rochlitz T, Csiszár A, Préda I: Preprocessing Method to Determine Parameters of Body Surface Potential Maps. Proc. 11th International Congress on Electrocardiology. Caen, 1984 (to be published).
11. Massey FJ: Distribution table for the Deviation between Two Sample Cumulatives. Ann. Math. Stat. 23: 435, 1952
12. Préda I, Kozmann GY, Rochlitz T, Mertz J, Tóth K, Antalóczy Z, Szilvási I, Balogh I: Left Bundle Branch Block and Chronic Myocardial Infarction: Isointegral Analysis of Body Surface Maps. Proc. 11th International Congress on Electrocardiology. Caen. 1984 (to be published).

Chapter 23

THE DISPLAY OF BODY SURFACE MAPS

A. HERINGA, G.J.H. UIJEN, R.TH. VAN DAM, J.P.J. DE VALK

1. INTRODUCTION

At present the measurement of body surface maps is rather easy because of the progress in the technology of amplifiers and microcomputers. A number of small systems which can measure body surface maps in clinical practice have been published in literature. Before body surface mapping will be a normal clinical tool its significance for diagnostic purposes has to be proven. The manner of presentation of the measured data is an important aspect for the clinical acceptance of this new technique. This contribution treats two aspects of the presentation of body surface data: 1. the interpolation of the data as measured at a coarse, irregular grid to data at a dense, regular one; 2.the display of these interpolated data both in black and white and in colour.

2. INTERPOLATION

2.1. Interpolation to a regular grid.

In general the body surface potentials are measured at sites irregularly distributed over the body surface because of the large gradients close to the heart and the smaller ones far from the heart. For ease of comparison the Standard 12 lead recording sites are often a subset of the body surface map recording sites. For the display of the measured data in a map extrapolation to a regular grid is necessary. One feasible method is to compute the data at the not measured points from the values at the measured ones by their correlations obtained from measurements of all grid points in a large population containing both normals and abnormals. The data bases which are appropriate for the computation of these correlation matrices are available at a few institutions only. From their meaurements and computations it can be concluded that the potential distribution at the body surface can adequately be constructed from 24-32, not homogeneously distributed, measurement points [1,2]. When the correlation matrices are not available and one does not want to measure at a substantially larger number of measurement sites another approach seems more adequate. We have chosen to measure at 64 sites being about twice the minimum number, distributed according to the suggestions derived from the large data bases. The interpolation is done by modelling the body as a resistor network at the surface of a cylinder (fig.1) as has been proposed by Van Oosterom [3]. In this network the measured voltages are applied at corresponding node points indicated by dots and the voltages at the not measured points result from either a hardware realization of this network or from computer computation. This interpolation is satisfactory when enough points are measured. However, when using a small number of measurement points an inadequate display will result since extreme values of the voltages will be at the measured points only.

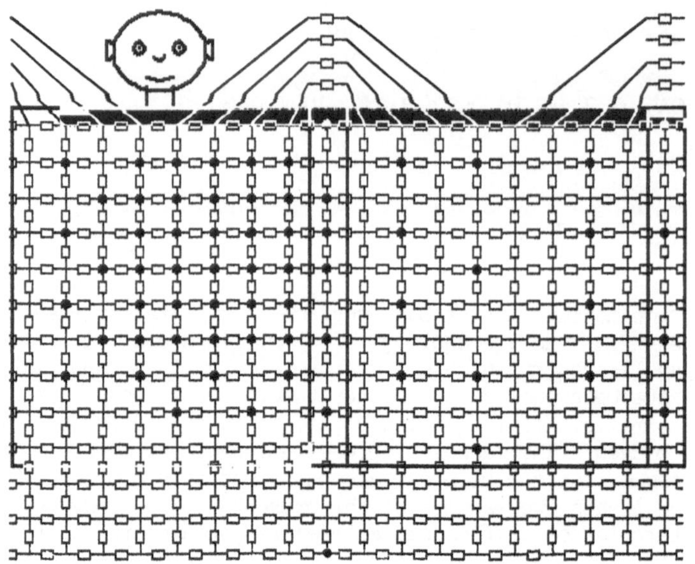

Fig.1 The body simulated by a resistor network at the surface of a cylinder which is, for the display, cut at the right arm. The measurements were done at the sites indicated by the heavy dots.

2.2.Interpolation between grid points.

The display of the full potential distribution at the body surface derived from the values at the regular grid can be performed by quasi 3D figures [4], by isofunction lines [5] or by intensity or colour coding[6,7]. A good display needs a fine sampling of the data and a clear distinction between negative, near zero and positive voltages. For a fine sampling interpolation between the grid points is necessary. A simple interpolation method which results in unique values V(x,y) of the voltage in a point (x,y) within four node points is the bilinear interpolation method which is given by

$$V(x,y) = a + b.x + c.y + d.x.y$$

in which the coefficients a,b,c and d are computed from the voltages at the node points. In fig.2 the results of this interpolation applied to a rectangle with the values V(0,0)=3, V(1,0)=-2, V(0,1)=-1 and V(1,1)=2 (leading to a=3, b=-5, c=-4 and d=2) is shown by both an isofunction line display and by a quasi 3D display.

3.MAP DISPLAY

In a map display it is arbitrary whether one chooses to display the body surface cut at the spine or cut at the right arm. A standard display obviously facilitates the interpretation of data from other groups and for tnis purpose we have conformed to the display with the frontal view to the left and the posterior view to the right. In the display of maps an easy discrimination between negative, near zero and positive values is necessary. In contrast to the quasi 3D display the isofunction line display in fig.2 clearly fullfills these requirements. In this display the positive area is displayed as white with black isofunction lines, the negative area as black with white isofunction lines and near zero as a grey dot pattern. In fig.3 body surface data from a normal at 38 and 62 ms after onset of the QRS-complex are displayed in this manner, with a 0.2 mV distance between the isofunction lines and a grey zone of 0.05 mV. For the major percentage of maps this display is satisfactory because the potential distributions are relatively smooth without isolated peaks or valleys. Moreover this type of display can be produced by inexpensive printers and can be reproduced (photocopied) easily.

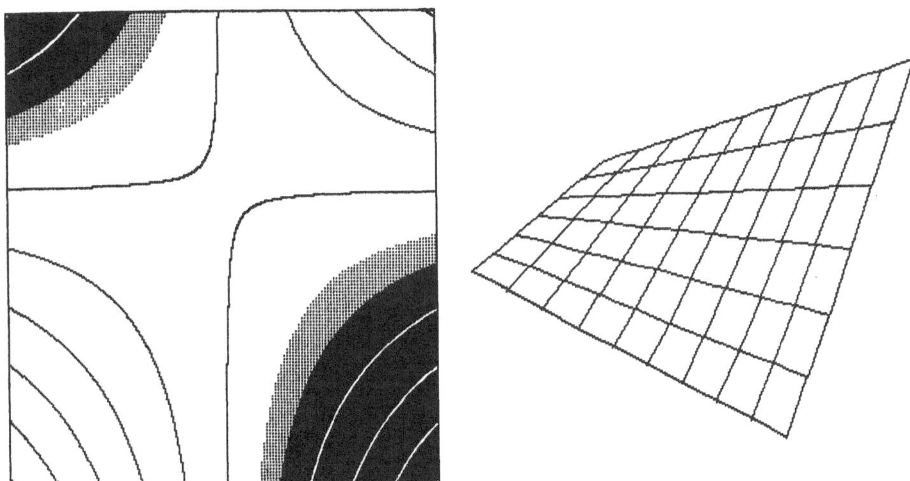

Fig.2. The bilinear interpolation in a rectangle with its vertices at $\begin{matrix} -1 & 2 \\ 3 & -2 \end{matrix}$ displayed (right) in a quasi 3D display and also (left) by isofunction lines with black lines on a white background for positive values, white on a black background for negative values and grey for near zero values.

A more attractive display is possible by colour coding of the potential data which can be realised even by small microcomputers. In this display one has to choose a sensible coding of the potential values into colour [6]. We have chosen to code positive voltage values as red, green as near zero and blue as negative in such a way that the amplitude is used for coding intensity. With this coding the desired tripartition of voltage values results and the intensity amplitude coding is a quite natural one. For body surface maps the blue-red coding has been advocated by Musha [8]. We have added the green zero zone as was proposed by Van Oosterom [3] in 1978. Body surface maps in colour have been published by e.g. Liebman et al. [7], in which a nonunique colour coding was chosen using a colour scale for positive and the same scale in reverse order for negative potentials. In fig.4 we show maps at 24, 38 and 62 ms after QRS onset in the Liebman et al. coding next to the coding as proposed by us. The scale with our unique colour coding clearly facilitates the interpretation of the map data.

4.CONCLUSION

Body surface maps measured from a limited number of electrodes can be expanded to a body surface map at the whole body surface by reliable

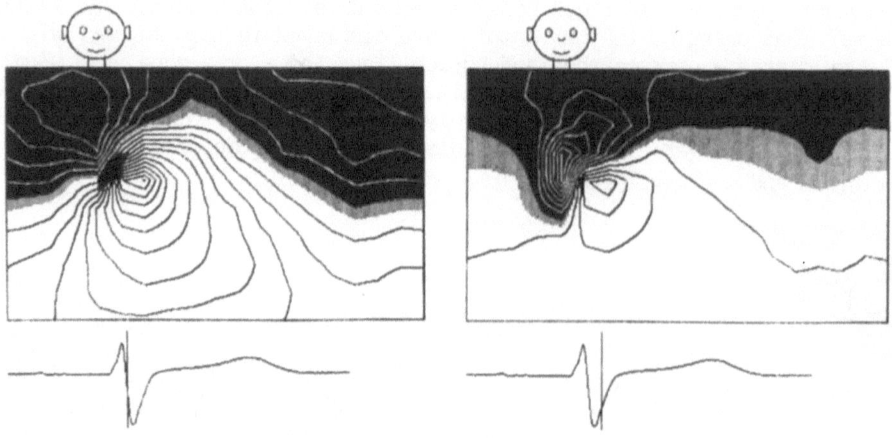

Fig.3 Body surface maps taken from a healthy subject at 38 and 64 ms after QRS onset. The displayed moment is indicated by the vertical line in the precordial V2 lead below the map. In the maps the distance between isofunction lines is 0.2 mV, black lines at white is positive, white lines at black is negative and the grey zone is 0.05 mV around zero. Zero reference is the Wilson Central Terminal.

methods. These total maps can be displayed in a form that can be understood easily by an inexperienced observer when the voltage values are partitioned in positive, near zero and negative. An attractive display is obtained when this tripartition is colour coded. For printing purposes a black and white display is quite satisfactory.

5.REFERENCES

1.RL Lux, CR Smith, RF Wyatt, JA Abildskov, Limited lead selection for estimation of body surface potential maps in electrocardiography. IEEE BME-25,270,1978

2.RC Barr, MS Spach, GS Herman-Giddens, Selection of the number and positions of measuring locations for electrocardiography. IEEE BME-18, 125,1971

3.A v Oosterom, Real time mapping in colour of the electrocardiographic body surface potentials, In: Adv. in Cardiology, vol 21,153, F Kornreich ed., Karger, Basel 1978

4.NC Flowers, LG Horan, Body surface maps in primary myocardial disease, In: Adv. in Cardiology, vol 10,270, S Rush, E Lepschkin eds., Karger Basel 1974

5.A Heringa, GJH Uijen, R Th v Dam, A 64-channel system for body surface potential mapping, In: Electrocardiology '81,297, Z Antaloczy, I Preda eds., Akademiai Kiado, Budapest 1982

6.JPJ de Valk, WJM Epping, A Heringa, Colour representation of biomedical data, Med.Biol.Eng.Comp. 23,343, 1985

7.J Liebman, C Thomas, Y Rudy, R Plonsey, Electrocardiographic body surface potential maps of the QRS of normal children, J.Electroc. 14, 249,1981

8.T Musha, Discussion In: Advances in body surface potential mapping, 293, K Yamada, K Harumi, T Musha eds., Nagoya Press, Nagoya 1983

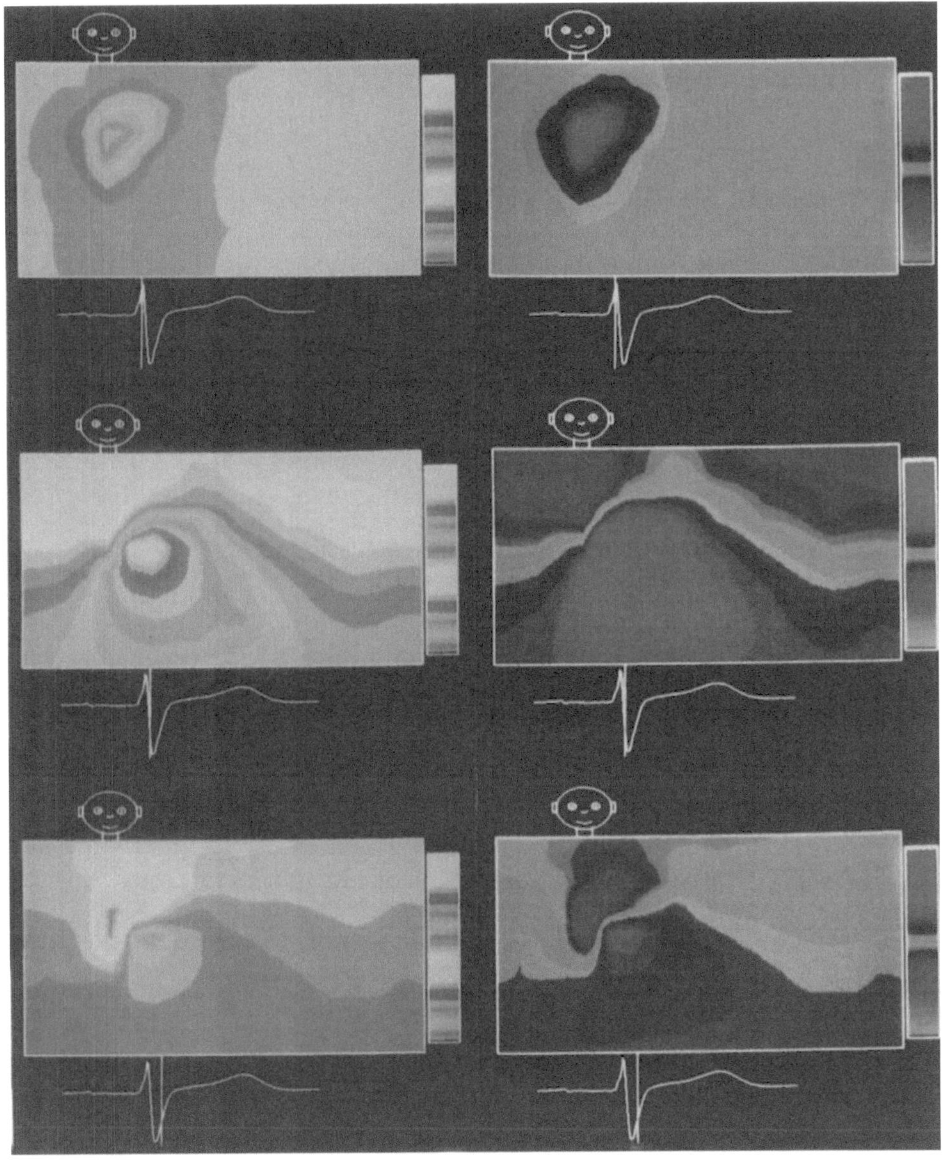

Fig.4. Body surface maps taken from a healthy subject at 24,38 and 62 ms after QRS onset. The displayed moment is indicated by the vertical line in the V2 lead below each map. At right of the maps the total colour scale is given ranging in a linear scale from -3 mV to +3 mV. At left the maps are displayed in the Liebman scale, at right in the NIJMEGEN scale.

PART 5

D A T A A N A L Y S I S

Chapter 24

USE OF ORTHOGONAL EXPANSIONS FOR REPRESENTING BODY SURFACE POTENTIAL MAPS

R.L. LUX, L.S. GREEN, C.W. HAWS, M.J. BURGESS, J.A. ABILDSKOV

1. INTRODUCTION

Applications of body surface potential mapping to clinical electrocardiography have increased, but only slowly in comparison to other, contemporary, non-invasive tests for heart disease. Some of the reasons for this are technical in nature, such as the number and placement of leads, sampling rates and methods of display. Other reasons are concerned with the expense and time of setting up a map acquisition and procesing facility. These technical considerations are not insurmountable and practical solutions exist to all of them. However, there are scientific reasons, more responsible for the slow progress of clinical mapping, which deal with the very nature of the electrocardiographic problem.

A primary consideration is that surface potential maps must be identified as observations of a process, highly random in nature. There are a great many physical and physiological variables which have strong effects on the observed potentials. As such, the sequence of potential distributions which characterizes a patient's physiological state may change in time due to physical or physiological changes within the patient, and may or may not be similar to those observed in other patients having similar electrophysiological states.

Another important consideration is the lack of a universally accepted method of describing or interpreting maps. It is relatively straight forward to view potential distributions, identify distinguishing features such as the location, magnitude and trajectory of extrema, and categorize patients according to independent documentation of disease. However existence or absence of a feature, tentatively identified as important in distinguishing between classes of patients, is highly dependent on the physical and physiological variation of the feature and its origin. For example, it is well documented that, in normals, a pseudopod of negative potential forms over the upper-right anterior chest at 30 - 40 ms into the QRS and has been identified as the body surface manifestations of right ventricular breakthrough. In some patients, two relative minima are observed within the global minimum. Should the presence of the 2 minima be interpreted as originating from a physiological event such as a particular activation sequence, or might it be caused by location, orientation or size of the heart, or perhaps the size and shape of the body?

A related consideration is the fact that most features used by clinicians for interpreting maps have been those having large magnitude and discriminating power by visual means when multiple groups are compared. For example, the orientation of dominant extrema in the QRS and distribution of ST segments in acute MI may be interpreted to indicate infarct location. Necessarily, the conventional 12 lead ECG will also reflect aspects of these features so little is gained from the map. On the other hand, little has been done to identify low level, less obvious features which might be of utility in characterizing subtle but significant disease states such as coronary disease without prior infarction.

A final reason for the slow progress of clinical mapping is the lack of sufficiently large map data bases which include a variety of heart disease classes. This has prevented the development of statistical approaches to map interpretation which will be a necessary part of utilizing map data on a large scale.

In this paper, we shall focus on a method of quantitatively representing body surface potential maps which we have developed and used on over 5000 maps in our library. The technique offers a vehicle for classifying large numbers of maps and provides a common basis for comparing maps serially within one patient, between patients within a group, or across patients in multiple groups.

2. ORTHOGONAL EXPANSIONS

The mathematical theory of signal representation permits the characterization of signals (data) by transformations which are reversible. The data on which the transformations operate may be deterministic or random in nature and a variety of approaches are possible, though the underlying theory is similar. Given a signal, $a(x)$, of an independent variable, x, and an infinite set of signals $\{b_i(x)\}$, both defined over a range $x \varepsilon \chi$, and if

$$\langle b_i(x) | b_j(x) \rangle = \delta_{ij} \quad \forall i,j \qquad \text{Eq. 1}$$

a statement of orthonormality of the $\{b\}$, then it may be shown that

$$a(x) = \sum_{i=1}^{\infty} c_i b_i(x) \qquad \text{Eq. 2}$$

where

$$c_i = \langle a(x) | b_i(x) \rangle \qquad \text{Eq. 3}$$

Thus, the original signal, $a(x)$, may be mathematically represented or characterized exactly by the infinte set of "parameters", $\{c_i\}$ in the sense that they, along with the set of functions, $\{b_i\}$, may be used to reconstruct the original signal according to the expansion given in

Eq. 2. If the expansion of Eq. 2 is carried out over a finite number of terms, then an approximation may be made

$$a_N(x) = \sum_{i=1}^{N} c_i b_i(x) \qquad \text{Eq. 4}$$

where a representation error results:

$$e_N = |a - a_N|. \qquad \text{Eq. 5}$$

The theory is applicable, whether the signal is deterministic or random, continuous or discrete.

There are two basic classes of representation functions, {b}, namely mathematical and statistical. In the former, the functions are deterministic, mathematically tabulated, orthogonal functions such as sines and cosines (Fourier Series), Tchebychev, Legendre or Bessel polynomials. In the latter case, the functions are derived from the data which they will represent. It is this class of representation techniques which we shall discuss in this paper, paraticularly as it pertains to the representation and classification of body surface maps.

3. APPLICATION TO BODY SURFACE MAPS

Mathematical representations have been applied to problems in electrocardiography over the past 20 years. Young and Huggins utilized complex exponentials to represent vectorcardiograms.[1] Brody[2] and Geselowitz[3] utilized the multipole series to characterize the cardiac source. Scher[4] and Horan[5] utilized factor analysis to extract temporal and spatial features which could explain most of the observed variability in electrocardiograms and body surface potential distributions. Barr[6] utilized principal components analysis as a vehicle for deriving estimation transformations in limited lead applications. More recently, Haliday[7], Lux[8], Evans[9], and Uijen[10] have applied the Karhunen-Loeve technique to the problem of representing body surface maps.

The major benefits to be derived from utilizing orthogonal representations include: 1) Data are converted from dependent samples to a sequence of independent parameters, 2) It is possible to order the parameters by importance in characterizing the data, and also to estimate the representation error from a given subset of paramters - this allows one to represent a set of data as accruately as desired, 3) Since the coefficients are independent, classification of data is greatly simplified because conventional techniques apply, and 4) All data may be represented using the same set of basis functions, hence data comparisons become simple and quantitative. For these reasons, we have developed a two step approach to quantitatively characterize each of over 5000 maps in our data base.

The two step procedure involves representation, first of the spatial and then of the temporal information. Prior to applying the representation, it was necessary to derive the sets of spatial and temporal basis functions to be used for all patient maps. For this purpose, each QRS and every 5th STT distribution from 192 lead body surface maps on each of over 200 patients were used to calculate a 192x192 covariance matrix, K. Over half the maps were from normal subjects with the remainder taken from patients with old myocardial infarcts, conduction disturbances, or hypertrophy. The twelve most significant eigenvectors, $\{\Phi_i\}$, were used as a spatial representation basis. Then, each potential distribution, P(k), was represented as

$$P(k) = \sum_{i=1}^{12} \alpha_i(k)\Phi_i \qquad \text{Eq. 6}$$

where

$$\alpha_i(k) = \langle P(k)|\Phi_i\rangle \qquad \text{Eq. 7}$$

In order to represent the resulting temporal "coefficient" waveforms, $\{\alpha_i(k)\}$, two sets of temporal basis functions (QRS and STT) were extracted from covariance matrices formed from the time normalized segments of each $\alpha_i(k)$. The 12 most significant eigenvectors of the QRS and 6 of the STT temporal covariances were used in the representation as:

$$\alpha_i(k) = \sum_{j=1}^{n} \beta_{ij}\xi_j(k) \qquad \text{Eq. 8}$$

where

$$\beta_{ij} = \langle\alpha_i(k)|\xi_j(k)\rangle \qquad \text{Eq. 9}$$

In summary, a patients body surface map, P(k), may be represented as

$$P(k) = \sum_{i=1}^{12} \Phi_i \sum_{j=1}^{12} \beta_{ij}\xi_j(k) \qquad \text{Eq. 10}$$

Since the spatial $\{\Phi_i\}$, and temporal $\{\xi_i(k)\}$ bases are common to all patients, the representation coefficients, β_{ij}, may be compared between patients or groups of patients. Each coefficient is tied to one spatial distribution and one temporal waveform, hence differences in parameters between patient maps or groups of maps convey important information regarding underlying physiological differences. Since the β_{ij} are independent, a consequence of the fact that the map data are represented along statistically orthonormal bases, powerful techniques may be brought to bear on problems of discriminating between classes of patient maps.

To illustrate the applicability of this representation to classification of maps, we selected 50 maps from our database. Twenty-five patients had one, two or three vessel coronary artery disease (CAD1, CAD2, CAD3) as determined by ventricular angiography and defined by 50% or greater stenosis. All patients in this group had **normal** resting, 12 lead ECGs. A group of normal patients, age and sex matched to each of the 25 patients, was selected as a control group (NRML). These patients were judged to be normal on the basis of history and physical, normality of the 12 lead ECG, and absence of abnormal cardiac symptoms. Each patient's map was represented using the above technique, which resulted in a 216 dimensional vector **β**. Average and variance of each of the 216 variables were calculated for each of the four groups. For each dichotomy of class pairs, the variables were ordered according to the t-test. Mean vectors and covariance matrices of the n features having the greatest discriminating power were determined and used in a parametric, nonlinear classifier. The value of n was always less than half the smaller of the number of samples in the groups compared. Using jackknifing, each of the 50 patients was classified into one of the four possible categories. In this approach, the influence of the patient's parameters on the mean vector and covariance matrix was removed and then the patient classified, thus removing bias in classsification. The resulting classification matrix

	CAD1	CAD2	CAD3	NRML
CAD1	4	0	0	2
CAD2	0	8	1	0
CAD3	0	0	9	1
NRML	0	0	2	23

Total Error: 12%

demonstrates the power, both of body surface mapping and the representation scheme to provide important, non-invasive diagnostic information. Although the maps on the abnormal patients were grossly similar to those of normals, it is clear in this case that low amplitude map features are significant in their ability not only to differentiate normal and abnormal, but also to stratify the abnormals into severity of disease.

4. REFERENCES

1. Young, T.Y., Hugginss, W.H., On the representation of electrocardiograms, IEEE Trans. **10**: 86 - 95
2. Brody, D.A., Bradshaw, J.C., Evans, J.W., A theoretical basis for determining heart-lead relationships of the equivalent cardiac multipole, IRE Trans. Biomed. Electron. **BME8**: 139, 1961
3. Geselowitz, D.B., Multipole representation for an equivalent cardiac generator. Proc. I.R.E. **48**: 75-79, 1960
4. Scher, A., Young, A. Meredith, W., Factor analysis of the electrocardiogram, Circ. Res. **8**: 519-525, 1960

5. Horan, L., Flowers, N., Brody, D., Principal factor waveforms of the thoracic QRS complex, Circ. Res. **15**: 131-138, 1964
6. Barr, R.C., Spach, M.S., Herman-Giddens, G.S., Selection of the number and positions of measuring locations for electrocardiography, I.E.E.E. Trans. Biomed. Eng. **18**: 125-138, 1971
7. Halliday, J.S., The characterization of vectorcardiograms for pattern recognition, Master's Thesis, M.I.T., Boston, 1973
8. Lux, R.L., Evans, A.K., Burgess, M.J., Wyatt, R.F., Abildskov, J.A., Redundancy reduction for improved display and analysis of body surface potential maps. I.#Spatial Compression, Circ. Res. **49**:#186-196, 1981
9. Evans, A.K., Lux, R.L., Burgess, M.J., Wyatt, R.F., Abildskov, J.A., Redundancy reduction for improved display and analysis of body surface potential maps. II.#Temporal compression, Circ. Res. **49**:#197-203, 1981
10. Uijen, G.J.H., Heringa, A., van Oosterom, A., van Dam R.Th., Infarction detection from QRS body surface potential maps or the standard ECG using several methods for feature extraction, Proc. Computers in Cardiology, Park City, Utah, p.255, 1984

Chapter 25

MULTIVARIATE ANALYSIS OF BODY SURFACE POTENTIAL MAPS FOR THE DIAGNOSIS OF MYOCARDIAL INFARCTION BEFORE AND AFTER TEMPORAL AND SPATIAL DATA REDUCTION

F. KORNREICH, M. KAVADIAS, J. WARREN, P. RAUTAHARJU, T. MONTAGUE, M. HORACEK

There is little doubt today that body surface potential maps (BSPM) contain diagnostic information not present in conventional lead systems (1, 2, 3). However, the need of specialized hardware and the large amounts of data to process and to analyze have hampered their widespread use.

The necessity of data reduction has been recognized as early as 1971 (4) and several strategies for achieving this goal have since been suggested (5, 6, 7, 8, 9).

The described procedures reduced the amount of data :

- by reducing the number of leads for optimal signal representation at unmeasured sites;
- by limiting the recordings to those leads found useful diagnostically;
- or by compressing the entire map- wether actually recorded from large electrode arrays or reconstructed from limited lead sets-along temporal basis functions and/or spatial basis distributions.

The present study investigates the diagnostic content of body surface potential maps and determines how much of this information is still available after applying data reduction schemes to the original data.

MATERIAL AND METHODS

Study populations

Four hundred and forty-four subjects were studied. Group A consisted of 184 normal control subjects; group B consisted of 177 patients who had suffered MI, and group C consisted of patients belonging to three other diagnostic categories. Group A subjects had no evidence of heart disease on history, physical examination, 12-lead ECG and echocardiogram; they ranged in age between 20 and 50 years (mean 34 years).

Group B patients had a typical history of cardiac chest pain and characteristic enzyme changes, and in most cases the MI diagnosis was substantiated by coronary angiography and ventriculography; the age range of this group was 34 to 71 years (mean 55 years). Group C consisted of 44 patients with isolated aortic valve disease and left ventricular hypertrophy assessed clinically, radiographically and by cardiac catheterization; 13 patients with ECG patterns characteristic of Wolff-Parkinson-White syndrome; and 26 patients with coronary artery disease demonstrated by coronary angiography, but without any evidence of MI.

Body surface potential mapping

For each individual, we recorded simultaneously on digital tape the ECG signals from 117 torso and 3 limb electrode sites, sampling each channel 500 times per second and using the Wilson central terminal as a reference potential. The tracings' quality was monitored visually during the recording. Later the data were processed by performing selective averaging, and again carefully inspected and edited. The QRST interval was then time-normalized over 250 points; we also time-normalized separately the QRS waveform and the STT waveform and represented them by 70 and 180 points, respectively.

Feature extraction

We examined three sets of ECG waveform features : instantaneous amplitude measurements (I.M.) obtained by sampling time-normalized QRS and STT at equal intervals (35 samples for QRS and 45 samples for STT i.e. 9600 variables per individual) and coefficients obtained by expanding the data either in terms of orthonormal time-functions or in terms of orthonormal spatial distributions. Details of the method used for the computation of the latter sets of features are described elsewhere (7, 8, 9).

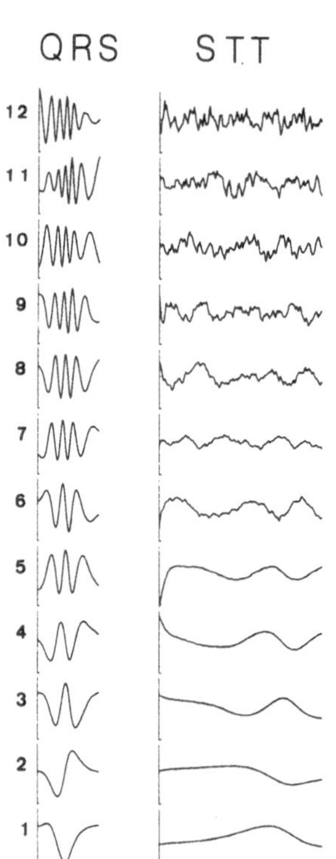

Briefly, temporal coefficients were obtained by expressing each ECG as a linear combination of orthonormal basis functions extracted from the ensemble of waveform of all 444 subjects of the study population by using the Karhunen-Loeve (K-L) expansion; similarly, spatial coefficients resulted from the expansion of each map frame, at each instant, along a set of orthonormal map distributions, computed from all the map frames of all individuals. (figs 1 and 2).

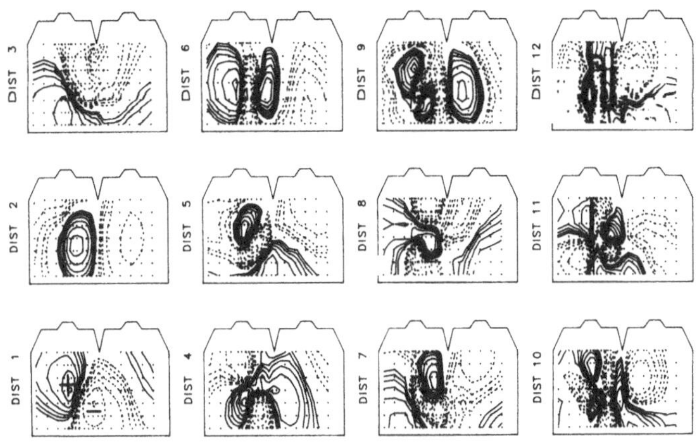

A linear combination of basis functions, when computed separately for QRS and STT segments, could represent any ECG waveform in the ensemble down to the noise level (the goodness of fit was expressed in terms of root mean square (RMS) residue); at most 10 QRS and 8 STT basis functions were needed to represent the respective segments, yielding 2160 features or time coefficients (T.C.) per individual.

The number of basis distributions, linearly combined, used to represent each map at each instant was kept at 12 as suggested by the Salt Lake City group. This in turn resulted in 12 x 250 i.e. 3000 features or spatial coefficients (S.C.)

Discriminant leads and discriminant maps

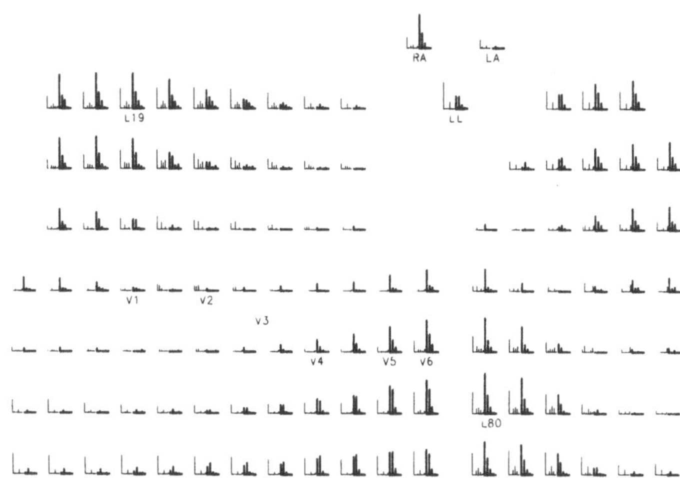

The diagnostic capabilities of temporal expansion coefficients are depicted in figure 3 : at each electrode site, the differences between the respective averaged normal and MI coefficients are divided by the corresponding pooled standard deviations; the resulting values are strictly proportional to Student's t-tests and consequently provide information about the capability for each feature in each lead to separate the MI group from the normal group (for each lead 6 QRS and 4 STT T.C. are plotted).

This representation provides clues for the selection of optimal leads and the extraction of optimal features for any bigroup or multigroup differentiation.

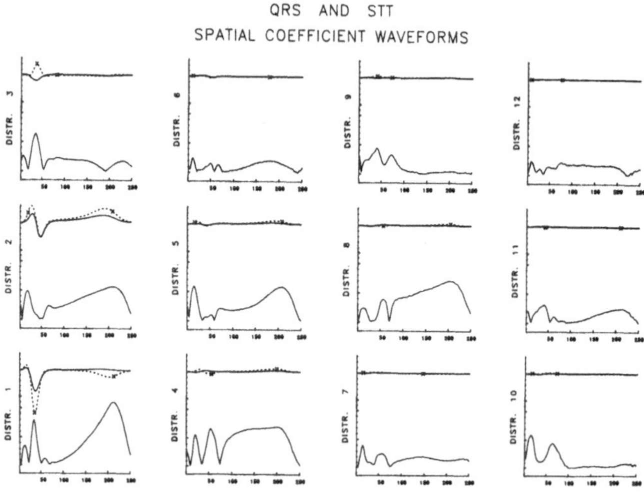

Figure 4, similarly, illustrates the discriminant power of particular map distributions. For each basis pattern, the associated expansion coefficients (S.C.) are depicted as they vary in time both in the normal and in the MI populations (superimposed upper tracings in each box); the bottom curves result from the substraction, at each instant, of the averaged normal and MI spatial coefficients, again weighted by the corresponding pooled standard deviations.

This representation points to those instants at which the amount of each characteristic map pattern is diagnostically different in normals and in any other pathological entity.

Statistical analysis

Separation of normal ECG recordings from those of patients with myocardial infarction was sought, using the three sets of features, alternately.

The statistical procedure involved 2 successive steps : first, the best classifiers were selected from the total number of available features by a stepwise selection, then these selected classifiers were combined into properly weighted linear discriminant functions; both steps were performed by programs from the Biomedical Computer Program library (BMDP 7 M) (18).

Because of the very large number of variables to process (9600 I.M., 2160 T.C., 3000 S.C.), the program entered 80 variables at a time and selected the 20 best from each batch, repeating the procedure until it obtained a final set of 20 optimal classifiers. Varying the composition of the batches and their order of entry did not affect the first 8 classifiers selected.

In order to investigate the repeatability of the diagnostic results, we divided the available population into a training set (100 N and 100 MI) and a testing set (84 N and 77 MI). New linear discriminant functions were computed for the 3 sets of features in order to separate the two groups of the training set. Running the thus calculated discriminant functions on the testing set permitted the classification of the remaining patients. A moderate deterioration of about 2 % was noticed for any of the 3 sets.

RESULTS

Figure 1 displays the normalized sets of (temporal) basis functions for QRS and STT separately.

Figure 2 shows the normalized set of (spatial) basis distributions for QRS.

TABLE 1

COMPARISON OF ORTHONORMAL BASIS FUNCTIONS AND BASIS DISTRIBUTIONS IN TERMS OF TOTAL SIGNAL REPRESENTATION

	TEMPORAL BASIS (% TRACE)		SPATIAL BASIS (% TRACE)	
	QRS	STT	QRS	STT
1	58.1	77.0	50.4	65.0
2	88.5	96.6	80.0	82.5
3	94.5	98.6	92.3	93.3
4	97.8	99.6	94.1	95.5
5	98.7	99.8	95.6	96.8
6	99.3	99.9	96.7	97.5
7	99.5	99.9	97.2	98.0
8	99.7	100.0 *	98.2	98.6
9	99.8	100.0	98.2	98.6
10	99.9	100.0	98.4	98.8
11	99.9	100.0	98.6	98.9
12	99.0	100.0	98.8	99.0

* 99.98

Table 1 indicates the cumulative amounts of signal accounted for by the first 12 eigenvectors of both bases expressed as percentages of the trace of the corresponding covariance matrices. One notes a more efficient representation of the original information with temporal basis functions, for both waveforms; while 10 QRS functions and 6 STT functions account 99.9 % of the trace, 28 distributions are required to achieve the same degree of fit for QRS and STT maps. Both bases, however, account for over 90 % of the total voltage information with the first 3 eigenvectors.

TABLE 2

RECONSTRUCTION OF BODY SURFACE POTENTIAL MAPS USING ORTHONORMAL TEMPORAL OR SPATIAL BASES.

		TEMPORAL BASIS FUNCTIONS	SPATIAL BASIS DISTRIBUTIONS
AVERAGE RMS ERROR (μV)	QRS	13.6 ± 19.1	53.2 ± 75.3
	STT	5.5 ± 8.2	21.0 ± 26.5
PEAK RMS ERROR (μV)	QRS	40.5 ± 58.4	97.2 ± 94.6
	STT	9.8 ± 18.6	35.5 ± 34.7

Table 2 lists the average and peak RMS errors computed from the difference between measured and reconstructed BSPM data using temporal and spatial bases, respectively. As expected from Table 1, larger residues are observed for both waveforms when spatial distributions are used.

Inspection of figure 3 reveals three clusters of leads with high discriminant capabilities : these are the right subclavicular area, the lower left anterior/posterior area and the upper dorsal region; isolated leads such as RA and LL also exhibit high discriminant ability. Except for V5 and V6, the precordial leads have lower discriminatory capacity than peripheral leads. One further notes that the overall discriminant power of the T wave is higher than that of the QRS complex. Finally, the discriminant ability of the "best" leads is practically restricted to the first coefficient for QRS and the first two coefficients for STT.

Figure 4 shows that the map patterns which occur in significantly different amounts in normals and in MI patients are of lower order (distributions 1 to 5) although discriminant patterns can be identified as far as in distribution 10. The highest discriminant spatial coefficients are associated with the first eigenvector map during the STT interval, reaching a maximum after the T wave's peak. That same pattern is also quantitatively different during depolarization with a maximum at the peak of QRS.

Linear discriminant functions were computed for the separation of normal individuals (N) from patients with MI, using 3 sets of measurements in turn.

Because of the very large number of measurements available for statistical analysis (250 samples per lead times 120 leads i.e. 30000 variables per individual), we arbitrarily represented and considered these measurements as representative of the total available signal information.

TABLE 3

SELECTED MEASUREMENTS FOR THE SEPARATION OF 184 NORMALS FROM 177 PATIENTS WITH MYOCARDIAL INFARCTION. (THE FIRST 6 VARIABLES ARE LISTED)

TEMPORAL EXPANSION COEFFICIENTS			SPATIAL EXPANSION COEFFICIENTS		
LEAD	COEF.	WAVE	DISTRIB.	WAVE	TIME*
80	1	STT	1	STT	212
VF	1	QRS	1	QRS	34
19	4	STT	10	QRS	16
77	1	STT	4	QRS	124
19	1	STT	7	QRS	16
87	4	STT	4	QRS	22

* THE TIME-SCALE IS NORMALIZED OVER 70 POINTS FOR QRS AND 180 POINTS FOR STT; TIME IS INDICATED FROM ONSET OF QRS

Table 3 lists the results of the stepwise selection procedure. Only the first 6 variables are tabulated since little improvement was noticed beyond this point. One notices that most T.C. are extracted from leads from the areas previously described (fig. 3) as containing maximum diagnostic capability; STT features are usually selected.

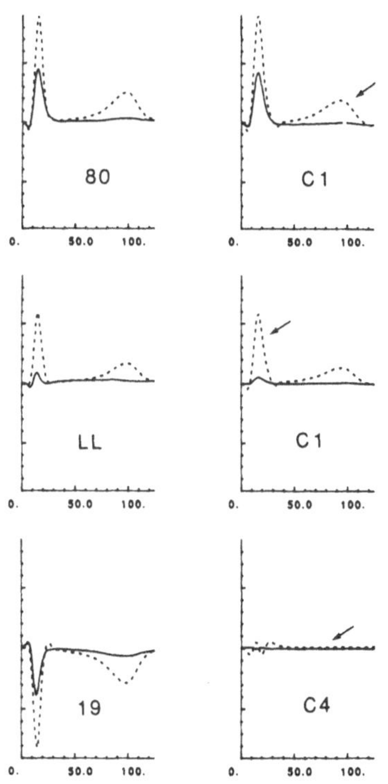

Figure 5 represents the 3 best temporal features of the linear discriminant function. The left column shows leads 80, LL and 19 from which the features are extracted. The N (dotted line) and MI (solid line) signals are averaged, time-normalized and superimposed. In the right column, opposite each lead, the corresponding averaged and superimposed N and MI orthogonal building blocks of interest are shown, namely the first (C1) for leads 80 and LL and the fourth (C4) for lead 19. The arrows point to that part of the ECG selected in the stepwise discriminant procedure.

The most potent S.C., associated with the first eigenvector map (fig. 4) were selected in the first 2 steps. Note the dominance of QRS features as well as the selection of higher order map patterns at the beginning of QRS.

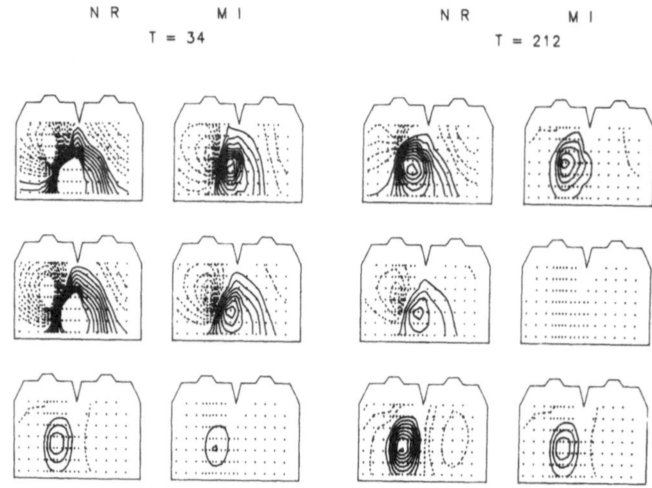

Figure 6 shows the best spatial features of the linear discriminant function. The upper row represents the original maps, averaged for N and MI at instants 34/70 for QRS (left pair of plots) and 142/180 for STT (right pair). The bottom rows depict the first (D1) and second (D2) eigenvector distributions associated with the respective N and MI S.C. at corresponding instants.

TABLE 4

DIFFERENTIATION BETWEEN 184 NORMALS AND 177 PATIENTS WITH MYOCARDIAL INFARCTION USING 3 SETS OF FEATURES*
(THE SPECIFICITY IS KEPT AT 95 %)

	SENSITIVITY (%)	MISSED CASES (NB)
INSTANTANEOUS MEASUREMENTS	97	14
TEMPORAL COEFFICIENTS	96	16
SPATIAL COEFFICIENTS	94	20

* (6 VARIABLES WERE SELECTED FOR EACH SET)

Table 4 lists the diagnostic results achieved with the 3 sets of features. Little difference is observed between in stantaneous measurements and temporal expansion coefficients. For an equal number of selected variables a statistically ($p < .05$) deterioration of the classification occured after spatial compression of the original map data.

DISCUSSION

The present study addresses the problem of diagnostic information contained in BSPM and investigates the possible loss of this information resulting from the use of data reduction methods on the maps.

The eigenvalue approach to data compression of multiple surface leads is not new; several authors have used this property to estimate the dimensionality of the ECG (11, 12, 13), to reconstruct complete maps from a limited number of recording sites (4, 6), or to achieve data compression for storage and transmission (14). More recently, Lux et al. (7) and Evans et al. (8) designed a method for combined spatial and temporal compression of BSPM by which any individual's map could be represented by 216 coefficients, and they concluded that these coefficients might ultimately be used for diagnostic classification.

We chose to investigate separately temporal compression and spatial compression of BSPM because we felt that :

- the diagnostic results would be easier to interpret if the 120 lead data were viewed either as a set of surface ECGs or as a succession of map patterns;
- the 2 approaches could serve different purposes, namely identifying sites of optimal diagnostic leads on one hand and instants of surface distributions, characteristic of underlying cardiac events on the other hand.

Both compression stategies achieve data reduction of BSPM to some extent (14 : 1 for T.C. and 10 : 1 for S.C.); however not with the same degree of conservation of signal and diagnostic information. In order for the spatial basis to represent the original data at the same error level, 28 patterns instead of 12 are required, resulting in a mere 4 : 1 data reduction.

As reported in the literature (8, 9), a further step in data compression can be achieved by representing the 12 spatial coefficient waveforms as a linear combination of temporal basis functions (10 QRS and 8 STT), computed either directly from the original 120 lead data or from the ensemble of S.C. waveforms themselves. It should be noted however that the representation error achieved with the thus obtained 216 temporo-spatial coefficients is still larger.

We tested the latter procedure on our data; the average RMS error obtained in approximating the original BSPM with 216 temporo-spatial coefficients, amounted to 63.8 μV for QRS and 21.6 μV for STT. Selecting the best 6 predictors from these coefficients in the discriminant analysis yielded a sensitivity of 93 % at a specificity level of 95 %.

The decrease in diagnostic performance of spatial and temporo-spatial coefficients (T.S.C.) can be ascribed to the less optimal representation of both signal and diagnostic information rather than to actual loss of information : indeed, the same level of diagnostic classification was reached when more measurements are used for S.C. (9 instead of 6) and for T.S.C. (11 instead of 6).

In practice, reduced lead sets consisting of 24 or 32 leads

(4, 6) and arrived at on the basis of optimal signal representation, are used in order to produce 150 or 192 point maps with an average RMS error ranging from 35 μV (32 leads) to 82 μV (24 leads); subsequent data compression of thus approximated BSPM will further increase the residual error and might in turn, result in further loss of diagnostic information.

In fact the pros and cons of the various data reduction procedures have to be evaluated in the light of acceptable loss of diagnostic information (cost) versus degree of data compression achieved (benefit). In addition, the problems of the interpretation of the diagnostic results have to be taken into account in order to promote the acceptability of the chosen procedure : while both temporal and spatial coefficients can be rather easily and directly related to ECG patterns or instantaneous map distributions, temporo-spatial coefficients do not allow such straightforward interpretation.

In the present study, the less efficient and less accurate representation of the signal information with 12 spatial coefficients could be compensated by utilizing more discriminant variables for diagnostic classification; this was possible, in part, because of the clear-cut nature of the diagnostic groups. Separation of more complex entities might require better representation of the data. The latter can be achieved by using more basis patterns and functions. It is probable that the number of coefficients resulting from combined temporal and spatial data compression needed for the representation of BSPM within the noise level might reach as much as 504 (e.g. 28 map patterns and 18 basis functions), which is still perfectly manageable for data storage, retrieval and transmission.

That compact set of coefficients can be used directly for statistical purposes; it can also be transformed in either temporal or spatial coefficients prior to the analysis, in order to facilitate the interpretation of the results in terms of "best" discriminant leads or optimal instantaneous map patterns. The larger number of variables resulting from the transformations can also be handled statistically provided some selection is performed (e.g. on the basis of t-tests) before the actual discriminant analysis.

1. F. Kornreich and P.M. Rautaharju : The missing Waveform and Diagnostic Information in the Standard 12 Lead Electrocardiogram. J. Electrocardiol. 14 (4), 1981, pp 341-350.

2. G.M. Vincent, J.A. Abildskov, M.J. Burgess, K. Millar R.L. Lux and R.F. Wyatt : Diagnosis of Old Inferior Myocardial Infarction by Body Surface Isopotential Mapping Am. J. Cardiol, vol 39, April 1977, pp 510-515.

3. J. Asugi, T. Ohta, J. Toyoma, F. Takatsu, T. Nagaya and K. Yamada : Body Surface Isopotential Maps in Old Inferior Myocardial Infarction Undetectable by 12 Lead Electrocardiogram. J. Electrocardiol. 17 (1), 1984, p 55-62

4. R.C. Barr, M.S. Spach and G.S. Herman-Giddens : Selection of the Number and Positions of Measuring Locations for Electrocardiography. IEEE Trans. Bio-Med. Eng. vol BME-18 n° 2, March 1971, pp 125-138.

5. F. Kornreich : The Missing Waveform Information in the Orthogonal Electrocardiogram (Frank Leads).
I Where and How Can This Missing Waveform Information be retrieved ? Circulation, vol 48, Nov. 1973, pp 984-995.

6. R.L. Lux, M.J. Burgess, R.F. Wyatt, A.K. Evans, G.M.Vincent and J.A. Abildskov : Clinically Practical lead Systems for Improved Electrocardiography : Comparison with Precordial Grids and Conventional Lead Systems. Circulation, vol 59, n° 2, 1979, pp 356-363.

7. R.L. Lux, A.K. Evans, M.J. Burgess, R.F. Wyatt and J.A. Abildskov : Redundancy Reduction for Improved Display and Analysis of Body Surface Potential Maps : I Spatial Compression. Circulation Res. vol 49, n° 1, 1981, pp 186-196.

8. A.K. Evans, R.L. Lux, M.J. Burgess, R.F. Wyatt and J.A. Abildskov : Redundancy Reduction for Improved Display and Analysis of Body Surface Potential Maps : II. Temporal Compression. Circulation Res. vol 49, n° 1, 1981, pp 197-203.

9. G.J.J. Uijen, A. Heringa and A. van Oosterom : Data Reduction of Body Surface Potential Maps by Means of Orthogonal Expansions. IEEE Trans. Bio-MEd. Eng. vol BME-31 n° 11, nov. 1984, pp 706-714.

10. BMDP-79 Biomedical Computer Programs. P Series. Dixon W.J. and Brown M.B. Eds. University of California Press, Berkeley 1979.

11. A.M. Scher, A.C. Young and W.M. Meredith : Factor Analysis of the Electrocardiogram. Circulation Res. 8, 1960, pp 519-526.

12. T.Y. Young and W.H. Huggins : On the Representation of Electrocardiograms. IEEE Trans Bio-Med. Eng. BME-10, 963, pp 86-95.

13. L.G. Horan, N.C. Flowers and D.A. Brody : Principal Factor Waveforms of the Thoracic QRS Complex. Circulation Res. 15, 1964, pp. 131-138.

14. E.M. Womble, J.S. Halliday, S.K. Mittler, M.C. Lancaster and J.H. Triebwasser : Data Compression for storing and Transmitting ECGs/VCGs. IEEE Proc. 65, 1977, pp. 702-706.

Chapter 26

ORTHOGONAL EXPANSION OF EPICARDIAL AND BODY SURFACE ECG POTENTIALS

H. TANAKA, K. HIRAYANAGI, T. FURUKAWA

1. INTRODUCTION

The information contents and the relation of the body surface and epicardial potentials were investigated by using the singular value decomposition (SVD). The study is composed of two kinds of the analyses.

First, spacial information amounts of the body surface and epicardial potentials were calculated taking the noise RMS voltage as a reference level. SVD was used to decompose the total variance of the spacial potential pattern into the sum of the independent components. Total information amounts were calculated by evaluating the information amount of each component and summing all of them.

Second, the potential transfer process between the epicardial and body surface potential distribution is investigated by (1) constructing the transfer coefficients matrix between epicardial and body surface potential based on the boundary element method, (2) applying SVD to this matrix to obtain the orthogonal components of the potential transfer process.

This kind of the information-theoretic study would be of use to clarify the basic limitation of resolution of the inverse solution and the diagnostic ability of body surface mapping to detect the local ECG abnormality of heart.

2. METHODS

2.1. SVD of the body surface and epicardial potentials

Three kinds of electrocardiographic potential distribution were used for the SVD analysis to extract the independent components of the spacial potential variation; body surface potentials of the human subjects including the patients with cardiac diseases, epicardial potentials and body surface potentials of canines. For the human subjects, 96-lead body surface potential maps were recorded with 50 cases; 200 frames of the maps were collected within a cardiac cycle in each case. For the epicardial and body surface potentials of canine, animal experiments were conducted in which 60 electrodes were implanted on the epicardium and 128 electrodes were attached on the thoracic surface; both body surface potential and epicardial potentials were measured simultaneously. The measured potentials were averaged over 12 beats in the animal experiments.

SVD was applied to the potential data matrix M wherein rows show the differences of the lead position and columns show the differences of the frames and subjects. SVD transforms M into the following form:

$$M = U \Lambda V^t$$

where V,U are the orthogonal matrix, Λ is the diagonal matrix of the singular values. Statistically independent potential patterns constitute the column vectors of the U. The toal information amount (IT) can be calculated by summing that of each component. The following formula was obtained according to the Shannon's definition.

$$IT = \sum_{i=1}^{p} \log_2 \left(\frac{\lambda_i}{\lambda_{p+1}} \right)$$

2.2. The orthogonal components of:the potential transfer process

The boundary element method was used to construct the potential transfer process between epicardial and body surface potential. This method is based on the boundary integral equations derived from the Green's second identities. Numerical procedures consist of (1) descretizing the body and heart surface with the sum of triangles, (2) using Gauss-Legendre's quadrature to calculate surface integral, and (3) solving thus descretized simultaneous equations by Gauss' elimination method.

SVD was applied to the potential transfer matrix H. This time the singular potential patterns exhibits the epicardial and body surface potential values of the orthogonal transfer components and singular value shows the transfer ratio of the potential from the epicardium to body surface.

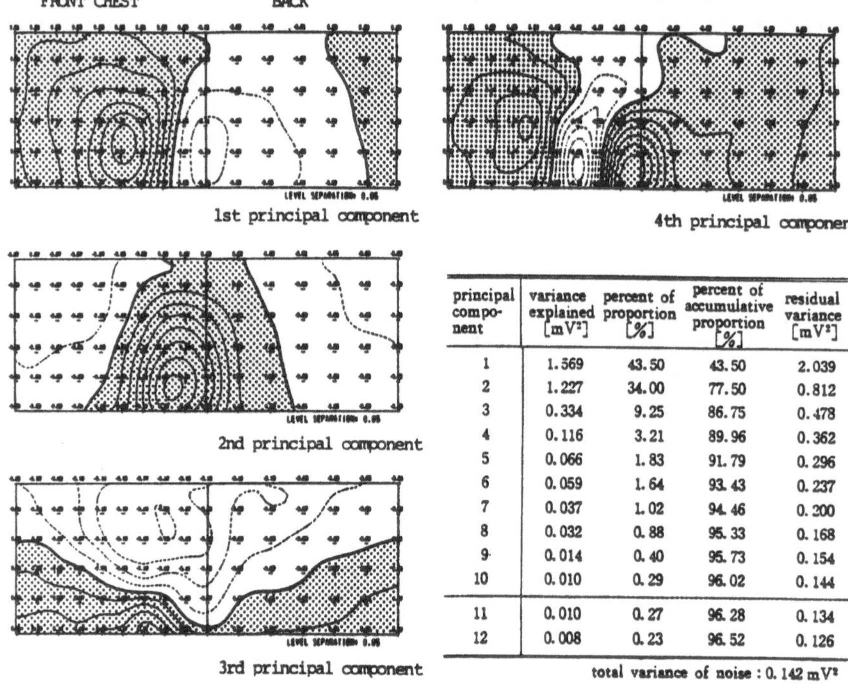

principal component	variance explained [mV²]	percent of proportion [%]	percent of accumulative proportion [%]	residual variance [mV²]
1	1.569	43.50	43.50	2.039
2	1.227	34.00	77.50	0.812
3	0.334	9.25	86.75	0.478
4	0.116	3.21	89.96	0.362
5	0.066	1.83	91.79	0.296
6	0.059	1.64	93.43	0.237
7	0.037	1.02	94.46	0.200
8	0.032	0.88	95.33	0.168
9	0.014	0.40	95.73	0.154
10	0.010	0.29	96.02	0.144
11	0.010	0.27	96.28	0.134
12	0.008	0.23	96.52	0.126

total variance of noise : 0.142 mV²

Fig. 1. Patterns of the Information Components

Table 1. Variaces of the Information Components

3. RESULTS

3.1. SVD of recorded human body surface potentials

Ten components were obtained as the effective information patterns containing greater variance than that of average noise (Table 1). The first three components accounted for 43.50%, 34.00% and 9.25% of the total variance of body surface potential distribution, respectively and were similar to dipolar patterns (Fig. 1). The fourth and the higher components show more complicated patterns indicating quadrupolar and the other multipolar components of body surface potentials. Up to these 10 components, 96.02% of the total variance was explained. The total information amount calculated based on the results of SVD and Shannon's formula was 16.08 bits if we took the average noise level as 0.038 mV.

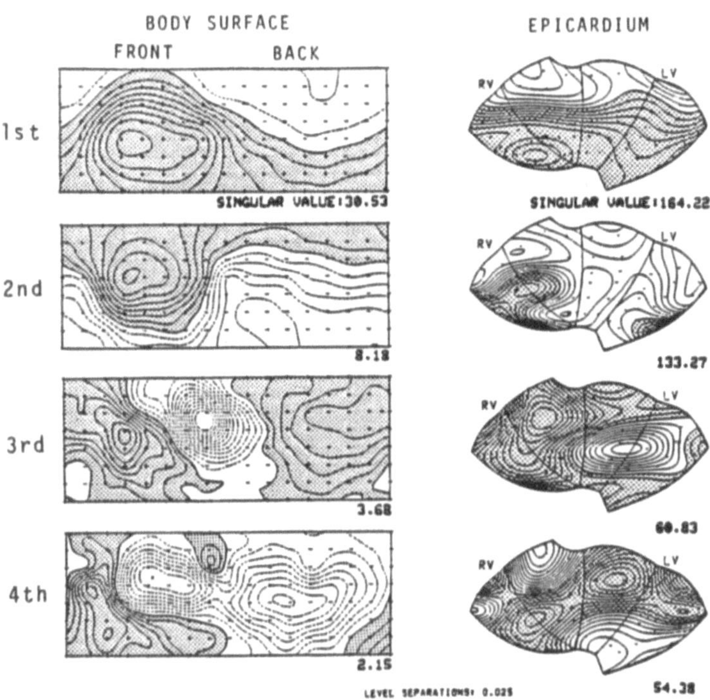

Fig. 2. SVD of the Canine Body Surface and Epicardial Potential Components

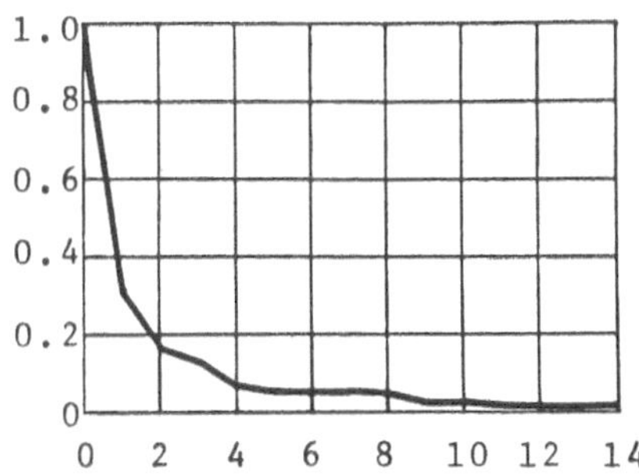

Fig. 3. Potential Transfer Characteristics

3.2. SVD of the recorded canine body surface and epicardial potentials

Seventeen components were extracted for the epicardial potential distribution as the independent components having greater variance than that of noise potential. The first component clearly showed the potential pattern of dipole along with the heart axis (Fig. 2), but the other higher components were relatively complicated. For the body surface potentials, the number of the independent components reduced much and was only 7. The total information amounts based on the SVD and Shannon's formula were 20.9 bits in the body surface and 40.7 bits on the epicardium.

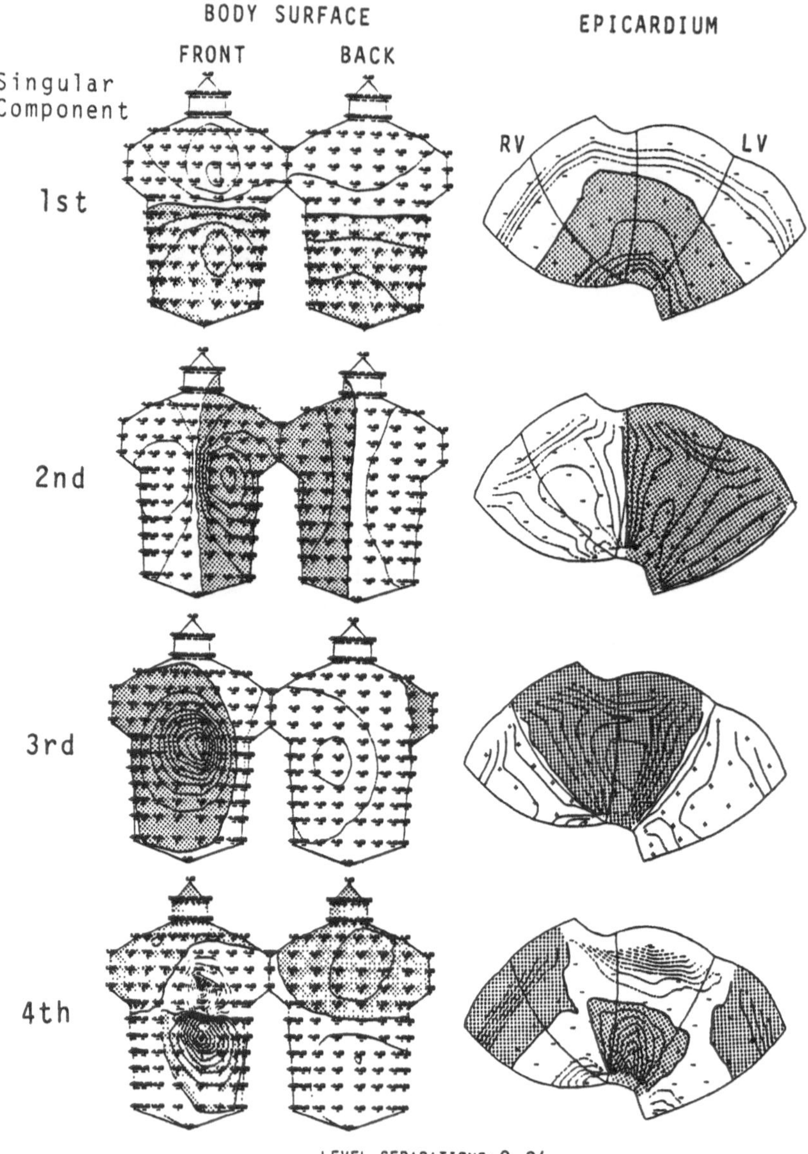

Fig. 4. Body Surface and Epicardial Potential Patterns of SVD Components of the computed transfer matrix H between canine epicardial and body surface potentials.

3.3. SVD of the potential transfer matrix

The potential transfer characteristics showed the exponentially decreasing patterns (Fig. 3); first component is a DC-like component, and the next three components showed dipolar patterns of three directions (Fig. 4). If we follow the statistics of the human body surface, admitting the 3.98% noise level and if the obtained covariance is assumed to be valid, then number of the effective components of the epicardial potential which have the greater variance on the body surface and which have the possibility to be recovered by the inverse calculation is 10-12.

Chapter 27

USEFULNESS OF TIME-INTEGRAL ANALYSIS OF BODY SURFACE POTENTIAL MAPS

L. DE AMBROGGI, T. BERTONI, C. RABBIA, E. LOCATI, F. NADOR

INTRODUCTION

Clinical investigations indicate that body surface potential maps (BSPM) provide diagnostic information undetectable by the conventional electrocardiographic leads in various heart conditions (1-6).

From the clinical point of view a major problem is the difficulty of extracting information of diagnostic value in given heart diseases from the large amount of data provided by the instantaneous BSPM.

We tackled the problem by using time integral analysis of the surface ECG tracings from which maps were generated. This technique greatly reduces the amount of data to be considered without substantial loss of information (2,4,7) and enables average maps for groups of subjects to be calculated without the problem of time-phase alignment.

METHODS AND STUDY POPULATION

BSPM were recorded from 140 lead points on the anterior and posterior chest surface. Groups of 35 ECG plus a reference lead were recorded at one time,using an instrument (Cardimap II) which performs on-line amplification,multiplexing (at 500 Hz per channel) and digital conversion of the signals. The blocks of data from 4 successive recordings,relating to 4 cardiac cycles at the end of a normal expiration,were processed together after time alignment on a Nova 4/C Data General computer connected to recording instrument.

The potential-time integral,relating to a given interval of the cardiac cycle,was calculated at each lead point as the algebraic sum of all potentials,from the instant of onset to the instant of offset,multiplied by the sampling interval. The values in µV•sec were transferred to a diagram representing the thoracic surface explored,then isointegral contour lines were drawn manually (Integral map, I-map).

For given time intervals,the mean I-map of the control group was subtracted from the I-map of each patient; the value obtained at each lead point was then divided by the standard deviation of the normal values for that point. The resulting values,indicating the standardized differences from normal values,were transferred to another map (Deviation Index - DI-map).

The following groups of subjects were studied: a) 15 patients,aged 35 to 65 years,with an old inferior myocardial infarction (MI) without ECG signs of necrosis; b) 14 patients,aged 27 to 71 years,with a non-transmural (non-Q) MI; c) 30 normal subjects,aged 20 to 57 years,as control group for MI patients; d) 18 patients,aged 8 to 45 years,with idiopathic long QT syndrome (LQTS); e) 18 normal subjects matched for age and sex as control group for LQTS patients.

RESULTS AND DISCUSSION

Myocardial infarction. In this group of patients we considered the integral maps of the first 40 msec of the QRS complex (Q-40) because,as is well known,the early phases of activation should reveal the greatest abnormalities due to MI,even though later phases can be altered.

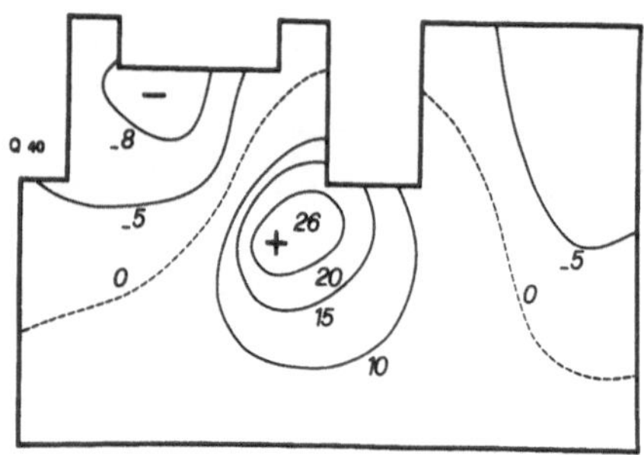

Fig.1 : Mean Q-40 I-map from 30 control subjects. Values are expressed in μV•sec. The left and right part of the map represent respectively the anterior and posterior chest surface.

To quantitate the differences in the individual I-maps between normals and MI patients,DI-maps were calculated by subtracting the mean Q-40 I-map of the control group (Fig.1) from the I-map of each patient.
An area where the Q-40 integral values were at least 2 SD lower than normal,was taken as an index of MI.

In 11 out of 15 patients with an old inferior MI (documented during the acute phase) without ECG evidence of necrosis,DI-maps showed an area of negative values (-2 SD) in the lower half of the trunk,either anteriorly or posteriorly (Fig.2)

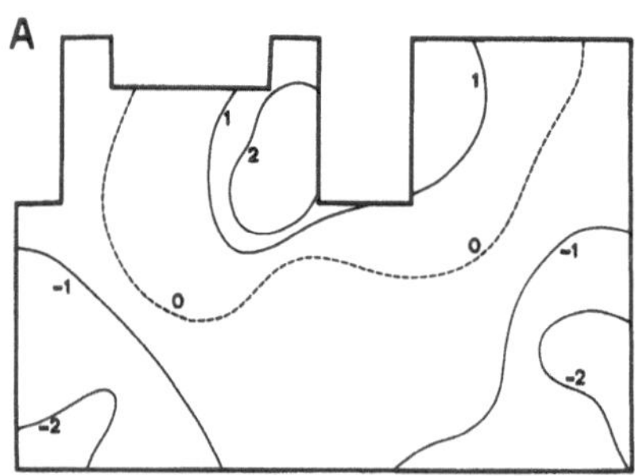

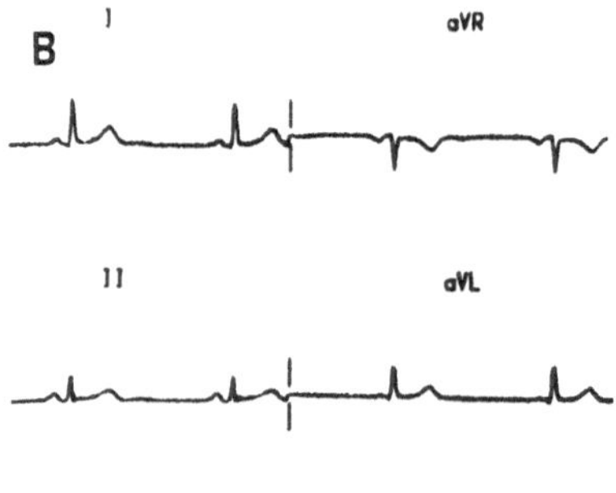

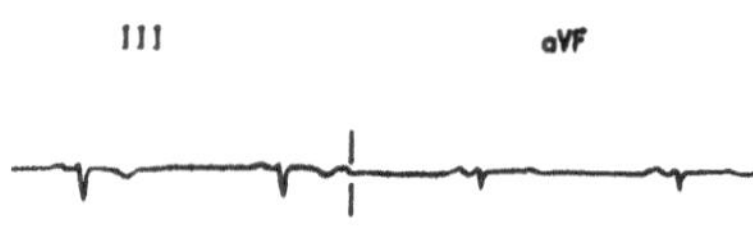

Fig.2 : DI-map (A) of a patient with inferior MI not revealed by the standard ECG leads (B).An area of integral values 2 SD lower than normal is evident on the inferior portion of the right thorax.

This pattern may be related to the presence of an infarcted zone in the diaphragmatic wall of the heart.

In 11 out of 14 patients with non-transmural MI,DI-maps showed negative areas(2 SD lower than normal),which were variously located on the chest surface. Figure 3 illustrates the Q-40 I-map and the relating DI-map of a patient with non-Q wave MI in whom the 2D-echocardiogram showed an antero-lateral and apical asynergy.

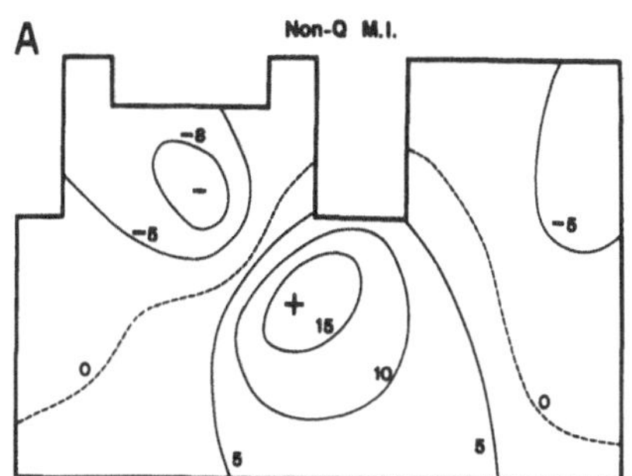

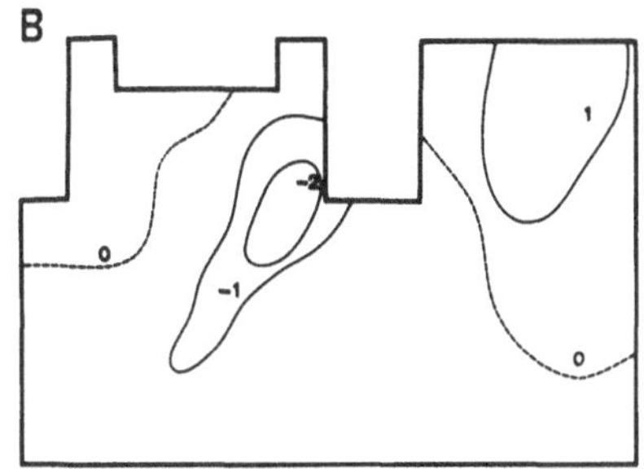

Fig.3 : I-map (A) and DI-map (B) from a patient with non-transmural MI.

In this case the location of the -2SD negative integral values was roughly in agreement with the topography of the asynergy in the heart. In 7 of 11 patients with abnormal DI-maps a relation was found between the surface location of the area of -2 SD negative values and the site of the infarct, as determined by 2D-echocardiograms.

Long QT syndrome. In LQTS,the normal sequence of ventricular repolarization may be altered,as a consequence of an imbalance of the cardiac sympathetic activity (8);thus electrical disparities may result among adjacent regions of the heart during the recovery process. In order to establish whether this complex intracardiac electrical situation could be revealed on the chest surface,we considered the integral maps of the ST-T interval.

The mean I-map of the ST-T interval calculated from 18 control subjects exhibited smooth bipolar distribution of the values,with a maximum located inthe left mammary region and a minimum in the right clavicular-upper sternal areas. The ST-T I-maps showed abnormalities in 14 out of 18 pa-

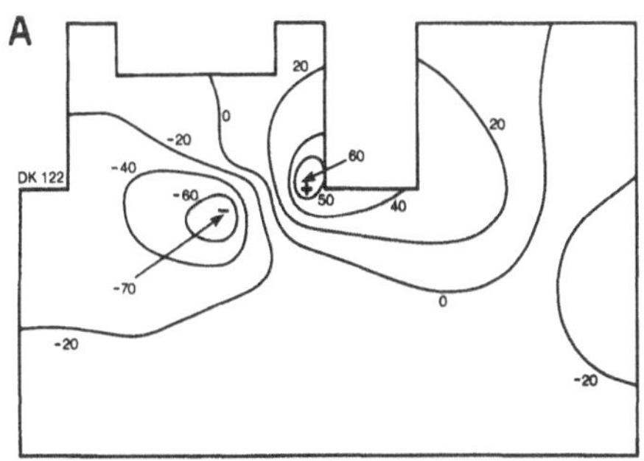

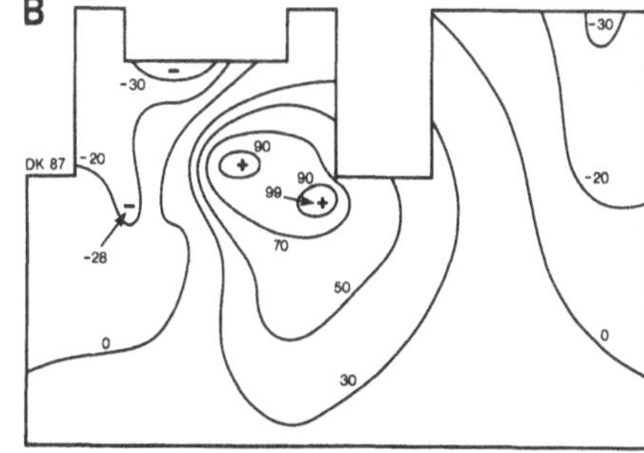

Fig.4 : Integral maps from two patients with idiopathic LQTS.

tients. The most frequent abnormal pattern was characterized by an area of negative values larger than normal,covering the anterior thorax and extending beyond the mid-sternal line (Fig.4 A). According to the hypothesis that in the idiopathic LQTS there is a lower-than-normal right cardiac sympathetic activity (8),the prominent negative area on the anterior chest surface could be ascribed to delayed repolarization of the anterior wall of the heart. In 5 patients the I-maps exhibited a complex distribution with multiple peaks of the potential-time integral values (Fig.4B). This pattern might be related to the presence of regional electrical disparities during the ventricular recovery,which could favour the occurrence of malignant arrhythmias.

CONCLUSIONS

Our results confirm previous reports (1-6) that BSPM have a greater information content than conventional ECG in various heart diseases. Moreover our studies demonstrate the usefulness of time integral analysis of BSPM,from which diagnostic quantitative criteria can be extracted with relatively simple methods. This kind of approach facilitates the evaluation of BSPM and can thus be expected to increase the clinical application of BSPM.

REFERENCES

1. Taccardi B.,De Ambroggi L.,Viganotti C.: Body surface mapping of heart potentials. In: Nelson CV and Geselowitz DB eds. The theoretical basis of electrocardiology. Clarendon Press,Oxford, 1976, p.436
2. Abildskov J.A.,Burgess M.J.,Urie P.M.,Lux R.L.,Wyatt R.F.: The unidentified information content of the electrocardiogram. Circ. Res. 40: 3, 1977.
3. De Ambroggi L.,Taccardi B.,Macchi E.: Body surface maps of heart potentials.Tentative localization of preexcited areas in 42 Wolff-Parkinson-White patients. Circulation 54: 251, 1976.
4. Montague T.J.,Smith E.R.,Spencer C.A.,Johnstone D.E.,Lalonde L.D., Bessoudo R.M.,Gardner M.J.,Anderson R.N.,Horacek B.M.: Body surface electrocardiographic mapping in inferior myocardial infarctions.Manifestation of left and right ventricular involvement. Circulation 67: 665, 1983.
5. Vincent G.M.,Green L.S.,Lux R.L.,Merchant M.H.,Abildskov J.A.: Use of QRST area distributions to predict vulnerability to cardiac death following myocardial infarction. Circulation 68: II-352, 1983.
6. Osugi J.,Ohta T.,Toyama J.,Takatsu F.,Nagaya T.,Yamada K.: Body surface isopotential maps in old inferior myocardial infarction undetectable by 12 lead electrocardiogram. J.Electrocardiol. 17:55, 1984
7. Montague T.J.,Smith E.R.,Cameron D.A.,Rautaharju P.M.,Klassen G.A., Felmington C.S.,Horacek B.M.: Isointegral analysis of body surface

maps: surface distribution and temporal variability in normal subjects. Circulation 67: 1166, 1981.

8. Schwartz P.J.,Periti M.,Malliani A.: The long Q-T syndrome. Am. Heart J. 89: 378, 1975.

Chapter 28

DO BODY SURFACE MAPS CONTAIN MORE INFORMATION THAN THE ECG?

G.J.H. UIJEN, A. HERINGA, R.TH. VAN DAM

1. INTRODUCTION

Both body surface maps (BSM) and the conventional clinical 12-lead ECG (ECG) are representations of the same electrical activity of the heart at the thoracic surface.

In two aspects BSM and ECG differ from each other.

1. Body surface maps are measured from many more recording sites than the conventional ECG.
2. BSM and ECG are presented in different ways: BSM are displayed as a series of maps of the thoracic potential distribution at consecutive time instants, while the ECG is displayed as a number of time signals.

Because of the first aspect more information on the electrical activity of the heart can be expected in the BSM than in the ECG from a technical point of view. For answering the question whether the diagnostic power is also increased by using BSM instead of ECG the second aspect is of importance, since usually different features are derived from BSM's and ECG's. Due to the different way of presentation a quantitative evaluation using these different features is hardly possible.

In this study we have tried to evaluate the diagnostic power in a statistical manner by processing both BSM and ECG by the same methods. Features that were selected from the BSM and ECG of normals and patients with a chronic infarction were entered in a classification procedure.

2. MATERIALS

BSM's were recorded from 139 subjects, consisting of a group of 54 normal subjects and a second group of 85 patients with a history of myocardial infarction. The ECG is as a subset present in the BSM.

The diagnosis of infarction was confirmed by the detection of left ventricular asynergy using ventriculography and/or echocardiography.

3.DATA RECORDING

64 leads were used in the recording system [1], which consists of 64 isolation amplifiers and a PDP 11/34 computer with peripherals. The standard ECG lead system is a subset of this mapping system. The recording sites are shown in figure 1. The 64 time signals were sampled simultaneously at 500 samples per second in time spans of 2 seconds. One representative heartbeat for each patient was selected. After linear baseline shift correction the onset QRS was determined.

For the evaluation single QRS complexes (till 100 ms from onset QRS) and Q-waves (till 30 ms from onset QRS) were used. By summing up the samples in the time direction, Q- and QRS-integrals were constructed and subsequently analyzed.

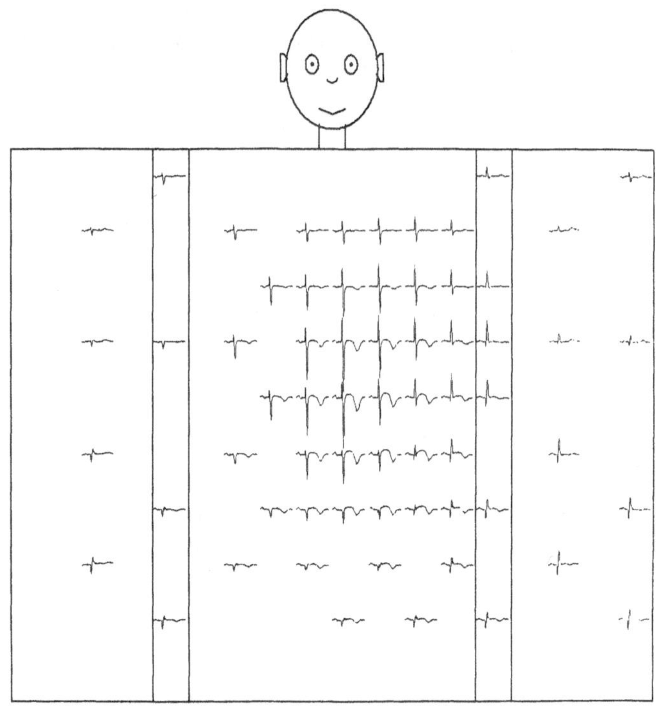

FIGURE 1.

4. DATA BASE

For each subject the data to be processed consists of L = p × t numbers with

p = the number of leads = 64 for the BSM,
= 8 for the ECG, because 8 of the 12 standard leads may be independent,

and

t = the number of time samples = 50 for the QRS,
= 15 for the Q,
= 1 for the integral data.

The numbers L of data representing the different cases are summarized in table I.

TABLE I. Number of data L representing a subject in different cases.

	QRS	Q	INTEGRAL
BSM	3200	960	64
ECG	400	120	8

5. DATA REDUCTION

For the classification procedure the number of parameters representing each subject has to be considerably lower than the number of subjects in a group (being 54 normals and 85 patients). This requirement has been met with in the present study.

In order to reduce the data the L number representation (i.e. BSM, ECG, integral BSM, integral ECG for both Q-interval and QRS-interval) of a subject is considered as one single vector. Depending on the type of representation the number of elements L of this vector ranges from 8 (ECG integral) to 3200 (QRS map).

The L-vector $\underline{y}(n)$ of subject n is expanded into a limited set of orthogonal L-vectors $\underline{u}(m)$ (m=1,...,M). The vector $\underline{y}(n)$ can approximately be represented by the M-vector $\underline{b}(n)$. When $\underline{u}(m)$ are the column vectors of a matrix U then

$$\underline{y}(n) = U\ \underline{b}(n)$$

The orthogonal vectors $\underline{u}(m)$ were computed from the singular value decomposition [2] of the matrix Y of which the columns are the vectors $\underline{y}(n)$ of all subjects involved [3]. The vectors $\underline{u}(m)$ are the eigenvectors of the covariance matrix YY^T.

At most 20 eigenvectors associated with the largest singular values were used for the expansion (so M=20), by which at least 97% of the power is represented in the coefficients. As an example a BSM recording in the single vector representation (L=3200) is shown in figure 2A. This vector is in fact a string of 64 QRS complexes. In figure 2B nine of its most prominent eigenvectors are shown.

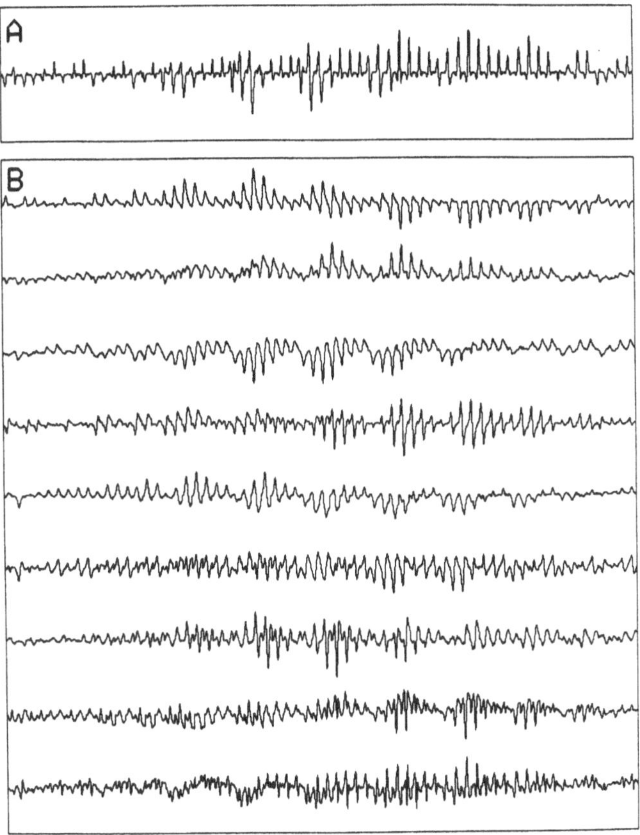

FIGURE 2.

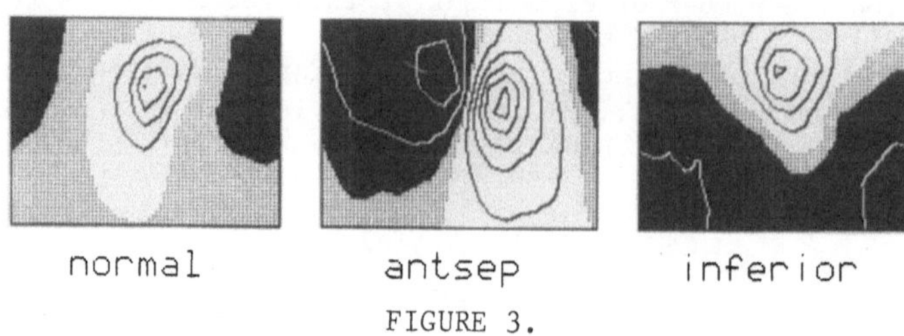

FIGURE 3.

In figure 3 Q-integrals (L=64) of 3 different subjects (normal, old anterior infarction and old inferior infarction) are shown, displayed as maps (white background is positive, black is negative and grey is zero borderzone).

The six most prominent eigenvectors as computed from the complete set of 139 Q-integrals are shown in figure 4, also displayed as maps.

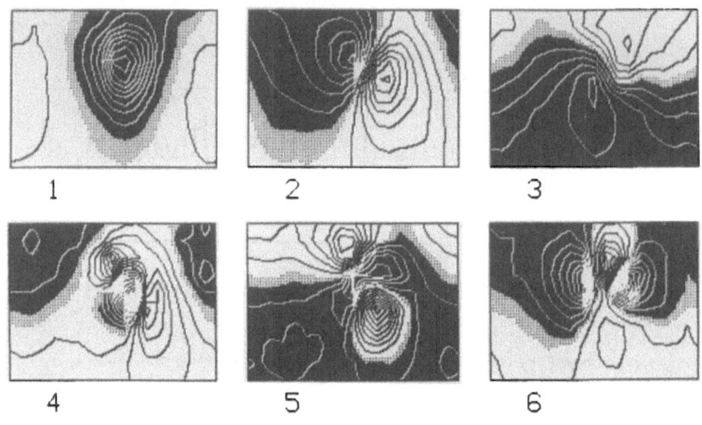

FIGURE 4.

6. CLASSIFICATION

A further reduction of features (expansion coefficients) was obtained in a stepwise discriminant procedure (SAS-STEPDISC) by selecting the features with the most discriminative power in discerning the normal subjects from the patients. Using these features discriminant functions were computed for each group or class of subjects. Since the number of subjects in the group is relatively low, the "jackknifing" evaluation procedure was carried out: all subjects except one are considered as the design set from which a discriminant function is derived; subsequently the subject left out is classified. This process is repeated for all subjects considered.

The diagnostic performance of the several data representations (QRS-BSM, QRS-ECG etc.) is defined as the total number of subjects correctly classified.

7. RESULTS

The summary of the overall results of the classification is shown in table II.

TABLE II. Diagnostic performance of BSM and ECG

	BSM			ECG		
	% correct classifications	L	M (number of features used)	% correct classifications	L	M (number of features used)
Q	91	960	3	91	120	4
QRS	91	3200	8	91	400	8
Q-integral	88	64	3	86	8	6
QRS-integral	82	64	6	77	8	3

For the Q-data the complete classification schemes with the number of subjects assigned to each class by the classification procedure are listed in table III.

TABLE III. Classification of subjects (Q-data)

	BSM (L=960;M=3) a posteriori		ECG (L=120;M=4) a posteriori	
	normal	MI	normal	MI
a priori				
normal	51	3	51	3
MI	9	76	10	75

8. DISCUSSION

Despite the inhomogeneity of the group of patients studied, consisting of subjects with old infarctions of different type, a rather high score (91%) can be obtained in distinguishing normals from infarctions. It is remarkable that this result can be obtained when the Q-data only are used which are represented by only 3 numbers. For the complete QRS, more features are required to reach the same result, which may be attributed to the larger variability of the depolarization pattern in the later QRS complex in the different persons. The minimum number of features for the QRS is comparable with the findings of others [4,5]. The lower figures for the integral data point to some loss of diagnostic information when the time samples are summed up, especially when the whole QRS interval is used.

An equal maximum result in this classification has been obtained both by the map and by the standard ECG. Therefore, the possible extra diagnostic information in the body surface map could not be demonstrated in this study. We think that the variability within groups of subjects as concerns the history of infarction, is much larger than the difference in information between the complete map and the standard ECG.

REFERENCES

1. Heringa A, Uijen GJH, Dam RTh van: A 64-channel system for body surface potential mapping. Electrocardiology '81, eds Z. Antaloczy and I. Preda, pp 297. Budapest: Akademiai Kiado; Excerpta Medica 1982.

2. Forsythe GE, Malcolm MA, Moler CG: Computer methods for mathematical computation, Ch. 9. Englewood Cliffs, N.J.; Prentice Hall. 1977.
3. Uijen GJH, Heringa A, Oosterom A van: Data reduction of body surface potential maps by means of orthogonal expansions. IEEE Trans. Biomed. Eng. 31: 706. 1984.
4. Kornreich F, Rautaharju P: The missing waveform and diagnostic information in the standard 12 lead electrocardiogram. J. Electrocard. 14: 341. 1981.
5. Lux RL, Green LS, Abildskov JA: Statistical representation and classification of electrocardiographic body surface potential maps. In: Computers in Card. '84, pp 251. Long Beach, Calif.: IEEE Computers Society. 1985.

Chapter 29

REPRESENTATION OF ELECTROCARDIOGRAPHIC BODY SURFACE MAPS BY CYLINDRICAL REGRESSION COEFFICIENTS

G. SCHOFFA, J. BÜRKELBACH

The representation of electrocardiographic body surface potential maps (BSPM) on the basis of an analytical function has several important advantages: The BSPM can be represented by a reasonably small number of coefficients, and these coefficients can be used for the calculation of an arbitrary number of values, e.g. for the graphical representation.

In our previous paper (1), we recommended the cylindrical model for the regression

$$y = X\beta + e$$

with
- y potential values vector
- X matrix of independent variables
- β regression coefficients vector, and
- e error vector.

The ordinary-least-square solution of the above function is

$$\beta = (X'X)^{-1} X'y'$$

Since the BSPM has y = 100 to 200 values, this solution leads to large matrices, and the inversion of matrices involves some rounding errors. Therefore, we have proposed (1,2) that the X matrix be replaced by $X_1 \times X_2$ Kronecker product. For the cylindrical model this leads to

$$\hat{\beta}(y) = (X'X)^{-1} X'y = ((X_1'X_1)^{-1} X_1' \otimes (X_2'X_2)^{-1} X_2')\, y$$

with (for 16 x 8 measurement points)

$$X_1 := \begin{bmatrix} 1 & \cos x_0 & \sin x_0 & \cdots & \cos px_0 & \sin px_0 \\ \vdots & \vdots & \vdots & & \vdots & \vdots \\ 1 & \cos x_{15} & \sin x_{15} & \cdots & \cos px_{15} & \sin px_{15} \end{bmatrix} \quad \text{and} \quad X_2 := \begin{bmatrix} 1 & z_1 & z_1^2 & \cdots & z_1^q \\ \vdots & \vdots & \vdots & & \vdots \\ 1 & z_8 & z_8^2 & \cdots & z_8^q \end{bmatrix}$$

in which

- p the degree of trigonometrical polynomial in the horizontal direction,
- x the angle in the horizontal plane (radians),
- q the degree of the ordinal polynomial in the vertical direction,
- z the vertical cordinate values, e.g. 1,2,....8 for equidistance.

For n x m = 16 x 8 = 128 BSPM values and p=q=4 it follows that
X_1 is an → n x (2p+1) = 16 x 9 matrix,
X_2 is an → m x (q+1) = 8 x 5 matrix.

The matrix multiplication

$$X = ((X_1'X_1)^{-1} X_1' \otimes (X_2'X_2)^{-1} X_2')$$

being the next operation, does not produce any appreciable rounding errors.

The regression coefficients are then

$$\beta = X.y'$$

with

$$y := (y_{01}, \cdots, y_{08}, y_{11}, \cdots, y_{18}, \cdots, y_{15,1}, \cdots, y_{15.8})',$$

For N=n.m

$$\beta((2p+1)(q+1)) = X(((2p+1)(q+1)) \times N).y(N)'$$

e.g. for 16 x 8 = 128 BSPM values matrix dimensions are

$$\beta(45) = X(45,128).y(128)'$$

The calculation of regression coefficients is just a matrix multiplication.

For the same number and position of electrodes and fixed polynomial degrees p and q, the matrix X remains the same - and thus may be calculated just once.

For equidistant angles in the horizontal plane, the matrix is diagonal

$$(X_1'X_1) = n/2 \text{ diag } (2,1,\ldots.,1).$$

The inversion of this matrix is very easy and free of rounding off errors.

In previous papers (1,2) was shown that a degree of p=q=4 may already be considered optimal, with the correlation coefficient R^2=0.99 .

The reconstruction of BSPM with regression vector β is given by

$$y' = (X_1 \otimes X_2).\beta$$

To calculate more points, i.e. for the graphical representation, X_1 and X_2 must be expanded for more values.

Because the regression is the best-fit least squares method, it is additionally a smoothing and filtering of the measurement matrix.

For the practical application of our method, we include a FORTRAN77 program which runs on IBM PC.

REFERENCES

1. Kasper L, Fieger W, Cremers H, Schoffa G: Body surface potential mapping based on cylindrical regression. IEEE Trans. BME-32: 237-239, 1985.
2. Kasper L: Das zylindrische Regressionsmodell. Diplomarbeit, Universität Karlsruhe, 1983.

```
C ** CYLINDRICAL REGRESSION PROGRAM - G.SCHOFFA/J.BÜRKELBACH
C ** X MATRIX, HERE FOR 16X8 BSPM ELECTRODES AND P=Q=4  (RUN ON IBM PC)
      INTEGER ANZW,ANZR,P,Q
      REAL*8 X1(16,9),X2(8,5),X1T(9,16),X2T(5,8),X(45,128)
      REAL*8 X1I(9,9),X2I(5,5),X1R(9,16),X2R(5,8),RING(8)
      REAL*8 WIN(16),C(9,9),B(9,9),CI(9,9),BI(9,9)
      DATA ANZW/16/,ANZR/8/,Q/4/,P/4/
      OPEN(10,FILE='X',STATUS='NEW')
      CALL INPUT(WIN,RING,ANZW,ANZR)
      CALL X1X2(P,Q,ANZW,WIN,ANZR,RING,X1,X2,2*P+1,Q+1)
      DO 10 I=1,ANZW
      X1T(1,I)=1.
      DO 10 K=2,2*P,2
      X1T(K,I)=X1(I,K)
 10   X1T(K+1,I)=X1(I,K+1)
      CALL MATMUL(X1T,X1,X1I,2*P+1,ANZW,2*P+1)
      CALL MATINV(X1I,2*P+1)
      CALL MATMUL(X1I,X1T,X1R,2*P+1,2*P+1,ANZW)
      DO 20 I=1,ANZR
      DO 20 K=1,Q+1
 20   X2T(K,I)=X2(I,K)
      CALL MATMUL(X2T,X2,X2I,Q+1,ANZR,Q+1)
      CALL MATINV(X2I,Q+1)
      CALL MATMUL(X2I,X2T,X2R,Q+1,Q+1,ANZR)
      DO 100 N=1,2*P+1
      DO 100 L=1,Q+1
      DO 100 M=1,ANZW
      DO 100 K=1,ANZR
 100  X((N-1)*(Q+1)+L,(M-1)*ANZR+K)=X1R(N,M)*X2R(L,K)
      WRITE(10,'(8F10.6)') ((X(I,K),K=1,128),I=1,45)
      END
C ** CALCULATION OF REGRESSION COEFFICIENTS AND RECONSTRUCTION
C ** FOR MORE VALUES (GRAFICS) EXPAND DIMENSIONS AND DATA
C ** MATMUL4=MATMUL,INPUT4=INPUT,X1X2R=X1X2 SUBR.,BUT FOR REAL*4
      INTEGER ANZW,ANZR,P,Q,MM
      DIMENSION X(45,128),SM(128),B(45),WIN(16),RING(8)
      DIMENSION X1(16,9),X2(8,5),X12(128,45),Y(128)
      DATA ANZW/16/,ANZR/8/,Q/4/,P/4/
      OPEN(10,FILE='X')
      OPEN(12,FILE='SM')
      READ(10,'(8F10.6)') ((X(I,J),J=1,ANZW*ANZR),I=1,(2*P+1)*(Q+1))
      READ(12,'(128F6.2)') (SM(I),I=1,ANZW*ANZR)
      CALL MATMUL4(X,SM,B,(2*P+1)*(Q+1),ANZW*ANZR,1)
      CALL INPUT4(WIN,RING,ANZW,ANZR)
C ** X1X2R=X1X2 SUBR.,BUT FOR REAL*4 AND DCOS=COS, DSIN=SIN
      CALL X1X2R(P,Q,ANZW,WIN,ANZR,RING,X1,X2,2*P+1,Q+1)
      DO 100 N=1,ANZW
      DO 100 L=1,ANZR
      DO 100 M=1,2*P+1
      DO 100 K=1,Q+1
 100  X12((N-1)*ANZR+L,(M-1)*(Q+1)+K)=X1(N,M)*X2(L,K)
      CALL MATMUL4(X12,B,Y,ANZW*ANZR,(2*P+1)*(Q+1),1)
      WRITE(*,'(8F6.2)') (Y(I),I=1,ANZR*ANZW)
      END
```

```
C ** INPUT SUBROUTINE FOR ANGLES AND ROW POSITIONS
      SUBROUTINE INPUT (WIN,RING,ANZW,ANZR)
      INTEGER ANZW,ANZR
      REAL*8 WIN(ANZW),RING(ANZR)
      WRITE(*,'('' INPUT ANGLES '')')
      READ(*,*) (WIN(I),I=1,ANZW)
      WRITE(*,'('' INPUT VERTICAL ROW NUMBERS'')')
      READ(*,*) (RING(I),I=1,ANZR)
      END
C ** MATRIX MULTIPLICATION
      SUBROUTINE MATMUL(A,B,C,M,N,L)
      REAL*8 A(M,N),B(N,L),C(M,L)
      DO 1 I=1,L
      DO 1 J=1,M
      C(J,I)=0.0
      DO 1 K=1,N
 1    C(J,I)=C(J,I)+A(J,K)*B(K,I)
      END
C ** MATRIX INVERSION WITH A SPECIAL ALGORITHM (SYM.MATRICES)
      SUBROUTINE MATINV(X,N)
      REAL*8 X(N,N),C(9,9),B(9,9)
      REAL*8 CI(9,9),BI(9,9)
      DO 1 I=1,N
      DO 2 J=I,N
      C(I,J)=X(I,J)
      IF (I.EQ.1) GOTO 2
      DO 3 K=2,I
 3    C(I,J)=C(I,J)+B(K-1,I)*C(K-1,J)
 2    CONTINUE
      DO 4 J=I,N
 4    B(I,J)=-C(I,J)/C(I,I)
 1    CONTINUE
      DO 10 I=1,N
      DO 20 J=1,I
      BI(I,J)=0
      IF (I.EQ.J) BI(I,J)=1.
      IF (I.EQ.1) GOTO 20
      DO 30 K=2,I
 30   BI(I,J)=BI(I,J)+B(K-1,I)*BI(K-1,J)
 20   CONTINUE
      DO 40 J=1,I
 40   CI(I,J)=-BI(I,J)/C(I,I)
 10   CONTINUE
      DO 50 I=1,N
      DO 50 J=1,N
      X(I,J)=0
      DO 50 K=1,N
 50   X(I,J)=X(I,J)-BI(K,I)*CI(K,J)
      END
C ** CALCULATE MATRICES X1 AND X2
      SUBROUTINE X1X2(P,Q,ANZW,WIN,ANZR,RING,X1,X2,N,M)
      INTEGER ANZW,ANZR,P,Q
      REAL*8 WIN(ANZW),RING(ANZR),X1(ANZW,N),X2(ANZR,M),PFAK
      DO 10 I=1,ANZW
      WIN(I)=3.141592*WIN(I)/180.
```

```
      PFAK=1.
      X1(I,1)=1.
      DO 10 K=2,2*P,2
      X1(I,K)=DCOS(PFAK*WIN(I))
      X1(I,K+1)=DSIN(PFAK*WIN(I))
10    PFAK=PFAK+1.
      DO 20 I=1,ANZR
      DO 20 K=1,Q+1
20    X2(I,K)=(RING(I))**(K-1)
      END
TEST DATA FOR ANGLES 0,22.5,45,...,337.5 AND VERTICAL DATA 1,2,...7,8
INPUT DATA FILE 12 "SM": ORIGINAL BSPM DATA
  -.06  -.18  -.19  -.19  -.36  -.38  -.52  -.56
  -.04  -.03  -.25  -.42  -.67  -.66  -.65  -.50
  -.12  -.23  -.49  -.68  -.80  -.78  -.78  -.53
  -.04  -.10  -.34  -.95 -1.03  -.78  -.66  -.49
   .26   .04  -.18 -1.41 -1.61  -.90  -.67  -.50
   .33   .77  1.08  1.39   .55  -.30  -.37  -.21
   .53   .57  1.38  1.85  1.11  -.06   .00   .21
   .66   .84  1.09  1.27   .72   .17   .14   .13
   .49   .66  1.04  1.18   .95   .47   .36   .28
   .46   .63   .91   .75   .40   .36   .25   .26
   .38   .48   .45   .52   .41   .16  -.01  -.17
   .23   .19   .12   .12   .03  -.06  -.27  -.23
   .03   .01  -.09  -.12  -.12  -.27  -.41  -.39
  -.06  -.24  -.22  -.21  -.37  -.33  -.48  -.54
  -.12  -.27  -.25  -.23  -.39  -.51  -.49  -.54
  -.19  -.30  -.22  -.38  -.42  -.54  -.49  -.53
OUTPUT DATA: X MATRIX (HERE ONLY THE FIRST ROW FOR CONTROL)
 .1953 -.1395 -.0837  .0502  .0904  .0055 -.0948  .0390
REGRESSION COEFFICIENTS
 .0840  .0491  .0427 -.0198  .0016 -.4429  .3508 -.3194  .0685
-.0043 -.3492  .6012 -.2187  .0258 -.0009  .3022 -.4792  .2771
-.0497  .0028 -.3885  .7270 -.4305  .0818 -.0048  .2537 -.4157
 .2523 -.0489  .0029  .5128 -.8323  .4146 -.0726  .0041 -.3735
 .6719 -.3523  .0635 -.0037 -.0099 -.0428  .0696 -.0168  .0011
BY REGRESSION COEFFICIENTS RECONSTRUCTED AND SMOOTHED DATA
  -.09  -.12  -.22  -.34  -.44  -.50  -.54  -.54
  -.07  -.11  -.15  -.25  -.41  -.57  -.65  -.50
  -.08  -.20  -.45  -.69  -.83  -.82  -.69  -.51
  -.02  -.10  -.68 -1.19 -1.32 -1.05  -.61  -.54
   .14   .31  -.15  -.67  -.94  -.85  -.56  -.43
   .35   .72   .88   .72   .28  -.26  -.56  -.13
   .50   .85  1.43  1.60  1.15   .28  -.40   .16
   .56   .80  1.23  1.37  1.08   .47  -.02   .30
   .52   .78   .91   .88   .70   .46   .26   .30
   .44   .71   .80   .74   .58   .38   .22   .18
   .35   .46   .57   .58   .44   .19  -.03  -.04
   .24   .15   .14   .12   .04  -.09  -.23  -.29
   .08  -.05  -.13  -.19  -.25  -.30  -.36  -.44
  -.09  -.17  -.17  -.18  -.25  -.38  -.49  -.48
  -.17  -.27  -.25  -.24  -.30  -.43  -.54  -.51
  -.15  -.24  -.33  -.40  -.46  -.49  -.51  -.56
```

Chapter 30

AUTOMATED QUANTITATIVE VECTORCARDIOGRAPHY: THE LOUVAIN VCG-COMPUTER PROGRAM

C.R. BROHET, C. DERWAEL, R. FESLER, A. ROBERT, L.A. BRASSEUR

INTRODUCTION

In the last 10 years, we have developed a computerized system for the analysis and interpretation of Frank orthogonal electrocardiograms and vectorcardiograms (VCG). As compared with other ECG-computer programs, the main characteristics of the Louvain program are: [1] a quantitative analysis of the spatial VCG in both adults and children, [2] criteria which take into account age and sex stratified normal limits of various parameters, [3] diagnostic classification by two complementary methods, i.e. deterministic (decision-tree) and statistical (multivariate). The Louvain program has been thoroughly evaluated by objective method, i.e. by comparing the automatic interpretation with the clinical diagnosis validated from ECG-independent evidence.

METHODS OF ANALYSIS AND CLASSIFICATION

Figure 1 shows the main areas covered by the Louvain VCG-program. The input is the same for the adults and the pediatric programs, i.e. 10 seconds of Frank XYZ leads digitized at 500/sec with 12-bit resolution. After removal of baseline drift and selective beat averaging, a noise-free "averaged" P-QRS-T complex is submitted to wave recognition techniques in which a mixture of threshold-crossing and template-matching methods is applied to filtered spatial velocity curves.

Fig. 1 THE LOUVAIN COMPUTER PROGRAM FOR THE ANALYSIS AND INTERPRETATION OF ORTHOGONAL ELECTROCARDIOGRAMS

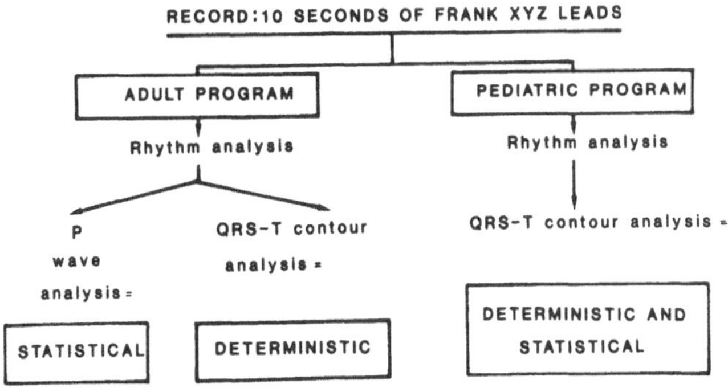

The rhythm analysis is similar in adults and in children, with some adaptation in the latter to accomodate for the higher heart rates and lower prevalence of rhythm disturbances in the pediatric age group. A total of 77 diagnostic statements is contained in the rhythm analysis section.

From the 260 vectorcardiographic parameters computed by the measurement program, about 80 are actually utilized for the diagnostic classification. More emphasis is placed on spatial parameters better able to quantify the severity of ventricular hypertrophy and to determine the location and extent of myocardial disease. Not only continuous variables (wave durations, linear and angular values of amplitude and area parameters) but also dichotomous variables such as direction of inscription of planar QRS loop are used in the diagnostic process.

The classification methods differ in the adult and the pediatric programs. In adults, normal age and sex ranges for VCG parameters were taken from the literature. The QRS-T contour analysis relies on the deterministic method in which the cardiologist's expertise is applied through Boolean algebra and decision-tree logic in order to reach a decision among a total of 199 diagnostic statements. The P wave contour analysis, by contrast, is performed by a multivariate statistical method which provides a probabilistic multigroup classification among 5 mutually exclusive diagnostic categories. In children, normal limits of pediatric VCG parameters were established from a local population. For the diagnostic interpretation of pediatric VCGs, both the deterministic and statistical methods are applied in sequence. The multiparameter - multithreshold procedure of the deterministic program (121 diagnostic statements) and the original multivariate statistical model for the multigroup diagnosis among 4 main diagnostic categories have been described (1-3).

RESULTS OF EVALUATION

Rhythm analysis (4)

In general, satisfactory results were found in the detection of most common cardiac arrhythmias. A correct diagnosis was obtained in 98% of cases with sinus rhythm, in 90% with atrial fibrillation, in 88% with premature ventricular complexes, in 86% of the electronic pacemakers and in 81% of the ectopic junctional rhythms. Existing algorithms have been improved for the detection of premature supraventricular complexes and of atrial flutter.

Analysis of adult VCGs (5,6)

The relative performance of the QRS-T contour analysis by the Louvain program (deterministic method) and the AVA program (7) (statistical analysis) on the same data set of 779 adult VCGs is shown in table 1. The higher sensitivity of AVA in most pathological categories was counterbalanced by a lower specificity.

Table 1: % CORRECT CLASSIFICATIONS IN MULTIGROUP DIAGNOSIS OF ADULT VCGs

	NORMAL (n=401)	LVH (n=135)	RVH (n=34)	COLD (n=16)	MI (n=193)	OVERALL (n=779)
AVA program	92	77	68	75	89	87
Louvain program	98	77	56	63	79	87
"Computer-assisted" physician	99	85	74	75	94	94

The overall diagnostic accuracy of 87% was identical for both programs. However, it was the so-called "computer-assisted" physician, i.e. the final decision made by the cardiologist using all pieces of information (12- and 3-lead tracings + computer print-out) which allowed to reach the highest degree of diagnostic accuracy (94% overall). The results of the multivariate analysis of P wave contours by the Louvain program have recently been reported (6). In a selected series of 260 records validated by ECG-independent means, using as best discriminators 6 linear and 1 angular P wave parameters, the percentages of correct multigroup classification were: 89% for the total group, 95% in normals, 79% in left atrial enlargement, 86% in right atrial enlargement, 64% in biatrial enlargement and 95% in intra-atrial conduction defect. Single differentiation between normal and abnormal P wave was correct in 96% of the cases with a sensitivity of 98% and a specificity of 95%.

Analysis of pediatric VCGs (8)
In children, the Louvain pediatric VCG-program was evaluated on a testing group of 500 unselected cases whose VCGs were prospectively collected as part of the daily routine load and, again, documented by means of ECG-independent data. Table 2 shows the results in terms of completely correct classifications by the deterministic (DET) and the statistical (STAT) methods. Both methods showed similar scores of overall diagnostic accuracy and specificity.

Table 2: AUTOMATIC INTERPRETATION OF PEDIATRIC VCGs BY THE LOUVAIN PROGRAM.

	LVH (n=113)	RVH (n=140)	BVH (n=83)	NORMAL (n=164)	TOTAL (n=500)
STAT correct:	62%	79%	47%	69%	66%
DET correct:	68%	73%	37%	70%	65%

The sensitivity of STAT was higher than that of DET in RVH and in BVH whereas that of DET was higher in LVH. Table 3 shows the diagnostic performance reached by the "computer-assisted" physician who could utilize both the visual analysis of the VCG and the 2 sets of computer-printout provided by the 2 diagnostic methods. The sum of partially correct and completely correct classifications reached the level of 86% without much variation between the various diagnostic groups.

Table 3: "COMPUTER-ASSISTED" INTERPRETATION OF PEDIATRIC VCGs WITH THE LOUVAIN PROGRAM

	LVH	RVH	BVH	NORMAL	TOTAL
1. Correct	57%	61%	52%	69%	61%
2. Partially correct	27%	29%	36%	16%	25%
3. Incorrect	16%	10%	12%	15%	14%
1 + 2	84%	90%	88%	85%	86%

DISCUSSION AND CONCLUSION

The choice of the Frank orthogonal lead system instead of the standard 12-lead ECG for processing by the Louvain computer program was determined by several reasons. First, without loss of basic information content, the 3 orthogonal leads provide for a 4-fold reduction in the amount of data being processed. Willems found that the multigroup accuracy of a logistic classification model was similar whether it be applied to the 12 lead-ECG or to XYZ data (9). Secondly, more quantitative data related to normal ranges of various parameters and better correlation with hemodynamic and anatomical data are available from the Frank leads than from any other lead system. Thirdly, orthogonality is essential to compute parameters which involve elements of spatial geometry. In the CSE study the measurement performance of XYZ programs was generally better than that of 12-lead programs (10). Furthermore, the contribution of VCG analysis to the increased accuracy in diagnostic electrocardiography has been documented in numerous studies. Among our clinicians, this automated VCG analysis is perceived as a complementary opinion supplementing that obtained from conventional ECG reading.

Characteristic features of the Louvain VCG-program include a quantitative analysis of the spatial VCG, the production of high resolution VCG loops for visual inspection, and the diagnostic classification by two different methods, leading to a complete interpretation in children from birth to adolescence, and in adults. The various parts of the Louvain VCG-program have been thoroughly evaluated with respect to the true clinical diagnosis determined from non-ECG clinical evidence. In the hands of experienced users, the Louvain system reaches a satisfactory level of diagnostic performance. It provides the user with pertinent information about the cardiac electrical activity as related to underlying anatomic and functional cardiac conditions. In the setting of non-invasive cardiac evaluation, we believe that it represents an important step toward "near-optimal" electrocardiography, both for the purpose of screening and for that of the differential diagnosis in a clinical environment with a high prevalence of cardiac diseases.

REFERENCES

1. BROHET CR, DERWAEL-BARCHY C, ROBERT A, FESLER R, STIJNS M, BRASSEUR LA, VLIERS A: Computer Interpretation of Pediatric Frank Vectorcardiograms in the evaluation of Congenital Heart Disease, Am J Cardiol 52: 127, 1983.
2. ROBERT A, DERWAEL-BARCHY C, FESLER R, STIJNS M, VLIERS A, BRASSEUR LA, BROHET CR: Computer Interpretation of Pediatric Vectorcardiograms by Multivariate Statistical Classification Techniques. IEEE 1984 Proceedings of Computers in Cardiology (Aachen, Germany, 1983).
3. BROHET CR, ROBERT A, DERWAEL C, FESLER R, STIJNS M, VLIERS A, BRASSEUR LA: Computer interpretation of pediatric orthogonal electrocardiograms: statistical and deterministic classification methods, Circulation, 70:255,1984
4. BROHET CR, DERWAEL-BARCHY C, FESLER R, BRASSEUR LA: Arrhythmia analysis by the Louvain VCG program, IEEE 1982 Proceedings of Computers in Cardiology (Florence, Italy, 1981).
5. BROHET C, DERWAEL-BARCHY C, FESLER R, BRASSEUR L: Computer-assisted interpretation of orthogonal electrocardiograms and vectorcardiograms by the Louvain system. Acta Cardiologica, Suppl. XXVI, 19:28, 1981.
6. BROHET CR, ROBERT A, DERWAEL C, FESLER R, BRASSEUR L: Computer interpretation of P wave contours in the orthogonal electrocardiogram by multivariate statistical analysis. IEE 1984 Proceedings of Computers in Cardiology (Salt Lake City, 1984).
7. PIPBERGER HV; The ECG computer analysis system developed in the U.S. Veterans Administration. Trends in Computer-Processed Electrocardiograms, North-Holland Publishing Co., 1977.
8. BROHET CR, ROBERT A, DERWAEL C, FESLER R, STIJNS M, VLIERS A, BRASSEUR LA: The Louvain computer program for the analysis and interpretation of pediatric orthogonal electrocardiograms. Proceedings of the Working Conference on "Computer ECG analysis" (Leuven, Belgium,1985) North-Holland Publishing Co, in press, 1985.
9. WILLEMS JL, LESAFFRE E, PARDAENS J, DE SCHREYE D: Multigroup logistic classification of the standard 12- and 3-lead ECG. Proceedings of the Working Conference on "Computer ECG analysis" (Leuven, Belgium, 1985), North-Holland Publishing Co, in press, 1985.
10. WILLEMS JL, ARNAUD P, VAN BEMMEL J et al: Assessment of the performance of electrocardiographic computer programs with the use of a reference data base. Circulation 71: 523, 1985.

Chapter 31

QUANTITATIVE VECTORCARDIOGRAPHY. A SPATIAL APPROACH AS THE BASIS OF A NEW DIAGNOSTIC LOGIC

P. ARNAUD

A spatial approach of the cardiac electrical field by the means of three corrected leads was proved as a powerful diagnostic method which provided valuable improvements. Indeed the Vectorcardiography allows a quantitative analysis of only one tracing, the VCG loop in space, which contains a large amount of information. Numerous parameters have been selected in order to constitute the basis of a new set of diagnostic criteria. A particular logic for automated interpretation was developed.

Furthermore the VCG data are easy to store. Large data bases may be collected for statistical analysis and for research studies. More recently sequential analysis was introduced and proved to be of great interest.

The fundamental characteristics of Vectorcardiography may be summarized briefly. The three corrected leads X,Y,Z are the axes of an orthogonal frame of reference having the electrical center of the ventricles, the point O, as origin. By computing these signals a spatial loop is constructed along time. It reflects most directly the cardiac electrical field, as well as the process of the ventricular activation and the intracardiac potentials.

It is well known that normal and pathological events bring about electrical forces that develop following a spatial pattern. The fundamental studies of DURRER and VAN DAM have shown this pattern in the human heart with very detailed maps. Thus by methods of spatial geometry, we may have, at each time, a vector which expresses the exact balance of opposite forces, according to the concept of the "single dipole".

The three orthogonal leads are supposed to be parallel with the respective axes of the thorax: transversal, vertical and sagittal axes. Of course such a frame of reference is quite different from the surface thoracic reference used in the body mapping approach.

Since the VCG leads are orthogonal to one another, no redundancy is to be expected.

More recently a new methodology was born: Quantitative Vectorcardiography. The spatial curve is well defined geometrically. So the mathematical analysis may be easy and very detailed as compared to the usual scalar ECG analysis. Valuable progress was made when a large number of spatial parameters along time could be derived by computer processing. For example 200 parameters are computed by the "Lyon program". We established many years ago a new set of diagnostic criteria, as follows:

The spatial VCG criteria of QRS may be sorted in four groups:

I. Certain criteria, namely amplitudes of the vectors, express the power of the different cardiac generators,

II. others point out the orientation of successive electrical forces and their spatial distribution.

III. others are related to the dynamics and to the timing of electrical forces,

IV. various criteria are related to the morphology, the pattern of the loop, its rotating direction, its planarity, etc.

Group I: This concerns the ELECTRICAL POWER OF THE GENERATORS. THE MAGNITUDE OF A RESULTANT VECTOR has the meaning of a specific state of balance between numerous generators at any given time. So the amplitude of the maximal QRS vector indicates the maximal gradient between opposite forces. It is decreased when the left ventricular function is depressed, as well as the ventricular work (for example in mitral stenosis). The amplitude is increased in left ventricular hypertrophy provided that the left ventricle keeps working in near normal conditions, that is to say normal cardiac metabolism, sufficient coronary perfusion, etc. In contrast, if a severe coronary insufficiency appears, the amplitude becomes normal or decreased.

The correlation between the left ventricular mass and the QRS amplitude in the cases of left ventricular hypertrophy has been proven to be stronger when VCG is used instead of ECG.

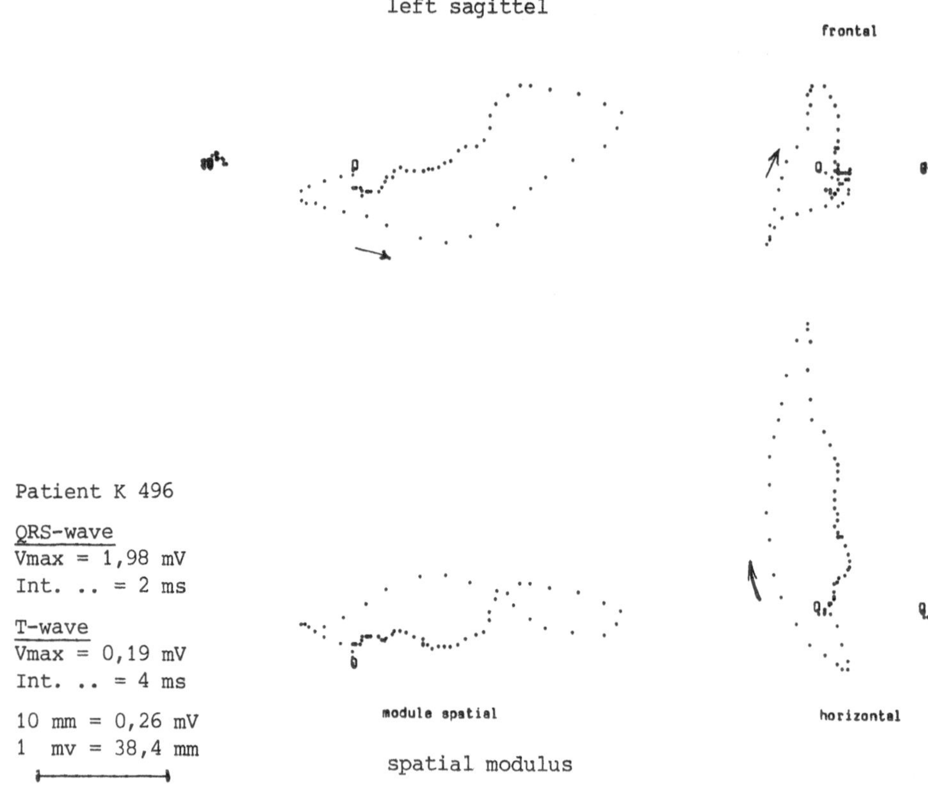

Fig. 1: An example of VCG projections, showing a pseudo-necrosis and some complex left ventricular conduction disturbances from a patient suffering a congestive myocardiopathy.

```
PATIENT: K      496                                        (COMPLEX 2,9 SEC.)

                  DURATIONS (MS) :      P      PQ      QRS     T      QT     QT C
                                                       128    172    360     417


                QRS WAVE                     I               ST-T SEGMENT
                                             I
                                             I
          OCT  AZI ELE AMPLIT R A  ST O D AREA I        OCT  AZI ELE AMPLIT  ST AREA
               (°) (°)  (MV)  (%) (MS)(MS)(%)  I             (°) (°)  (MV)  (MS)(%)
                                             I
MAX V   PDS +092 -11  1,980      050         I MAX V  AGS -006 -18   ,196 084
                                             I
H A V   PDS +092 -08  1,921 097 048          I
                                             I OJ V   PGI +027 +34   ,105
S A V   AGI -016 +36  1,287 070              I
                                             I
M O V   AGI -066 +27   ,490 025 016 020 004  I M O V  PGS +006 -24          076 058
        PDI +100 +02  1,411 071 042 022 034  I        AGS -006 -18          084 042
        PDS +092 -11  1,980 100 050 016 040  I        AGI    0   0          172 000
        PGS +088 -25  1,313 066 060 028 017  I
        PGI +070 +02   ,529 027 092 038 005  I SPATIAL AREA (MV2)               ,03
        AGI -018 +66   ,156 008 128 004 000  I
                                             I ANGLE QMAXV TMAXV  095
SPATIAL AREA (MV2)                     1,84  I ANGLE Q HAV TMAXV  096
                                             I
NOTCH               *0                       I ANGLE TMAXV T HAV  013
                                             I
ROTATION :                                   I ROTATION :
PLAN H :  HOR                                I PLAN H :  HOR
PLAN F :  HOR                                I PLAN F :  FH FH HOR
                                             I
                                             I
```

```
PATIENT: DIAT              LOUIS        M      52  ANS      52  KG      165 CM

K 496          28/06/83  09H05MN                          DEPARTMENT: DESCOS

                      ANALYSIS AND PROPOSED INTERPRETATIONS

                                     RHYTHM

ATRIAL FIBRILLATION. VENTRICULAR RATE ABOUT 81.

NON SATISFIED
CRITERIA (NB)                       QRS COMPLEX

   1   COMPLETE LEFT BUNDLE BRANCH BLOCK PROBABLY ASSOCIATED WITH SEPTAL NECROSI
       S AND WITH LEFT VENTRICULAR HYPERTROPHY (74-162-163-173-161-178)

   2   RIGHT VENTRICULAR HYPERTROPHY AND INCOMPLETE RIGHT BUNDLE BRANCH BLOCK (9
       2-110-83)

   3   COMPLETE LEFT BUNDLE BRANCH BLOCK PROBABLY ASSOCIATED WITH LATERAL NECROS
       IS AND WITH LEFT VENTRICULAR HYPERTROPHY (74-6-114-110-162-163-173-161-17
       8)

   3   RIGHT VENTRICULAR HYPERTROPHY (110-83-189)

   3   COMPLETE RIGHT BUNDLE BRANCH BLOCK POSSIBLY ASSOCIATED WITH SLIGHT RIGHT
       VENTRICULAR HYPERTROPHY (91-78-36)

   3   COMPLETE RIGHT BUNDLE BRANCH BLOCK AND LEFT VENTRICULAR HYPERTROPHY (92-9
       3-91-77)
                           VENTRICULAR REPOLARIZATION

   0   REPOLARIZATION ABNORMALITIES (IF ISCHEMIA , INFERIOR LOCALIZATION)

REVIEWED BY :
COMMENTS    :4 E ESPACE
```

Fig. 2 : Automated results (same patient as in figure 1). Top = the main parameters of QRS, ST and T. Bottom = rhythm analysis and contour interpretation. Concerning QRS only the first diagnosis of the list is to be considered.

If a left bundle branch block is associated with a left ventricular hypertrophy the maximal vector increase is then the only criterion which is able to reveal the presence of a left ventricular hypertrophy.

The values of the maximal spatial vector may be judged very low below 1mV, low below 1.35 mV, increased above 1.8 or 2 mV, and largely increased beyond 3 mV. So we may appreciate the degree of left ventricular hypertrophy.

THE TOTAL AREA OF THE SPATIAL LOOP is equivalent to the sum of gradients. It is a less accurate criterion because it is influenced by the shape more or less elongated of the loop. When it is larger than 2.8 mV^2 it suggests a left ventricular hypertrophy.

Group II: ORIENTATION OF THE SUCCESSIVE ELECTRICAL FORCES AND THEIR SPATIAL DISTRIBUTION.

If a part of the QRS loop deviates from the usual normal pattern, this fact is considered as the most important diagnostic criterion.

The orientation of the MAXIMAL VECTOR expresses the resulting balance in the middle part of the loop. In contrast, the HALF AREA VECTOR more clearly shows the general orientation of the entirety of the loop. Azimuth and elevation angles are measured. It may be noted that the elevation of a spatial vector is quite different from the angle calculated in the frontal plane from the ECG because the latter is distorded by a projection effect.

The spatial orientation of the FIRST ACTIVITY detected, provided it is recognized as significant, and of the FIRST VECTORS (0.01 s and 0.02 s) is of great interest. This approach of the Q waves problem is more accurate than with the scalar method, particularly in the cases of necrosis and pseudo-necrosis.

In order to appreciate the relative importance of electrical forces oriented to the left and the right, up and down, front and back, we utilize the method of octantal characterization. In each of the eight octants we measure:

- an OCTANTAL AREA, expressed as a percentage of the total QRS area,
- the AMPLITUDE of the MAXIMAL OCTANTAL VECTOR expressed in absolute value and as a percentage of the maximal maximorum vector amplitude.

These orientation parameters are very sensitive to pathological disturbances. They are applied in many diagnoses, such as: - Infarcts: anteroseptal necrosis is detected when the first QRS octant is left posterior. Inferior necrosis is concerned by the maximal vector in the superior left anterior octant which must be larger than 40% of the maximal maximorum vector. In posterior necrosis we use the left anterior area which must be larger than 48% of the total area, and the maximal vector which must be deviated forward with an azimuth of less than -30°. In antero-lateral necrosis, half-area vector orientation is used to appreciate the rightward deviation. - Right ventricular hypertrophy: in the second part of QRS the right posterior area is increased between 22% and 35% at an initial stage of overload. It is up to 35% at a medium stage of evolution. At an advanced stage it is the right anterior area which has to be considered: it is larger than 20%.

- Intra-ventricular blocks: we can observe posterior deviation of the entirety of the loop in left bundle branch block, right deviation in left posterior fascicular block, upper deviation in left anterior fascicular block, right anterior deviation of the terminal part of the loop in right bundle branch block associated with left anterior fascicular block.

GROUP III: DYNAMICS, TIMING AND CHRONOLOGICAL ORDER OF THE ELECTRICAL FORCES.

THE VELOCITY DIAGRAM as a function of time shows the linear velocity along the spatial trajectory. Its abnormalities, such as a slowing of the terminal part, proved to be of interest in daily practice.

Various parameters are calculated:

- THE MAXIMAL VELOCITY in the initial or in the terminal segment,
- THE DURATION OF THE ACTIVITY IN EACH OCTANT,
- THE TIME OF APPEARANCE OF THE VECTORS from the beginning of QRS,
- THE TIME ELAPSED BETWEEN TWO VECTORS.

These parameters are involved in the detection of either a lengthening of activation time, for example in left ventricular hypertrophy, or a slackening of activation process in a sector of a ventricle, in cases of infarcts or myocardiopathies, or a conduction defect: bundle branch or fascicular blocks, or preexcitation syndrom.

GROUP IV: MORPHOLOGY AND STRUCTURE OF THE SPATIAL LOOP.
The morphological features are fundamental characteristics of a given individual. They largely depend on constitutional factors particular to each heart. They remain very stable in any detail on the whole life. Conversely they are very sensitive if a cardiac trouble appears, even a minor one. Therefore the interest of analysing these parameters and repeating the records along time on the same subject.
Are analyzed:

- THE GENERAL MORPHOLOGY of the loop by comparing with the normal one.
- IRREGULARITIES, notches, changes in direction, curve developed in two parts.
- Presence of a CONCAVITY on the initial branch which is nearly always significant of myocardial infarct,
- the degree of PLANARITY of the spatial loop which is a very interesting criterion, as a nearly perfect planarity -at least 80% of the QRS area- suggests that the ventricles are normal. On the contrary almost all pathological situations distort QRS planarity to various degrees.
- THE DIRECTION OF ROTATION of the loop, namely on the horizontal projection, is an important criterion. It is observed: - counterclockwise in normal QRS and in isolated right bundle branch block. In this case a complementary criterion "no succession from the inferior left anterior octant to the right anterior octant" suggests a right bundle branch block without right ventricular hypertroply. - clockwise in left bundle branch block (the curve being developed in the left posterior quadrant), in lateral necrosis (right posterior quadrant), in severe right ventricular hypertrophy (right anterior quadrant).

THE T-WAVE is computed in the same way, but the parameters are more simple. The ST-SEGMENT is measured in space, as well as THE QRS-T ANGLE.

A new diagnostic logic
On the basis of these different types of criteria, a new methodology had to be elaborated, that means a strategy able to characterize all the diagnoses involving depolarization and repolarization following a particular logic in space. This logic no longer involves the signal recorded, but parameters at a second level, that is to say characteristics of an unique curve, that are related to notions of magnitude, orientation, timing and morphology. This approach is more complex than the traditional one, but it has the advantage of being in close relationship with our knowledge of pathophysiology. It is thus in principle more efficient and easy to understand. In addition it is easy to be utilized in an automated system of the type "expert system".

For each diagnosis A SPATIAL MODEL was established using a set of criteria judged as the most significant ones and closely related to the process of the ventricular activation. These criteria are listed on a table, like a table of decision. In average there are twelve criteria in each table.

It is important to note that each diagnosis is not only described in itself, but also contrasted with all the other diagnoses. It results in a COMPETITION between all diagnoses. So we have positive criteria (specific of the concerned diagnosis), discriminative criteria relatively to the other diagnoses, and in addition complementary ones which may be useful in bordeline tracings.

The STRUCTURE OF A CRITERION is either one parameter which must satisfy a particular condition, for instance a threshold value, or two or several criteria linked one with others by "and" or "or". Sometimes a criterion is repeated twice or more on the same table. These procedures are useful to introduce a certain PONDERATION of a criterion depending on its weight, more or less important, in such a diagnosis.

Such a methodology is performant enough not only to indicate the stage of evolution of a ventricular overload (see before the example of right ventricular hypertrophy), but also to allow the determination point by point of COMPLEX DIAGNOSES. It may be illustrated by two examples, as follows:

- A subset of five diagnoses is considered: complete right bundle branch block, either isolated or associated with different degrees of right ventricular hypertrophy which are: "possible and mild" "probable and moderate", "certain", "severe". In order to discriminate these diagnoses, two parameters are used together (see fig. 3), the right posterior area (as the ordinate of the graphic) and the right anterior area (as the abscissa). Various threshold values allow to delimit the intersections between the five diagnoses. In addition they are supported by other criteria such as magnitude and orientation of certain vectors, direction of rotation, etc. (see fig. 4).

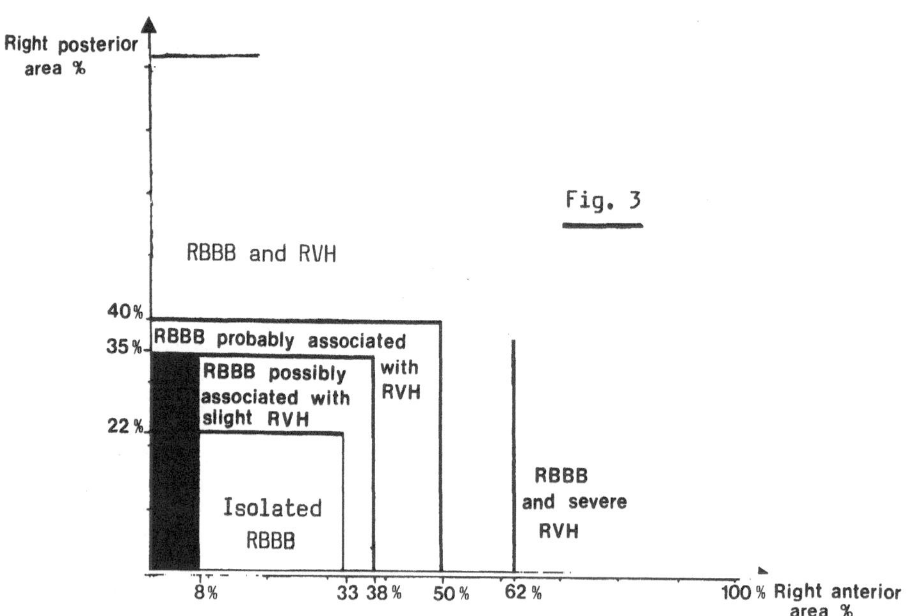

Fig. 3.

QRS parameters		Isolated RBBB	RBBB possibly associated with slight RVH	RBBB probably associated with RVH	RBBB and RVH	RBBB and severe RVH
Half-area vector orientation		Inferior left anterior or inf. left posterior or inf. right posterior		/	/	/
Maximal spatial Vector	Octant	Inferior left posterior or * Inferior left anterior		Inferior left posterior or right posterior or * inferior left anterior		Inf. left ant. or right ant. or right post.
	Azimuth	*< 40°				/
	Magnitude	< 2 mV		< 2.1 mV		/
Maximal inf. left anterior vector Magnitude (%)		> 47%	/	/	/	/
Right posterior area %		< 22	22 - 35 / < 35	35 - 40 / < 40	> 40 / /	/
Right anterior area %		8 - 33	8 - 38 / 33 - 38	< 50 / 38 - 50	< 62 / 50 - 62	> 62
Rotation horizontal projection		NO CLOCKWISE				/

Fig. 4: Each column represents a diagnostic table. The five diagnoses, involving RBBB and RVH, are the same as in figure 3.

C LBBB+probably AL N+LVO

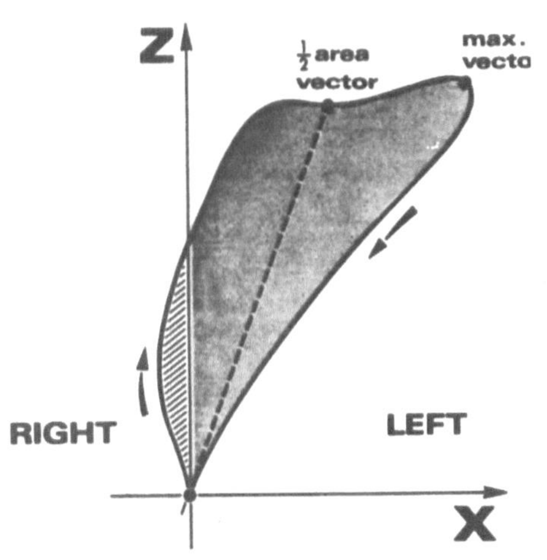

Fig. 5.

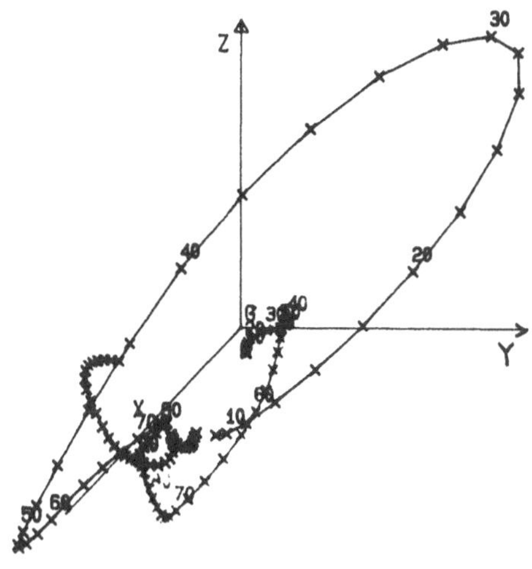

Fig. 6: Two successive loops of the same patient in space: the first (bigger one) with inferior necrosis and right bundle branch block, the second one with anterior necrosis and left anterior fasicular block in addition.

CONCLUSION

The major interest of the Vectorcardiography is not the data reduction (only 3 leads by using 7 electrodes) but the progress introduced by A PARTICULAR STRATEGY OF DIAGNOSIS. Indeed with the SPATIAL CRITERIA all the information we need in daily practice seems to be available. An in-deep analysis and a good understanding of electrical mechanisms may be obtained.

The DIGITAL METHODS are able to process this information in a better way than traditional ones. They may provide valuable improvements. So the aid to diagnosis is more efficient.

Another point to be debated is the present state of STANDARDISATION. Some procedures are well standardized and currently accepted by the cardiologists, namely:

- lead system, as the Frank's system is widely used,
- data acquisition techniques and digital methods,
- graphic display of the curves.

But we do not have yet any standardisation of the diagnostic criteria.

There remains the problem of the DATA BASES: large data bases well documented and validated exist in several centers, but they have to be still increased in order to develop new research projects.

PART 6

MODEL STUDIES

Chapter 32

FORWARD PROBLEM SIMULATIONS OF THE WOLFF-PARKINSON-WHITE SYNDROME WITH A MULTIPLE-DIPOLE HEART MODEL

R.M. GULRAJANI, M. LORANGE, F.A. ROBERGE

1. INTRODUCTION

This paper begins with a brief review of the different types of computer models of the heart, then touches upon solution methodologies for solving the forward problem of electrocardiography, and finally describes the results obtained with forward problem simulations of the Wolff-Parkinson-White syndrome using a particular example of a computer model of the heart.

2. COMPUTER MODELS OF THE HEART

2.1. Types of models

In general, two broad categories of heart models may be defined: those models that use element-to-element propagation to automatically generate activation isochrones, and those that simply postulate a set of fixed activation isochrones corresponding to normal excitation. The fixed-isochrone category of model is obviously of more restricted applicability, since cardiac abnormalities that involve an altered activation pattern are not easily simulated. Both types of models are considered here.

2.1.1. Propagation-type heart models. Strangely enough, some of the earliest computer heart models were of the propagation type (1, 2, 3). These models of necessity employ rather large-scale models of the ventricular myocardium, consisting of several thousands of cell elements, in order that the simulated activation isochrones be sufficiently smooth. The points of initial activity on the endocardium are either specified manually, or are determined from a prior simulation involving a similar cellular model of the His-Purkinje system. The basic principle of propagation-type heart models was described by Solomon and Selvester (2), and is a computer implementation of the so-called Huygens' wavefront construction. In one form of computer implementation of this construction, spherical wavelets of radius $r = vt$ are described around every initially activated point. Here v is the assumed-isotropic myocardial-wavefront propagation velocity, and t the isochrone interval. Those unactivated model points that fall within these spheres are deemed to be activated at time t. These newly-activated points then serve as the centers for the spherical wavelets determining the points activated at time $2t$, and so on, till the entire model heart is activated. Other assumptions are a faster, but again isotropic, propagation velocity within the His-Purkinje system and usually an absolutely refractory cell-element so that only one cardiac excitation cycle is simulated.

An interesting variant of the basic propagation-type model described above has been developed by Eifler et al. (4). This model uses 24,413 excitable elements to represent the ventricles. Each element is of rhombododecahedral shape and has four distinct states - resting, depolarizing, absolutely refractory, and relatively refractory. Activation is simulated using a set of state-dependent transition rules between elements. With all types of propagation models, because the isochrones are self-generated, conduction abnormalities are easily simulated.

2.1.2. Fixed-isochrone heart models. As already mentioned, these models (5, 6, 7) postulate a set of normal activation isochrones, usually those first described for the isolated human heart by Durrer et al (8). Because no propagation has to be simulated, a smaller number of cell elements may be used. The limitation with respect to simulating conduction abnormalities has already been mentioned.

2.2. Converting isochrones to equivalent dipoles

Once the entire heart model is activated, i.e. the isochrones determined, for computation of the surface potentials the usual step involves replacing the isochrones with equivalent dipoles. There are two methods to achieve this, either by replacing the wavefront area by a layer of dipoles, or by replacing the volume of active myocardium by a dipole moment density.

2.2.1. Two-dimensional dipole layer. Here the vector area of the activation wavefront during QRS is replaced by a dipole layer of strength proportional to this area and oriented normal to the wavefront (3, 6). More recently, to take into account the anisotropy of myocardial conductivity, Colli-Franzone et al. (9) have advocated the use of oblique dipole layers to represent the front. The disadvantage with this essentially two-dimensional equivalent dipole layer approach is that it is only valid when sharp wavefronts are present, i.e. during QRS and not during ST-T.

2.2.2. Three-dimensional dipole moment density. Here the volume of active myocardium is replaced by a dipole moment density $\vec{p}$, given by (7, 10),

$$\vec{p} = -\left(\frac{g_i\, g_e}{g_i + g_e}\right)\nabla V_m , \qquad [1]$$

that acts in the extracellular myocardial space. Clearly $\vec{p}$ exists only where the spatial gradient of the transmembrane potential distribution V_m is non-zero. The quantities g_i and g_e are respectively the effective intracellular and extracellular conductivities of the network of myocardial cells. The transmembrane potential distribution V_m at every model point is determined from the isochrones and an assumed transmembrane cardiac action potential waveform. This approach was used by Miller and Geselowitz (11) to conveniently simulate myocardial ischemia, by appropriately varying the action potential waveform allotted to "ischemic" model points. Whichever approach is used to obtain the equivalent dipoles, for greater computational tractability in calculating the surface potentials the smaller elemental dipoles are summed according to heart region, and the resultant 20 to 30 equivalent dipoles assumed to act at the region centroids, resulting in the well-known "multiple-dipole" heart model.

2.3 A heart model for the eighties

Given the computing power readily available today, clearly any heart model for the eighties must be a propagation-type model with dipole moments computed via equation [1]. Such a model may well be able to simulate all major cardiac abnormalities, those involving action potential waveform changes such as ischemia as well as those involving altered conduction such as bundle branch blocks. One model with this versatility was the one developed by Eifler et al. (4). A second was recently described by Lorange and Gulrajani (12), who implemented a modified Huygens' wavefront construction into the fixed-isochrone Miller-Geselowitz model (7, 11). The modification entailed attempting to account for anisotropic myocardial conductivity, and hence anisotropic propagation velocities, by employing ellipsoidal instead of spherical wavelets in the Huygens' construction. Lorange and Gulrajani assumed that the anisotropic effects of the parallel layers of differing

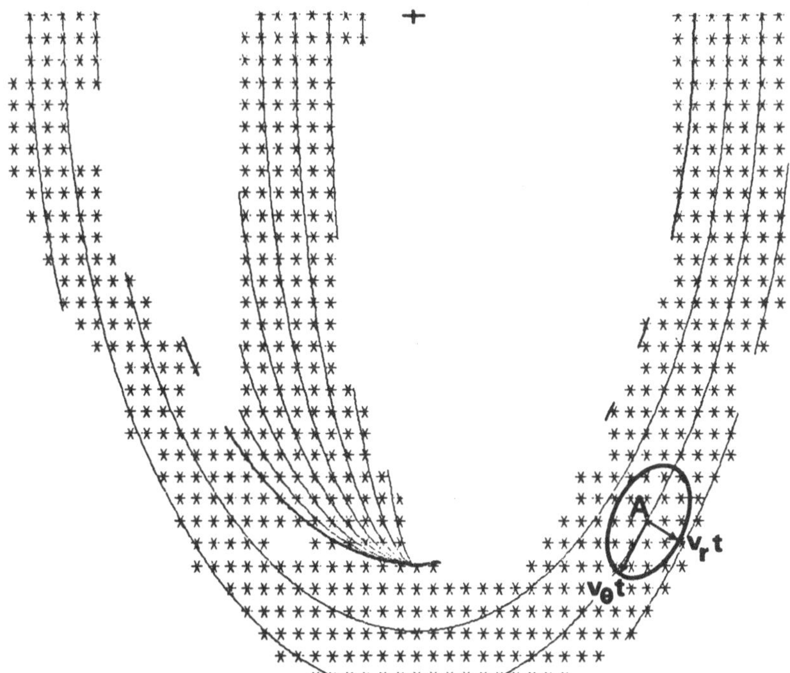

FIGURE 1. Longitudinal view of the heart model showing segments of the ellipsoids of revolution that approximate the model geometry, as well as an ellipsoidal Huygens' wavelet around point A. From Ref (12), © IEEE.

fibre orientations from endocardium to epicardium could be represented, in a macroscopic sense, by a thick block of anisotropic tissue, with one axis of low electrical conductivity oriented from endocardium to epicardium and with the other two perpendicular axes of equal but higher conductivity. The low conductivity value was simply the effective electrical conductivity across cardiac fibres, whereas the higher conductivity was an average value of the effective conductivities across and along cardiac fibres. Accordingly propagation from a model point A (see Fig. 1) was characterized by an ellipsoid of revolution with semi-axes $v_r t$, $v_\theta t$, $v_\theta t$, oriented so that the direction of slower velocity v_r coincided with the endocardium to epicardium direction at A. This direction was approximated by first fitting the geometry of the heart model with a family of ellipsoids of revolution (thin lines in Fig. 1), and then taking the gradient of the analytic equation describing the particular ellipsoid of revolution passing through A.

Starting from initiation sites on the endocardial surface of the Miller-Geselowitz heart model, Lorange and Gulrajani were able to automatically generate the activation isochrones corresponding to normal excitation of the human heart (see Fig. 2). To generate smooth isochrones, it was found necessary to double the density of model points in each direction, thereby increasing the number of model points, from 4000 in the original Miller-Geselowitz model, to over 25,000. The numbers in Figure 2 represent the activation times in tens of milliseconds, e.g. a 1 represents points activated 10 msec into QRS, a 2 those additional points activated between 10 and 20 msec into QRS, etc.

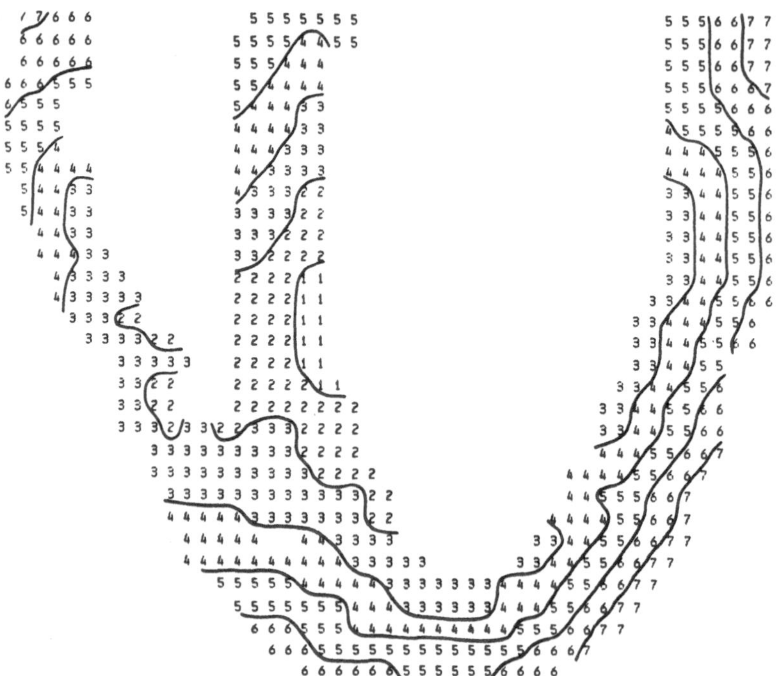

FIGURE 2. Simulated isochrones corresponding to normal excitation. The velocities used were v_r = 38 cm/sec and v_θ = 72 cm/sec.

3. SOLUTION METHODOLOGIES FOR THE FORWARD PROBLEM

Once the activation isochrones have been converted to equivalent dipoles, the forward problem of electrocardiography needs to be solved to obtain the body surface potentials. It is well known that quasi-static conditions apply to the forward problem due to the fact that propagation, capacitive and inductive effects may be neglected (13). Under these conditions the potential is governed by Poisson's equation, with the added boundary conditions of continuity of potential, as well as that of the normal component of current, across conductivity interfaces. To date the most common approach to numerical solutions of the forward problem has been to solve integral equation formulations derived from Poisson's equation and the boundary conditions. Recently, however, the solution of Poisson's equation via a variational principle is rapidly gaining greater acceptance.

3.1 Integral equation formulations

Either of two integral equation formulations may be used, and as yet there is no consensus as to which of the two is the better approach from a computational standpoint. The first approach solves for the single-layer secondary charges, induced on each surface element separating conductivity interfaces in the torso model employed in the forward problem. The desired potentials on each surface element are obtained in a subsequent step from the calculated charges. An iterative procedure for obtaining these charges, based on intuitive physical arguments, was first proposed by Gelernter and Swihart (14). The underlying intergral equation for the charge, on which the procedure was based, was described later by Rush et al. (15). The second integral equation approach was proposed by Barr et al. (16), and directly derives the potential on each surface element without the need to compute its surface charge. Solution procedures for both integral equation formulations first involve obtaining approximate matrix representations of the respective integral equations (17). However, the usual forward problem employing current dipoles as heart sources is indeterminate to within an additive constant for the potential, leading to singular coefficient matrices, and solution procedures that are far from straightforward (18, 19). One advantage with integral equation approaches is that because only surface elements between interfaces are involved, as opposed to three-dimensional volume elements spanning the entire torso geometry, smaller matrix dimensions result.

3.2 Variational or finite-element formulation

Here a variational principle is used to show that the solution to Poisson's equation, together with the above-mentioned boundary conditions, is obtained by finding a potential function that minimizes an appropriate energy functional (20, 21). The approach is more commonly termed the finite-element method, because it employs a three-dimensional volume representation of the torso employing finite volume-elements, unlike integral equation formulations that only characterize the torso by its two-dimensional conductivity interfaces. Solutions via the finite-element method can also result in singular matrix equations, and the same techniques are used to circumvent this as with integral equation approaches.

In the past the main drawback of the finite-element method applied to electrocardiography was the large dimensions of the resulting coefficient matrix. With the ever-decreasing cost of computing power, and with special computational algorithms (22) designed to take advantage of the sparseness of the finite-element coefficient matrix, this is no longer a problem. Moreover the finite-element method can, in principle, handle anisotropies and varying inhomogeneities within the torso geometry. Finally, a recent simulation study by Pilkington et al. (23) suggests that the finite-element method results in slightly improved accuracies for the computed surface potentials than those obtained with integral equation formulations. More dramatic improvements in solution accuracy were noted when inverse electrocardiographic solutions were attempted with the two approaches, promising to give an increased impetus to the finite-element method.

4. SIMULATIONS OF THE WOLFF-PARKINSON-WHITE SYNDROME

This final section depicts the use of the modified propagation type Miller-Geselowitz heart model described earlier in simulating one type of conduction disturbance, namely the Wolff-Parkinson-White preexcitation syndrome. Here, as is well-known, preexcitation of the basal ventricle occurs ahead of normal His-Purkinje excitation, and the QRS complex is a fusion beat characterized by an early delta wave

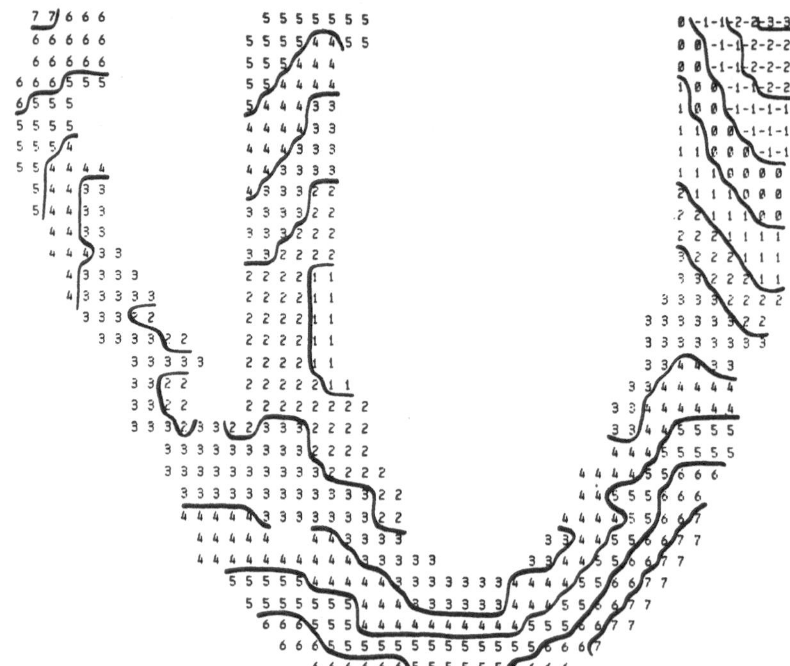

FIGURE 3. Simulated isochrones corresponding to preexcitation from a left lateral site.

reflecting preexcitation. An anomalous accessory pathway bridging the auricles and ventricles underlies the preexcitation. Occasionally this pathway can act as the substrate for a circus tachycardia, in which case its surgical excision is indicated. Precise determination of the accessory pathway site is only possible via open-heart epicardial mapping protocols prior to excision, though the pattern of the body surface potential maps (BSPMs), during the delta wave reflecting preexcitation, and during the early ST-segment reflecting repolarization of the preexcited region, has proved a useful non-invasive index of the approximate site of the accessory pathway. In fact, Benson et al. (24) have published characteristic BSPMs during the delta wave of QRS and during the early ST-segment for each of eight preexcitation sites around the atrioventricular ring. Lorange and Gulrajani (12) used the modified Miller-Geselowitz model to simulate these surface maps for different assumed preexcitation sites, and compared these simulated maps with the clinically-measured maps of Benson et al.

To simulate preexcitation, an additional initiation site corresponding to the assumed location of the accessory pathway was activated, approximately 30 msec prior to the onset of normal activation. The resulting isochrones corresponding to a preexcitation site in the left lateral ventricle are shown in Figure 3. Comparisons with the normal isochrones of Figure 2 reveal the preexcitation wavefront in the left ventricular free-wall, and its fusion with the normal excitation wavefront. Isochrones were obtained for each of eight preexcitation sites closest to those of Benson et al. These sites are

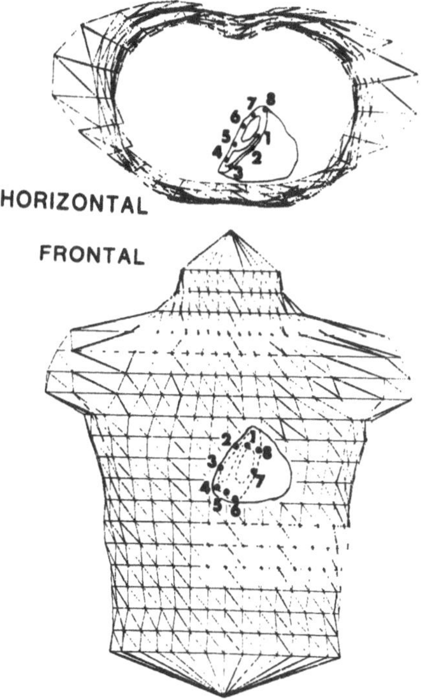

FIGURE 4. Two views of the heart model in the torso model. The numbers refer to the location of the eight preexcitation sites chosen. From Ref (12), © IEEE.

identified in Figure 4, which depicts the heart model properly positioned and oriented within a torso model. For clarity the torso model is depicted as homogeneous, although all computations were done with an inhomogeneous version of the model that includes regions of altered conductivity to represent the intraventricular blood masses, the lungs and a skeletal muscle layer at the surface (25). Calculation of the surface potentials was done using the integral equation for the potential (16).

Figure 5A shows the simulated BSPMs during the delta wave of the QRS and the early ST-segment, for all eight preexcitation sites. The left half of each simulated map corresponds to the anterior chest, and the right half to the back. The positions of the maximum and minimum potential are identified by the plus and minus signs. Alongside, in Figure 5B, are presented for comparison the BSPMs observed by Benson et al. (24) in patients with the same preexcitation site. Note that here the left two-thirds of each measured map represents the anterior chest, owing to a non-uniform horizontal scale. In general, the agreement between simulated and experimental map patterns is very good for all eight sites, and for both QRS and ST maps. The discrepancies are minor, and take the form of slight alterations in the position of the zero potential line demarcating positive and negative potential areas, and also small shifts in the positions of the extrema. The largest such shift was in the position of the minimum in the QRS map for preexcitation in the posterior septum (site 5), which moved from the lower back in the measured map to the lower right-anterior chest in the simulated one.

A characteristic of the QRS maps, both experimental and simulated, is the relative stationarity of the maximum on the anterior chest. This is because irrespective of the exact location of the preexcitation site, the preexcitation front originates at the base of the heart and subsequently moves towards the apex, i.e., towards the same point on the anterior chest. It is the position of the minimum that varies according to the region preexcited, and thus identifies the approximate location of the accessory pathway. The ST- segment maps, as noted by Benson et al., are generally mirror images, about the zero potential line, of the corresponding QRS maps. This too was verified in the simulations (Fig. 5). Also evident is the similarity in the measured QRS and ST maps for sites in the anterior septum and anterior right ventricle respectively. This similarity was also noted in the simulated BSPMs , and confirms the observation by Benson et al. that distinguishing between these two sites on the basis of BSPMs alone is difficult.

The Wolff-Parkinson-White syndrome simulations not only demonstrate the power and flexibility of simulation studies utilizing realistic heart and torso models, but also attest to the correctness of the Benson et al. classification scheme. The modified Miller-Geselowitz model, as described here, is essentially a stepping stone to a more complete heart model, incorporating additional features such as representation of the auricles, a separate His-Purkinje conduction system, and a parameter specifying element refractoriness. Given enough time and computer resources, these improvements are eminently feasible, and such an improved model may well be versatile enough to simulate a broad spectrum of cardiac abnormalities, occurring either singly or in combination, as

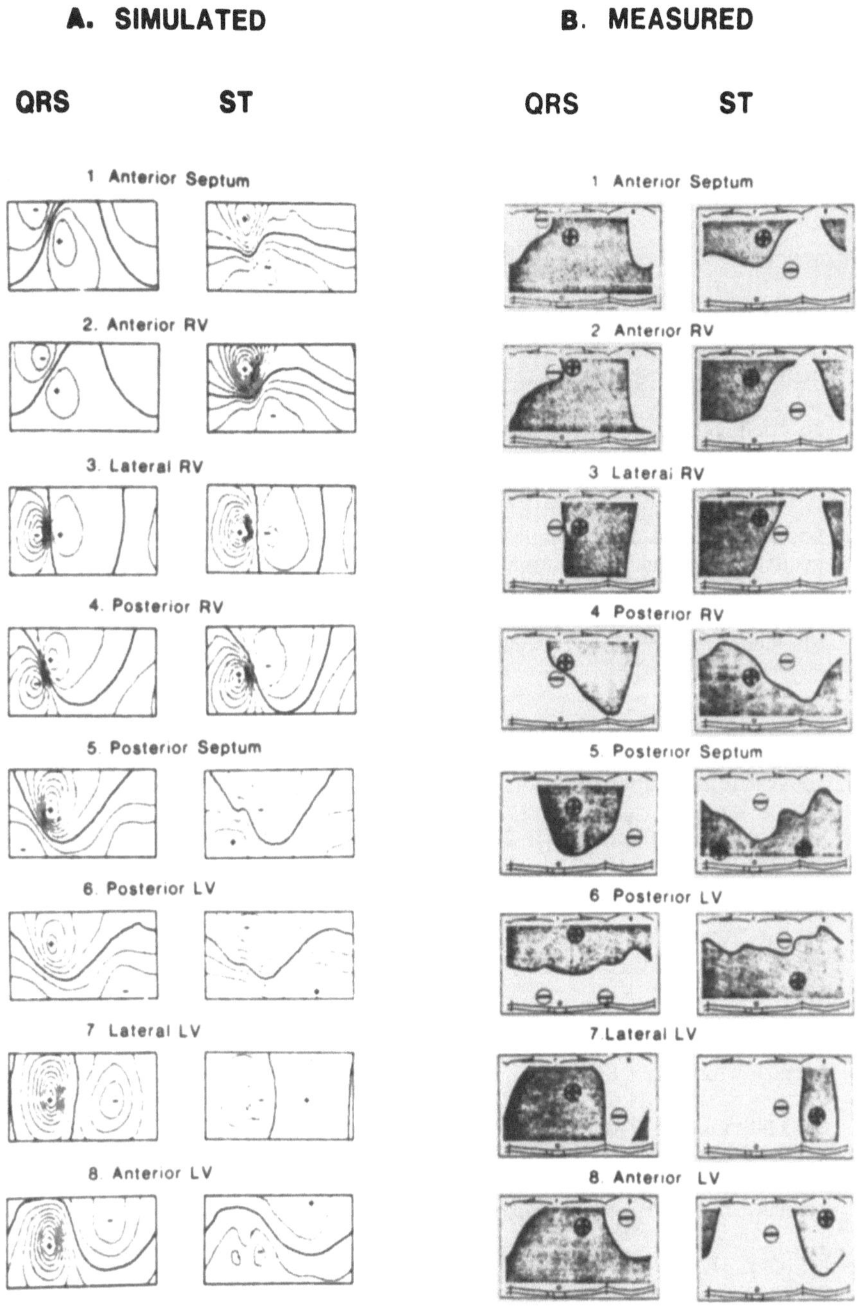

A. SIMULATED

B. MEASURED

QRS ST

QRS ST

1 Anterior Septum

2. Anterior RV

3. Lateral RV

4. Posterior RV

5. Posterior Septum

6. Posterior LV

7 Lateral LV

8. Anterior LV

FIGURE 5. A) Simulated BSPMs for the eight sites in Figure 4, compared with B) the experimental BSPMs published by Benson et al. (24) for the same sites. From Ref (12), © IEEE.

for example the simultaneous presence of myocardial infarction and bundle branch block.

ACKNOWLEDGEMENTS

This work was supported by the Medical Research Council of Canada, the Quebec Heart Foundation and the Fonds de la recherche en santé du Québec.

REFERENCES

1. Okajima M et al: Computer simulation of the propagation process in excitation of the ventricles. Circ Res, 23: 203-11, 1968.

2. Solomon JC and Selvester RH: Myocardial activation sequence simulation. In Hoffman I(ed): Vectorcardiography 2. Amsterdam: North-Holland Publishing Co, 175-82, 1971.

3. Solomon JC and Selvester RH: Simulation of measured activation sequence in the human heart. Am Heart J, 85: 518-23, 1973.

4. Eifler WJ et al: Mechanism of generation of body surface electrocardiographic P-waves in normal, middle, and lower sinus rhythms. Circ Res, 48: 168-82, 1981.

5. D'Alché P et al: Computer model of cardiac potential distribution in an infinite medium and on the human torso during ventricular activation. Circ Res, 34: 719-29, 1974.

6. Cuffin BN and Geselowitz DB: Studies of the electrocardiogram using realistic cardiac and torso models. IEEE Trans Biomed Eng, 24: 242-52, 1977.

7. Miller WT and Geselowitz DB: Simulation studies of the electrocardiogram. I. The normal heart. Circ Res, 43: 301-15, 1978.

8. Durrer D et al: Total excitation of the isolated human heart. Circulation, 1: 899-912, 1970.

9. Colli-Franzone P et al: Potential fields generated by oblique dipole layers modeling excitation wavefronts in the anisotropic myocardium. Comparison with potential fields elicited by paced dog hearts in a volume conductor. Circ Res, 51: 330-46, 1982.

10. Plonsey R: Quantitative formulations of electrophysiological sources of potential fields in volume conductors. In Proceedings - Sixth Annual Conference IEEE Engineering in Medicine and Biology Society. New York: IEEE Press, 367-74, 1984.

11. Miller WT and Geselowitz DB: Simulation studies of the electrocardiogram. II. Ischemia and infarction. Circ Res, 43:

315-23, 1978.

12. Lorange M and Gulrajani RM: Computer simulation of the Wolff-Parkinson-White syndrome. In Proceedings - Sixth Annual Conference IEEE Engineering in Medicine and Biology Society. New York: IEEE Press, 461-4, 1984.

13. Plonsey R: Bioelectric Phenomena. New York: McGraw-Hill Book Co, 202-11, 1969.

14. Gelernter HL and Swihart JC: A mathematical physical model of the genesis of the electrocardiogram. Biophys J, 4: 285-301, 1964.

15. Rush S et al: Computer solution for time-invariant electric fields. J Appl Phys, 37: 2211-17, 1966.

16. Barr RC et al: Determining surface potentials from current dipoles with application to electrocardiography. IEEE Trans Biomed Eng, 13: 88-92, 1966.

17. Barnard ACL et al: The application of electromagnetic theory to electrocardiology. II. Numerical solution of the integral equations. Biophys J, 7: 463-91, 1967.

18. Lynn MS and Timlake WP: The use of multiple deflations in the numerical solution of singular systems of equations with application to potential theory. SIAM J Numer Anal, 5: 303-22, 1968.

19. Salu Y: Implementing a consistency criterion in numerical solution of the bioelectric forward problem. IEEE Trans Biomed Eng, 27: 338-41, 1980.

20. Huebner KH: The Finite Element Method for Engineers. New York: John Wiley, 1975.

21. Norrie DH and de Vries G: An Introduction to Finite Element Analysis. New York: Academic Press, 1978.

22. Kim Y: A Three-Dimensional Modifiable Computer Body Model and its Applications. Madison, Wisconsin: The University of Wisconsin, dissertation, 1982.

23. Pilkington TC et al: A comparison of finite element and integral equation formulations for the calculation of electrocardiographic potentials. IEEE Trans Biomed Eng, 32: 166-73, 1985.

24. Benson DW et al: Localization of the site of ventricular preexcitation with body surface maps in patients with Wolff-Parkinson-White syndrome. Circulation, 65: 1259-68, 1982.

25. Gulrajani RM and Mailloux GE: A simulation study of the effects of torso inhomogeneities on electrocardiographic potentials, using realistic heart and torso models. Circ Res, 52: 45-56, 1983.

Chapter 33

THE RELATIONSHIP BETWEEN BODY SURFACE AND EPICARDIAL POTENTIALS: A THEORETICAL MODEL STUDY

Y. RUDY

1. INTRODUCTION

As a result of the electrical activity of the heart, electrical potentials appear throughout the torso volume conductor. Of particular interest are the potential distributions over the body surface and on the epicardial surface of the heart. The body surface potential distribution provides the data for non-invasive electrocardiography. While standard ECG techniques sample these data at only a small subset of points, the more recent body surface mapping techniques measure the potential distribution over the entire torso and permit, in some cases, the detection and identification of regional electrical events in the heart (1). The ability to localize cardiac events from body surface data is limited, however, since the surface potential is an integrated, smoothed-out, low resolution reflection of the underlying cardiac electrical activity. In contrast, experimental studies (2-9) demonstrate that epicardial potentials contain a considerable amount of detailed, high resolution information about the underlying intramural electrophysiological events, and permit a direct interpretation of these events in a fashion that is not possible from body surface distributions. As a result of these properties, epicardial potential mapping has become an important experimental tool in the study of normal and abnormal excitation (in particular the detailed study of reentrant arrhythmias), as well as an intraoperative clinical tool used to determine the site of origin of arrhythmias prior to surgical ablation.

Both body surface potentials and epicardial potentials are modified by properties of the torso volume conductor and do not reflect the cardiac sources alone. In this paper selected effects of the torso inhomogeneities on body surface and epicardial potentials are discussed and compared (10). The effects of variations in important torso geometry and volume conductivity parameters on the accuracy of recovering epicardial potentials from body surface potential distributions (the "inverse problem") is examined. In addition, results relating inaccuracies in the surface data ("noise") to errors in the recovered epicardial potentials are reported.

2. A COMPARISON OF VOLUME CONDUCTOR EFFECTS ON BODY SURFACE AND EPICARDIAL POTENTIALS

The effects of variations in geometry and volume conductor properties (conductivities of the various torso compartments) were studied using the idealized eccentric spheres model of the heart-torso system (11,12). This model is simple enough to be solved analytically, yet sufficiently sophisticated to include all important torso inhomogeneities (blood cavity, pericardium, lungs, skeletal muscle, and subcutaneous fat). The analytic nature of the model permits the easy manipulation of the conductivities and dimensions of these compartments, and allows adjustment of the location of the heart and its size. Results of these forward simulations contrasting the effects on body surface and epicardial potentials were reported in detail (10). A summary of some of the results follows:

2.1 The "Smoothing Effect" of the volume conductor

As mentioned above, the ability of body surface potential distributions to clearly reflect regional electrical events in the heart is limited. In contrast, epicardial potentials accurately mirror details of the myocardial electrical events with high resolution. This property is demonstrated in Figure 1. In this simulation, when two activation fronts in the anterior part of the spherical myocardium are separated by less than 100°, two discrete maxima arise on the epicardium, whereas a single broad maximum appears on the body surface. For a spearation greater than 100°, two discrete maxima are apparent on the body surface as well. Note, however, that the fact that the single surface potential maximum shown in Figure 1,I originated from a specific multiple source configuration is reflected in its specific amplitude and shpae (spatial extent of the maximum and low level "tails"), in contrast with the single maximum in 1, II, which arises from a different multiple source configuration. Even when two maxima appear on the surface (Figure 1, III), their location does not correspond to the location of the wavefronts. In contrast, the location of the epicardial maxima accurately reflects the location of the underlying activation waves so that in this example, the epicardial potential map is an accurate reflection of the myocardial sources.

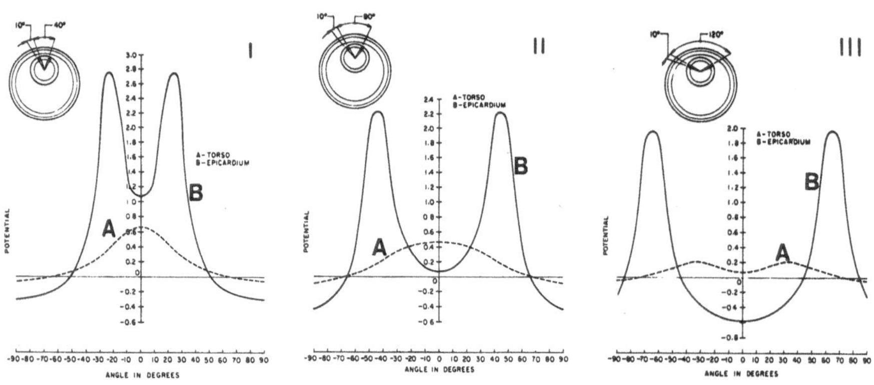

FIGURE 1. Comparison of body surface (A) and epicardial (B) potentials originating from two discrete activation wave fronts located in the myocardium. The central angles of the two activation waves are 10°. The separation between the wave fronts is I-40°, II-80°, III-120°. The geometry is illustrated by the cross section of the model in the left upper corner of each graph.

2.2 The effects of heart position

Another property of epicardial potentials is demonstrated in Figure 2. Our simulations show that these potentials (Figure 2B) are almost completely independent of the location of the heart within the torso, while surface potentials (Figure 2A) are greatly affected by heart position. When the eccentricity (distance from heart center to torso center) is increased from 1 to 5 cm, the torso potential is almost doubled (97% increase). In contrast, the same change in eccentricity produces a potential increase of only 3.8% at the epicardium. This implies that epicardial maps are not sensitive to variations in the location of the heart caused by different postures of the subject, and are almost completely free from effects of body shape and size.

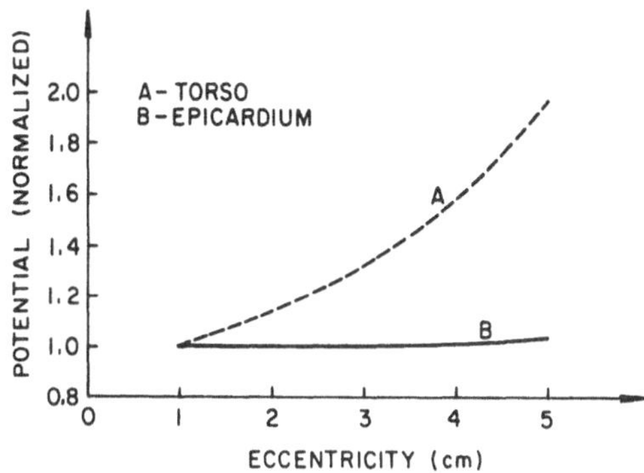

FIGURE 2. The effects of variations in the eccentricity of the heart on body surface (A) and epicardial (B) potentials. The potentials are normalized to unity at an eccentricity of 1.0 cm.

2.3 Effects of variations in conductivities of the torso inhomogeneities

2.3.1. Lungs The effect of the lung inhomogeneity on body surface potentials is different from its effect on epicardial potentials. Whereas epicardial potentials decrease monotonically with increasing lung conductivity, torso potentials attain a maximum at a conductivity that is very close to typical physiological values. The behavior of surface potentials is bell-shaped with low amplitudes obtained for high as well as low conductivity values (13). By comparing the potentials obtained for typical lung conductivity to the values obtained when the conductivity is set equal to that of the myocardium, it is seen that the lung inhomogeneity augments the epicardial potentials by 85%, whereas the augmentation factor for surface potentials is only 19%. Consequently, the lung inhomogeneity is very important in determining the epicardial potential distribution but has a much smaller, though significant, effect on the body surface distribution.

2.3.2. Surface Muscle Layer The high conductivity skeletal muscle layer plays an important role in determining the troso surface potential distribution; in particular it determines the bell-shaped behavior of surface potentials as a function of lung conductivity (in the absence of the muscle layer, the surface potential increased monotonically as the lung conductivity decreases). In contrast, the functional dependence of epicardial potentials on lung conductivity is independent of the presence of the surface muscle layer in the model. The muscle layer attenuates surface potentials; the decrease in potential caused by this layer is 22.5% (relative to the case in which the surface muscle layer has the same conductivity as the underlying lung region). The surface potential decreases with increasing muscle conductivity, and a 5-fold increase in the conductivity causes the potential to decrease by 40.5%. In contrast, the epicardial potential distribution is not strongly affected by the presence of the surface muscle layer. A 5-fold increase in muscle conductivity causes a slight increase of only 8% in epicardial potential.

2.3.3. Subcutaneous Fat The effect of this outermost layer on torso potentials is small; a 10-fold increase in fat conductivity causes the potential to decrease by only 15%. The epicardial potentials are even less affected by variations in fat conductivity; in fact, the effect of the subcutaneous fat layer on these potentials can be completely ignored.

3. EFFECTS OF GEOMETRY AND INHOMOGENEITIES ON THE INVERSE RECONSTRUCTION OF EPICARDIAL POTENTIALS

The results described above demonstrate that epicardial potentials provide a high resolution picture of the underlying cardiac electrical activity modified only slightly by torso effects. Epicardial potentials permit, therefore, a direct interpretation of electrical events within the heart in a fashion that is not possible from body surface distributions. A non-invasive method of reconstructing epicardial potentials from body surface data is therefore highly desirable both for basic in-vivo studies of the normal and abnormal electrical activity of the heart, and as a clinical tool with the potential ability to non-invasively obtain useful diagnostic information concerning local cardiac events. The objective of the work described in this section is to characterize the effects of variations in important torso geometry and volume conductivity parameters on the accuracy of inverse-recovered epicardial potentials, independently of the effects of noise, regularization techniques, and other distortions. For this purpose synthetic, noise-free surface potentials data generated by the eccentric spheres model was used. The inverse procedure utilized surface integration (Gaussian Quadrature) to construct a spherical harmonics series expansion of the torso potential. Using appropriate boundary conditions at internal inhomogeneity interfaces, the potential distribution on the epicardium is recovered. Excellent convergence was obtained with 20 terms in the series expansion (less than 3% error). The availability of the accurate epicardial potentials generated by the forward model provides a basis for comparison and permits an evaluation of the performance and accuracy of the inverse procedure.

3.1 Reconstructing and localizing discrete cardiac events

During a normal cardiac cycle, multiple activation fronts appear within the ventricular walls. This electrical activity, accurately reflected as multiple maxima and minima in the epicardial potential distribution, projects to the body surface with much less resolution. The epicardial and torso potential distributions shown in figures 3 and 4 demonstrate the ability of the inverse procedure to reconstruct multiple epicardial maxima and to identify and locate simultaneous sites of activity from a smooth, single-maximum potential distribution on the body surface. Figure 3 (left panel) depicts inverse-computed epicardial potentials together with the surface potentials from which they are computed. The actual epicardial potential, computed from the underlying sources, is shown in the right panel of the same figure. The calculations are for an anterior dual-source configuration with two discrete activation fronts in the anterior heart wall. The activation fronts are separated by 40 degrees, and each is 10 degrees in extent (from +20 to +30 degrees, and from -20 to -30 degrees relative to an axis that connects the heart center and the mid-point of the anterior chest wall). The agreement between the inverse-computed and the actual (forward-computed) epicardial potentials is excellent. Note that the inverse-computed epicardial potential distribution has two clearly separated peaks, reflecting the exact location and extent of the underlying activation fronts. In contrast, the surface potential from which these epicardial potentials are computed is much smoother, displays only one peak, and does not reflect the dual-front nature of the underlying myocardial sources.

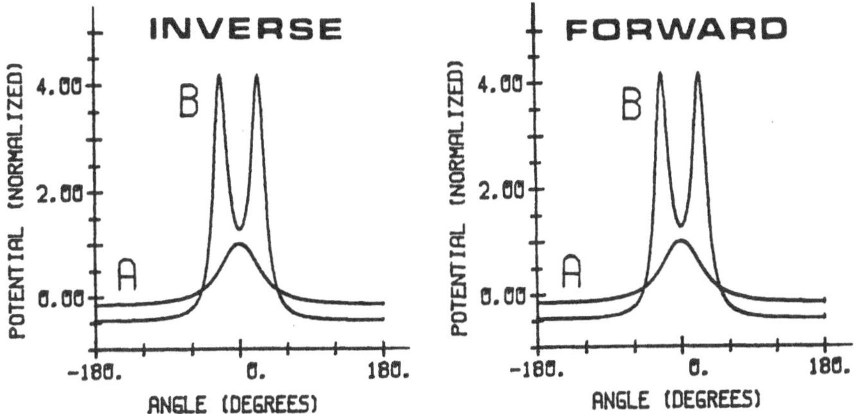

FIGURE 3. Inverse reconstruction of separate anterior epicardial maxima.

The smoothing effect of the torso volume conductor is even greater for posterior myocardial activation. Because of the greater distance between the posterior of the heart and the torso, potential gradients on the torso surface are small and different posterior source configurations result in very similar surface potential distributions. Figure 4 shows body surface and epicardial potentials for two posterior source configurations. The upper panel is for a double activation front configuration: one at +120 to +130 degrees and the other at -120 to -130 degrees. The lower panel is for activation fronts at +150 to +160 and a -150 to -160 degrees. Note how similar the torso potential distributions are despite the very different source configurations. It is clear that by simply observing the surface potentials it is impossible to distinguish between the two source configurations. The inverse procedure, however, accurately recovers the epicardial potentials in both cases and depicts the exact location and extent of the underlying activation fronts.

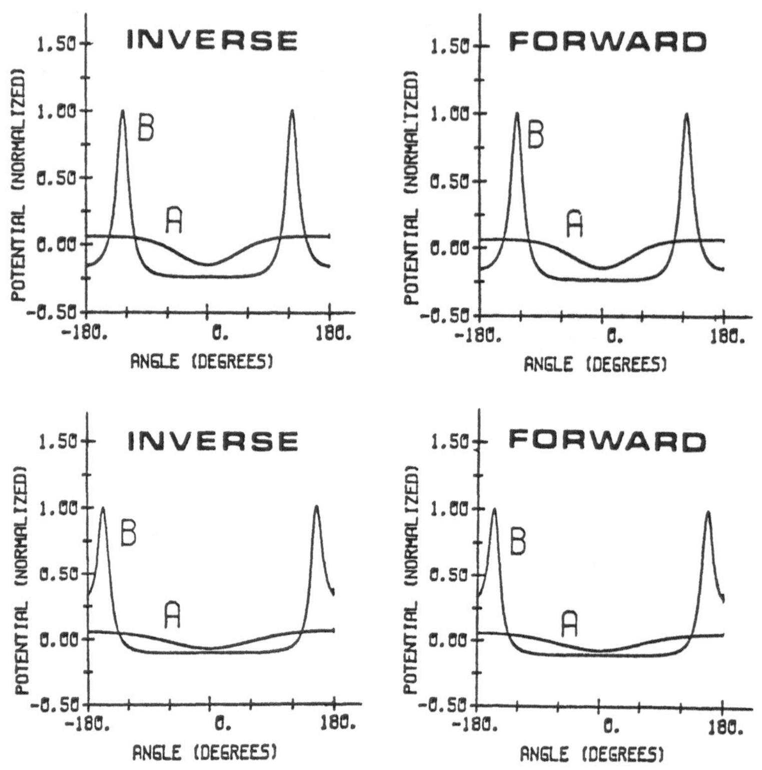

FIGURE 4. Reconstrucing separate posterior epicardial maxima

3.2. The homogeneous approximation

In the simulations above (section 3.1) the geometry and conductivity parameters of the torso volume conductor were known precisely. Realistically, these parameters can only be estimated. In addition, it is desirable to simplify the inverse procedure as much as possible. The "homogeneous approximation" is an attempt to simplify the inverse solution by assuming the torso to be homogeneous. The effects of this simplification are shown in Figure 5. All forward computed potentials are obtained in a model which includes all the torso inhomogeneities. The computed torso potentials

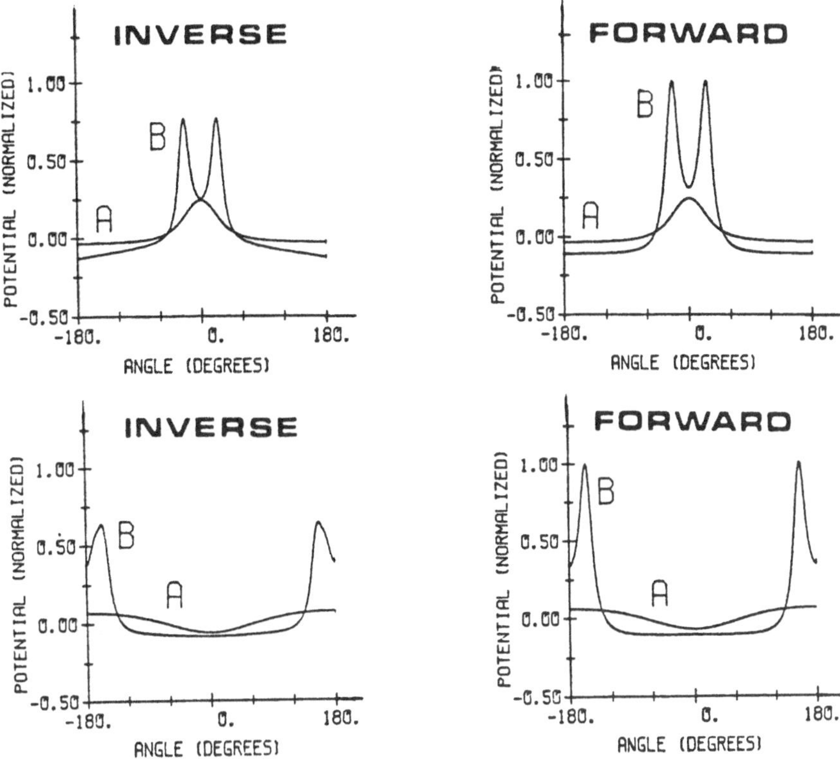

FIGURE 5. Effects of the "homogeneous approximation" on the inverse reconstruction of epicardial potentials

are therefore the analogue of actual surface potentials that are measured on a subject, and the forward-computed epicardial potentials represent the actual epicardial potential distribution of that subject. The inverse-reconstructed epicardial potentials were computed from the surface data using the "homogeneous approximation". Two different source configurations are considered: two separate activation fronts in the anterior ventricular wall (upper panels), and two separate activation fronts in the posterior ventricular wall (lower panels). In both cases the inverse-reconstructed epicardial potentials under the homogeneous simplification (left panels) display a significantly diminished amplitude relative to the actual epicardial potentials (right panels), but the location and extent of the potential maxima are only slightly affected. For the anterior activation fronts the peak to peak potential is decreased by 23.8%, and the resolution (defined as the ratio of the local minimum between the peaks to the global minimum far from the peaks) is reduced from 0.64 to 0.57. For the posterior activation fronts the peak to peak amplitude drops by 36.7%, and the resolution with which the potential maxima can be separated decreases significantly from 0.59 to 0.35 (a 40.7% decrease).

Utilizing the same model, the effects of variations and inaccuracies in estimation of the conductivity of the individual torso inhomogeneities on the inverse-reconstruction of epicardial potentials were analyzed. The following results were obtained:

3.3 Skeletal Muscle

The recovered epicardial potentials are significantly affected by overestimation of the skeletal muscle conductivity. For anterior sources, at twice the normal (physiological) conductivity, the recovered peak potential relative to the actual forward-computed value is 1.5 (50% increase); at five times the normal conductivity, the relative recovered epicardial peak potential is 3.1. In contrast, underestimating the conductivity has a much smaller effect with a maximum decrease of 28% in the recovered peak potential relative to the actual one. Potentials associated with posterior soucrces behave in a similar fashion. However, due to the greater heart-torso distance, the effects of inaccuracies in the estimated muscle conductivity on the recovery of epicardial potentials are more pronounced. Greater deviations of amplitudes from the actual ones are observed for the same estimation errors in muscle conductivity. In addition, a 50% drop in resolution of dual peaks is observed.

3.4 Lungs

Recovered epicardial potentials increase as the estimated lung conductivity decreases from the normal physiological value of 0.0005 mho/cm. At one fifth the normal conductivity, the recovered peak potential (for anterior sources) is 3.4 relative to the actual one. For this range, the resolution of two maxima is not significantly affected. For overestimated lung conductivities the inverse-recovered epicardial potentials are smaller than the actual ones. A 4% decrease in amplitude is observed for a lung conducitivity which is estimated to be five times the actual value. As with the skeletal muscle, the effects are greater for posterior sources, resulting in larger changes in amplitude and a decrease in resolution.

3.5 Subcutaneous Fat

The effects of errors in estimating the fat conductivity on the inverse-recovery of epicardial potentials are minimal. With an estimated fat conducitivity one fifth the normal value, the recovered peak epicardial potential is reduced by only 8%, and no significant change in resolution is observed. For comparison, similar variations in skeletal muscle conductivity can cause as much as five times more change in the amplitudes of recovered epicardial potentials.

3.6 Location of the heart

The proximity of the heart to the anterior chest wall is an important property of the heart-torso system. It is incorporated into the model by the eccentricity parameter, indicating the distance between the heart center and the torso center. Using anterior myocardial sources, the model demonstrates that an error of 0.5 cm in the eccentricity estimate causes a 35% decrease in the amplitude, and the resolution drops by 50%. An error of 4.5 cm in the estimate of the heart position causes an 86% reduction in amplitude and the two potential maxima can no longer be distinguished (resolution drops to zero). Obviously, the inverse procedure is very sensitive to inaccuracies in estimated heart position.

3.7 Size of the heart

The size of the heart is another important geometrical parameter that has to be estimated for the inverse procedure. The model simulations maintained the distance between the anterior heart wall and the chest wall constant. For an anterior source position, the effect of overestimating the heart size on the amplitude of recovered epicardial potentials is small, with only 18% reduction for an estimation error of 3 cm. The resolution of the two anterior epicardial maxima drops by only 10% over this range. However, a significant error (18 degrees) in the location of the potential maxima is introduced. It should be emphasized that errors in recovered anterior epicardial potentials are small as a result of the constraint on the distance of the anterior epicardium from the chestwall. When this constraint is removed, variations in recovered potentials are much greater. Since the posterior wall of the heart is not fixed, its position within the torso changes as the heart size increases. Under these conditions for an overestimation of heart size by 1 cm the amplitude of recovered posterior epicardial potentials drops by 70%, and the peaks nearly merge.

4. EFFECTS OF INACCURACIES IN THE BODY SURFACE POTENTIAL DATA

The formulation of the inverse problem in terms of epicardial potentials has several advantages over the equivalent generator approach. Epicardial potentials are real, physically measurable quantities that can be related to the underlying physiological events. The formulation in terms of potentials does not require restrictive assumptions regarding the nature of the sources to be made. The intracavitary blood inhomogeneity is taken into account implicitly in the potential formulation. In addition, inverse solutions in terms of potentials can be evaluated by a direct comparison with epicardial measurements, such as those obtained simultaneously with surface potentials in an exprimental animal.

The formulation of the inverse problem in terms of potentials leads to a Cauchy problem for the Laplace's equation. As such the problem is ill-posed (14) in the sense that small variations in the data (surface potentials) can cause very large variations in the solution (epicardial potentials) and hence the solution is unstable. The understanding of the nature of this instability is essential since in the actual application the data is always affected by noise (noise in the body surface potential measurements, as well as errors in the torso and heart geometry).

To study the dependence of error in the inverse solution on noise in the surface potential data we developed a deterministic, integral-operator approach to the solution of the Cauchy problem. The solution is constructed in three steps: (1) analytic continuation of the data to cover a desired domain; (2) an integral transformation of the continued data to construct a holomorphic function in a complex domain $B(n_2)$; (3) use of the Bergman operator (15) to construct a harmonic function which provides the solution to the Cauchy problem in a cylindrical volume, and in particular on the epicardial face of this volume. Analysis of this procedure identifies the instability with the analytic continuation step, and as a result permits the use of the Hadamard 3-spheres theorem (16) to obtain the following stability estimate (*) where M is an a-priori bound on the solution (epicardial potential magnitude), and α is a logarithmic function of the heart-torso geometrical relationship. This expression provides an

$$(*) \qquad \|\zeta\| \leq M^{1-\alpha}\|\chi\|^{\alpha}$$

estimate of error in the inverse-recovered epicardial potential (ς) resulting from small fluctuations (noise) in the body surface potential data (χ). Note that by restricting the solutions to those satisfying a prescribed a-priori bound on epicardial potentials (M), continuity is restored. For relaistic heart-torso geometrical relationships the following results were obtained using expression (2):

(1) A reduction in the body noise from 100 μV to 10 μV (a 10-fold decrease) brings about a reduction of epicardial error by only a factor of 1.75

(2) The epicardial error is reduced by a factor of five for a 10-fold decrease in the a-priori epicardial bound M.

(3) An increase in the distance of the epicardial surface by 7 cm (from 1 cm to 8 cm) causes a 50% increase in the error, pointing to the fact that solutions for remote areas of the heart (posterior wall, diaphragmatic surface) are expected to be less accurate.

A comparison of the results (1) and (2) above calls attention to an important practical consideration regarding the solution of the inverse problem. It is clear that reduction in body surface noise (which is difficult to achieve) is unlikely to significantly improve computed epicardial potentials. In contrast, incorporating into the solution (through the use of regularization techniques) a-priori estimate of a bound on the epicardial potential should be the method of choice. The accuracy of the solution will be greatly improved if accurate epicardial bounds are specified for different regions of the heart, at different time intervals during the QRS-T, and for various abnormalities.

5. SUMMARY

The results of the eccentric spheres forward simulations (section 2 above) call attention to two important properties of epicardial potential distributions. (1) Epicardial potential maps mirror details of the electrical sources within the myocardium that may not be reflected in body surface distributions and allow more detailed examination of regional electrical events within the heart. (2) Epicardial potentials (in contrast to surface potentials) are almost completely independent of the location of the heart within the torso. This implies that epicardial maps are not sensitive to variations in the location of the heart, resulting from changes in posture of the subject, and are almost free from effects of body shape and size. In addition, the effects of the surface muscle layer and subcutaneous fat on the actual epicardial potentials are shown to be minimal so that, of all extracardiac secondary sources only those at the heart-lung interface affect significantly the potential distribution at the epicardium. In view of the above, a transformation which reconstructs epicardial potential maps from body surface potentail maps (the "inverse problem") serves to enhance the resolution with which intracardiac events can be detected, as well as to normalize the potential maps (to free them from the effect of body shape, so that they depend on cardiac sources alone).

The eccentric spheres model simulations also provide an insight to the sensitivity of the inverse problem in electrocardiography to variations in various geometry and conductivity parameters. The results demonstrate that knowledge of most of these parameters is important for an accurate reconstruction of epicardial potentials, and that posterior potentials on the epicardium are more sensitive to errors in estimating these parameters than are anterior potentials. Specifically, assuming the torso to be homogeneous results in a significant loss of resolution of posterior epicardial potential maxima, and errors in estimated lung and skeletal muscle conductivities significantly affect recovery of posterior epicardial potentials. In contrast, the effects of the subcutaneous fat layer are minimal suggesting that inverse computations can be simplified by eliminating this layer from the torso volume conductor model. The simulations demonstrate that the inverse procedure is quite sensitive to inaccuracies in estimating heart position and size. Both lead to large errors in recovered amplitudes and to a reduction in resolution. It is clear that a practical inverse procedure will have to incorporate a regularization technique that will minimize these effects. Finally, the stability estimates show that the accuracy with which epicardial potentials can be recovered depends strongly on the accuracy of a-priori prescribed bounds. This implies that specifying different bound for different regions in the heart and for different time instances during the cardiac cycle will improve the inverse solution. it also points to regularization techniques which incorporate a-priori prescribed bounds on the solution (17) as a method of choice.

ACKNOWLEDGEMENT

This work was supported by Grant HL 33343 from the National Institutes of Health.

REFERENCES

1. Rudy Y (1985) Critical aspects of the forward and inverse problems in electrocardiography. In: Sideman S, Beyar R eds. Simulation and Imaging of the Cardiac System. Martinus Nijhoff Publishers, The Netherlands, pp. 279-298.

2. Arisi G, Macchi E, Baruffi S, Spaggiari S, Taccardi B (1983). Potential fields on the ventricular surface of the exposed dog heart during normal excitation. Circ Res 52: 706.

3. King TD, Barr RC, Herman-Giddens GS, Boaz DE, Spach MS (1972). Isopotential body surface maps and their relationship to atrial potentials in the dog. Circ Res 20: 393.

4. Ramsey M III, Barr RC, Spach MS (1977). Comparison of measured torso potentials with those simulated from epicardial potentials for ventricular depolarization and repolarization in the intact dog. Circ Res 41: 660.

5. Spach MS, Barr RC (1975). Ventricular intramural and epicardial potential distributions during ventricular activation and repolarization in the intact dog. Circ Res 37: 243.

6. Spach MS, Barr RC (1975). Analysis of ventricular activation and repolarization from intramural and epicardial potential distributions for ectopic beats in the intact dog. Circ Res 37: 830.

7. Spach MS, Barr RC (1976). Origin of epicardial ST-T wave potentials in the intact dog. Circ Res 37: 830.

8. Spach, MS, Barr RC, Lanning CF, Tucek PC (1977). Origin of body surface QRS and T wave potentials from epicardial potential districutions in the intact chimpanzee. Circulation 55: 268.

9. Spach MS, Barr RC, Lanning CF (1978). Experimental basis for QRS and T wave potential distributions in the intact chimpanzee. Circ Res 42: 103.

10. Rudy Y, Plonsey R (1980). A comparison of volume conductor and source geometry effects on body surface and epicardial potentials. Circ Res 46: 283.

11. Rudy Y, Plonsey R (1979). The eccentric spheres model as the basis for a study of the role of geometry and inhomogeneities in electrocardiography. IEEE Trans Biomed Eng 26: 392.

12. Rudy, Y, Plonsey R, Liebman J (1979). The effects of variations in conductivity and geometrical parameters on the electrocardiogram, using an eccentric spheres model. Circ Res 44: 104.

13. Rudy, Y, Wood R, Plonsey R, Liebman J (1982). The effect of high lung conductivity on electrocardiographic potentials: Results from human subjects undergoing bronchopulmonary lavage. Circ 65: 440.

14. Tikhonov AN, Arsenin VY (1977). Solutions of Ill-Posed Problems. Winston, Wiley.

15. Bergman S, (1961). Integral operators in the theory of linear partial differential equations. Ergeb Math NS Vol 23. Springer, Berlin.

16. Titchmarsh EC (1979). The theory of functions. Oxford, Clarendon Press.

17. Twomey S (1965). The application of numerical filtering to the solution of integral equations encountered in indirect sensing measurements. J. Franklin Institute 27: 95.

Chapter 34

ACCURACY OF EPICARDIAL POTENTIALS INVERSELY RECONSTRUCTED FROM BODY SURFACE MEASUREMENTS

Y. YAMASHITA

1. INTRODUCTION

In this paper, we propose an inverse procedure using finite elements which solves directly the Cauchy problem to reconstruct epicardial potentials from the body surface map and carry out numerical experiments to evaluate the accuracy of reconstructed epicardial maps. It is well known that, due to the ill-posedness of the inverse potential problem in electrocardiology [1-4], the accuracy of reconstructed electrical activity of the heart depends greatly upon the number of body lead points as well as noise contained in body surface maps. We demonstrate the accuracy of reconstructed epicardial potentials under various measuring conditions of body surface maps. Finally, we apply the proposed inverse calculation procedure to real body maps collected using a body surface mapping system and show a possibility to detect the site and extent of the infarcted area by using the reconstructed epicardial map.

2. MATHEMATICAL FORMULATION OF THE INVERSE POTENTIAL PROBLEM

2.1. RECONSTRUCTION OF EPICARDIAL POTENTIALS

Assuming the body surface potentials v_B are known, then the inverse problem involves estimation of epicardial potentials by solving the following Cauchy problem for an elliptic operator of second order: Let R_T be the torso volume conductor between the body surface S_B and the heart surface S_H, and G(x) be known as the conductivity tensor in R_T. Find v(x) on S_H where v(x) satisfies

$$\begin{aligned} &\operatorname{div} G(x) \operatorname{grad} v(x) = 0 && \text{in } R_T,\quad x\varepsilon R_T \\ &-n\cdot G(x) \operatorname{grad} v(x) = 0 && \text{on } S_B \qquad (1) \\ &v(x) = v_B && \text{on } S_B \end{aligned}$$

2.2. FINITE ELEMENT SOLUTION OF THE CAUCHY PROBLEM

The finite element solution to this problem results in a system of matrix equations [3]

$$\begin{pmatrix} W_{BB} & W_{BH} & W_{BI} \\ 0 & E & 0 \\ W_{IB} & W_{IH} & W_{II} \end{pmatrix} \begin{pmatrix} v_B \\ v_H \\ v_I \end{pmatrix} = \begin{pmatrix} 0 \\ h \\ 0 \end{pmatrix} \qquad (2)$$

where vectors v_B, v_H and v_I stand for nodal values of potential on S_B, S_H, and in V_T, respectively, E is an identity matrix with appropriate dimensions, and h is the unknown epicardial potential, which works as a forced (Dirichlet) boundary condition. Since nodal points on S_B and S_H are not connected directly with each other, in practical cases for finite elements, W_{BH} will be null, so we drop this hereafter. To relate the heart and body potentials without explicitly considering the potentials of the internal nodes, v_I should be eliminated. From the third row of (2) we obtain

$$v_I = -W_{II}^{-1} (W_{IB}v_B + W_{IH}v_H). \tag{3}$$

Substituing (3) into (2) and separating v_B and v_H lead to

$$v_H = h(\text{unknown}) \tag{4}$$

$$(W_{BB}-W_{BI}W_{II}^{-1}W_{IB})v_B =(W_{BI}W_{II}^{-1}W_{IH})v_H \tag{5}$$

The matrix W_{II} in (5) is square and its inverse is well behaved.

2.3. REGULARIZATION OF THE ILL-POSED INVERSE PROBLEM

In order to estimate v_H(= h: unknown) from the measured body surface map v_B, we can rewrite (5) in the following manner:

$$v_H = W_{HB}^{*}(W_{BB}-W_{BI}W_{II}^{-1}W_{IB})v_B. \tag{6}$$

Here the the optimal inverse, W_{HB}^{*}, is defined as

$$W_{HB}^{*} = [(W_{BI}W_{II}^{*}W_{IH})^{t}(W_{BI}W_{II}^{-1}W_{IH})+kE]^{-1}(W_{BI}W_{II}^{-1}W_{IH})^{t}. \tag{7}$$

Note that, taking into account the ill-posedness of this inverse problem, the Moore-Penrose generalized inverse with the regularizing parameter k [1-7] is used for (7), where spatial frequency components, having small singular values below noise level, are damped. Stability and accuracy of the solution are dependent on the regularizing parameter. The optimal value of k can be determined iteratively using the a priori known information of the overall noise affecting the body surface data [3, 7].

3. NUMERICAL EXPERIMENTS FOR A REALISTIC TORSO MODEL

3.1. A GEOMETRICAL MODEL OF A HUMAN TORSO

In order to verify the solution method proposed as well as to clarify what degree of accuracy is possible in the inverse estimation of the epicardial map, we carried out a numerical experiment using a realistic torso model. Fig. 1 depicts the geometry of the torso volume conductor used in this numerical experiment. It shows a typical human thorax from the vertebral level T_1 to the vertebral body of L_5, and contains the heart, the lungs, and the thoracic wall. Each region has been assumed to be isotropic but different in conductivity: lungs=0.08 mho/m, thoracic wall=0.17 mho/m, and heart(intraventricular blood mass is included)=0.53 mho/m.

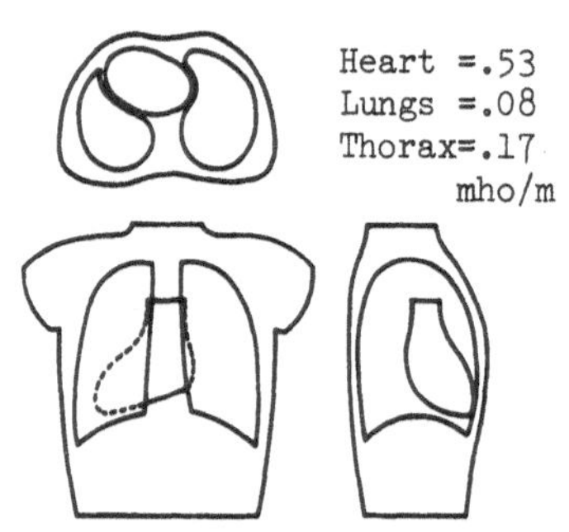

Fig. 1 A geometrical model of the torso volume conductor. This was used to compute epicardial potentials from body surface maps.

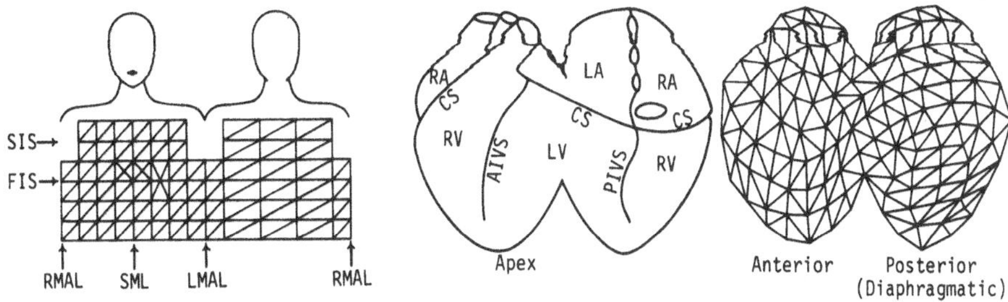

Fig. 2 Geometric models of the epicardial and body surface with associated triangulations. Body surface (left) and epicardial surface (middle & right). SIS & FIS=second & fifth intercostal space, RMAL & LMAL=right & left middle axillar line, SML=sternal median line. RV & LV=right & left ventricle, RA & LA=right & left atrium, CS=coronary sulcus, AIVS & PIVS= anterior & posterior intraventricular sulcus.

In the present study, the torso volume conductor was divided into a series of tetrahedra, in which each tetrahedron has four nodes at the vertices. The whole torso was composed of 13955 tetrahedral elements with 2768 nodes. The interfaces between different organs were also composed of a series of triangular planes. There were 110, 460, and 528 nodes assigned on the epicardial, lung, and body surface, respectively. Adjacent nodes on the epicardial surface were spaced as evenly as possible, but the distance between them ranged from 1.2 cm to 2.3 cm with the average being approximately 1.8 cm. Fig. 2 indicates the geometric models of the epicardial and body surface together with their anatomical features as well as their triangulation.

3.2. AN EXAMPLE OF SIMULATED CARDIAC ELECTRIC FIELD

Fig. 3 gives an example of the electric field induced by a quadrupole-like current generating source in the heart region. Such a source was obtained by fixing the potential at four points in the heart at ±100 mV. The equipotential contour line must be normal to the body surface as this is exposed to the air. This boundary condition is locally violated (but satisfied in the mean) at the posterior body surface where the division was coarser. Fig. 3 reveals that the absolute voltage rapidly decreases as the distance from the source gradually increases, so less than 7 percent of the peak-to-peak value of the source voltage can be observed on the body surface. Thus, assuming the absolute voltage of the source to be 100 mV, the absolute maximum values of epicardial and body surface potentials would be approximately 25 mV for the former and at most 7 mV for the latter. In addition to a decrease in voltage value, the isopotential lines become gradually smoother the farther away they are from the source, which means that the current pattern is much more diverse in the thoracic region. The smoothing property of the electrocardiographic field makes this inverse problem technically cumbersome (i.e., ill-posed or ill-conditioned), because we must reconstruct a detailed structure of the heart generators from smoothed distribution and reduced voltage values on the body surface.

3.3. EXAMPLES OF THE INVERSE CALCULATION FOR EPICARDIAL POTENTIALS

We show the epicardial potential distribution reconstructed from the body surface map indicated in Fig. 3. Random numbers which have a normal

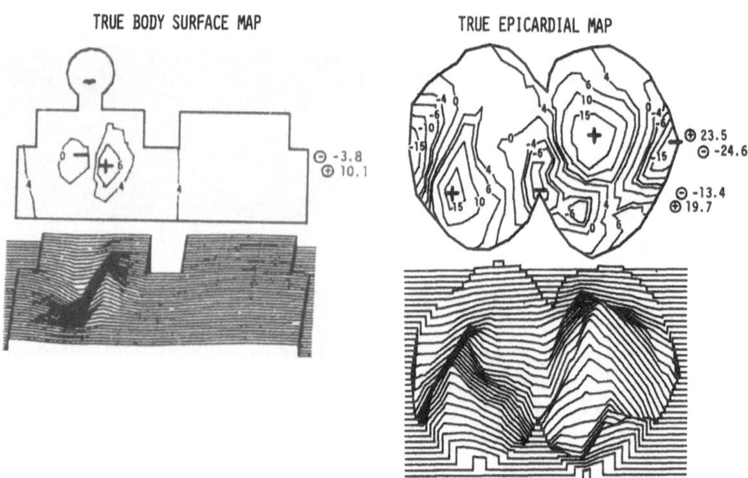

Fig. 3 An example of the epicardial and body surface potentials induced by a quadrupole-like current generating source placed within the heart. The electric field was calculated using the finite element method. Epicardial (right) and body surface (left) maps with their perspective plots. Voltage values are indicated on contour lines. The large plus and minus signs identify maxima and minima the values of which are shown to the right of the map.

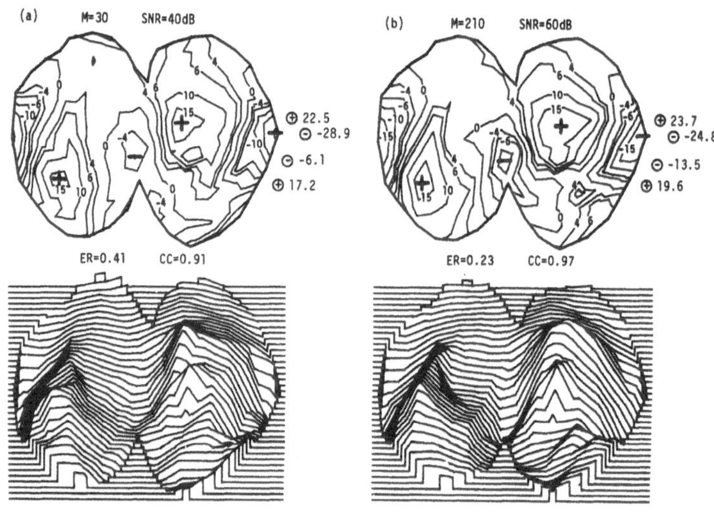

Fig. 4 The inverse epicardial potentials which were calculated from the body surface map shown in Fig. 3 under different conditions in measuring body surface potentials. M=number of body surface lead points, SNR=$20\log_{10}$(ratio of the peak-to-peak voltage value of body surface potentials to the rms value of measurement noise). ER=ratio of the rms differences between the inverse and true epicardial map to the rms true epicardial value, CC=correlation coefficient between the inverse and true epicardial maps.

distribution with zero mean were generated and added to the body surface potentials. Fig. 4 shows the inverse epicardial maps under different measuring conditions along with optimal choices of value of the parameter k in (7). The SNR is defined as the ratio of the peak-to-peak value of body surface potentials to the root-mean-square (rms) of measurement noise. SNR=40 and 60 will correspond to measurement noise equal to about 70 μV and about 7 μV in rms value, respectively, with the assumption that the peak-to-peak value of body surface potentials is about 7 mV. Fig. 4(a) is an underdetermined case, i.e., the number of body lead points M is only 30 while the number of nodes on the epicardial surface N is 110. The sites of major maxima and minima as well as the overview of distribution in the inverse maps resemble the "true" ones shown in Fig. 3. However, there is much difference in the detailed distribution. This result suggests that an appropriate regularization procedure can stabilize the inverse solution in the presence of noise but it is difficult to reconstruct the detailed distribution of epicardial potential. Fig. 4(b) shows one of the best cases we were able to attain in this numerical experiment. There is complete agreement on the anterior side but there are still some differences on the posterior/diaphragmatic side. An increase in the SNR as well as in the number of body lead points has more recognizable effects in improving the accuracy on the anterior side than on the posterior/diaphragmatic side. Thus, the inverse estimation will result in relatively low accuracy on the heart surface far away from the body surface.

3.4. EFFECT OF NUMBER OF BODY LEAD POINTS AND SIGNAL-TO-NOISE RATIO OF BODY MAP ON ACCURACY OF INVERSE EPICARDIAL DISTRIBUTION

From a standpoint of diagnostic application of the inverse procedure, the effect of the number of body lead points and the SNR values on the accuracy of the reconstructed epicardial map is a very interesting question. Here, we will investigate the estimation error in the inverse calculation under various measuring conditions. Fig. 5 shows a relation of the

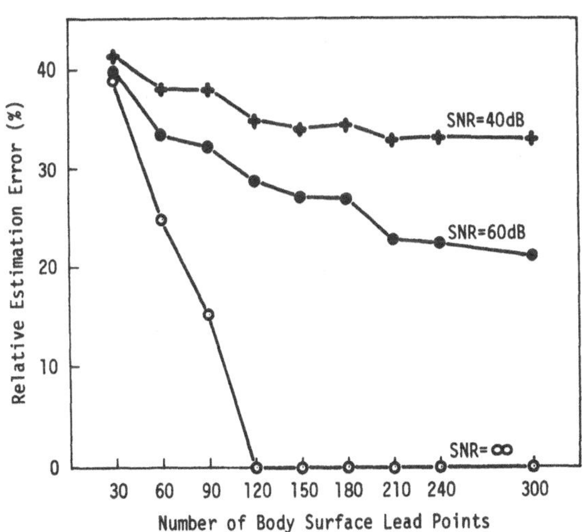

Fig. 5 Expected values of ER (see caption of Fig. 4) vs number of body surface lead points(M) at various SNR of body surface potentials.

rms error in the inverse epicardial map as a function of various numbers of body lead points M at various SNR's. In each case, almost two-thirds of the body lead points were located in the anterior chest and the rest on the back. The body lead points have been selected with almost equal spacing. In the case of M<=90 and SNR=∞, which means an ideal situation free from noise, the estimation error is directly dependent upon M. Meanwhile, M>N as well as SNR=∞ enables us to recover completely the epicardial potentials since in this numerical experiment the epicardial potentials have been assumed to be fully expressed by N=110 linearly independent functions.

In the presence of noise, the estimation error seems to become gradually smaller as M increases. Thus even if M>N, an increase in M will lead to improvement of the accuracy of the inverse estimation, particularly in a higher SNR case. On the other hand, the accuracy of the inverse epicardial map seems to be saturated in lower SNR cases. Thus, an increase in body lead points without suppressing measurement noise has little effect on improving the accuracy. If we consider the case of SNR=40 dB as a real situation, body lead points greater than about 210 will not improve the accuracy of the inverse estimation.

4. APPLICATION OF INVERSE CALCULATION PROCEDURE TO REAL BODY SURFACE MAPS

Taking into account the accuracy of inverse epicardial distribution under realistic measurement conditions, we applied the solution method proposed above to real body surface maps. These body surface maps were

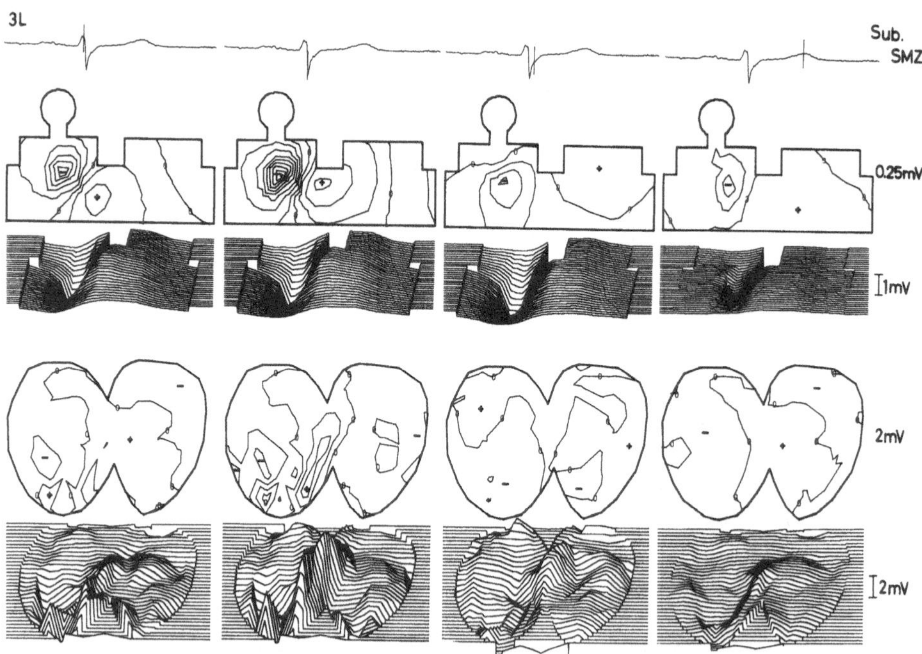

Fig. 6 An example of application of the inverse calculation procedure to real body surface maps. Measurement condition corresponds to M=90 and SNR=40 dB. This case has a small infarcted area on the anterior side of the right ventricular surface where we can observe no electrical activity.

measured using 90 body lead points which were located at crossing points of the triangulation of the torso surface indicated in Fig. 2. The SNR is about 40 dB since an estimate of the variance of measurement noise will be about 50 μV while the maximum peak-to-peak value of body surface maps is several mV. According to the numercal experiments described above, the accuracy of the inverse epicardial map is expected to remain fairly good on the anterior side of the epicardium but to be rather poor on the posterior/ diaphragmatic side. Fig. 6 shows a case of infarction on the right ventricle which has been diagnosed using scintigraphic findings. We can observe a small area on the right ventricular surface where the potential remains unchanged when the time change of the epicardial maps are carefully investigated. This fact suggests that there is no electrical activity in the infarcted region. Although the confidence of this fact may not be definite, a possibility of application of the inverse epicardial distribution to clinical use has been shown.

5. CONCLUSION

We proposed the inverse procedure using finite elements which solves directly the Cauchy problem for the elliptic operator of second order. Stability of the solution for this ill-posed inverse potential problem was accomplished by means of a regularizing parameter. The degree of accuracy attainable in the reconstructed epicardial map was dependent on the SNR of the body surface map as well as the number of lead points. If we consider as a realistic measuring condition the case such that SNR=40 dB and the number of body lead points is about 90, the accuracy of the reconstructed epicardial map is good over the anterior side of the epicardial surface but very poor over the posterior or diaphragmatic side. Bearing in mind low accuracy over the posterior/diaphragmatic side of the ventricular surface, we applied the proposed inverse procedure to real situations and suggested that the infarcted area shows no electrical activity.

REFERENCES

1. Yamashita Y, Takahashi T: A New Method of Solving the Inverse Problem in Electrocardiography Using the Finite Element Method, in Proc Int Symp Med Inform System (MEDIS)'78, Abe H(ed), 243-246. Tokyo:MEDIS Center, 1978.
2. Yamashita Y: Inverse Solution in Electrocardiography. Japan Circ J, 45, 1312-1322, 1981.
3. Yamashita Y, Takahashi T: Use of the Finite Element Method to Determine Epicardial from Body Surface Potentials under a Realistic Torso Model. IEEE Trans Biomed Eng, BME-31, 611-621, 1984.
4. Colli-Franzone P, Guerri L, Taccardi B, Viganotti C: The Inverse Potential Problem Applied to the Human Case, in Models and Measurements of the Cardiac Electric Field, Schubert E(ed), 19-33. New York:Plenum Press, 1982.
5. Tikhonov AN, Arsenin VY: Solutions of Ill-Posed Problems. New York:John Wiley & Sons, 1977.
6. Frieden BR: Image Enhancement and Restoration, in Picture Processing and Digital Filtering, Huang TS(ed), Chap 5. New York:Springer-Verlag, 1979.
7. Hunt BR: The Application of Constrained Least-Squares Estimation to Image Restoration by Digital Computer. IEEE Trans Comput, C-22, 805-812, 1973.

Chapter 35

COMPARISON OF SEVERAL SOLUTIONS OF THE FORWARD POTENTIAL PROBLEM FOR A FINITE CONDUCTING CYLINDER

E. NYSSEN, J. CORNELIS, P. BLOCK, O. STEENHAUT

1. INTRODUCTION

Several static solutions of the forward potential problem in homogeneous cylindrical volume conductors are described in the literature :

- the discretised integral equation method (DIEM) (1)
- the analytical solution for centric dipoles (ACD) (2)
- the analytical solution for arbitrary dipoles (AAD') (3)

When these solutions are compared, fundamental contradictions are found.

A mathematical proof of the incorrectness of the published and still generally accepted AAD' can be given and a correct rederivation of the AAD has been performed (4). In this paper the results will be summarized and discussed and the behaviour of the numerical implementation will be described. A more rigorous mathematical development is given in (4).

2. COMPARISON OF DIFFERENT SOLUTIONS

Regressing the potential map, obtained for a centered horizontal dipole in a finite length cylinder (figure 1a) by method AAD' (figure 1b), on the map obtained by DIEM (figure 1c) for the same source, reveals a difference by a scale factor 2. Moreover the maps are not perfectly correlated. The existence of a residual map (figure 1d) reveals the presence of non-dipolar components in one of both maps under the assumption that the other map is correct. Since a good agreement is found between the ACD and the DIEM solution, it is the AAD' solution which is suspected to be erroneous (figure 2).

This hypothesis can be proven mathematically (4). Starting from a dipole $\overline{P} = (p_x, p_y, p_z)^\tau$, on the cylinder axis, the AAD' equations may be evaluated for the points at the cylinder surface (solution of the forward potential problem).

The equations estimating the dipolar components of the sources inside a volume conductor from a potential distribution at its surface are (5) :

$$p_i = \sigma \int_S \Phi(\bar{r})\, dS_i(\bar{r}) \quad ; \quad i = x,y,z$$

(solution of the inverse potential problem).

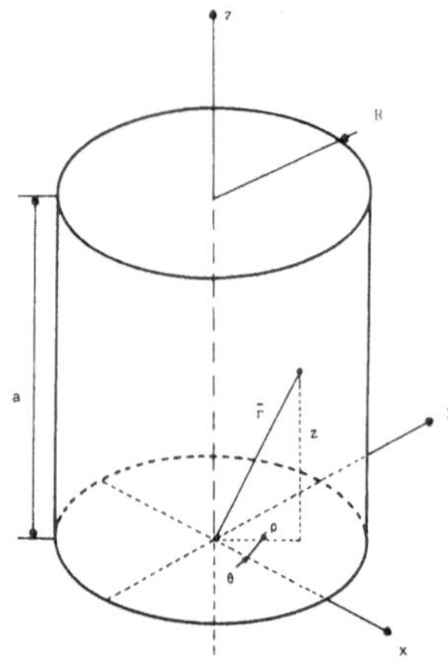

FIGURE 1.a homogeneous cylinder R = 0.190 ; a = 0.450; distance bottom-horizontal centric unitary dipole = 0.225; σ = 1.0

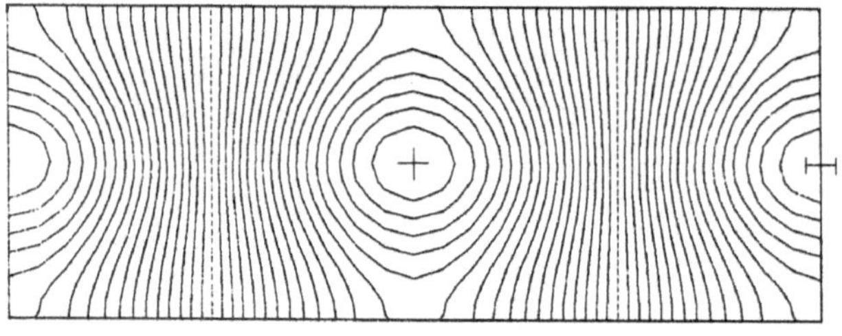

FIGURE 1.b MAP(AAD') : potential distribution on the vertical surface of the cylinder calculated by AAD' (increment between adjacent equipotential lines 0.5)

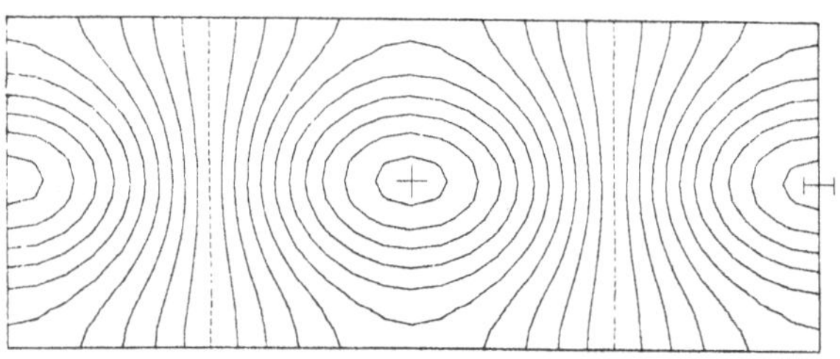

FIGURE 1.c MAP(DIEM)

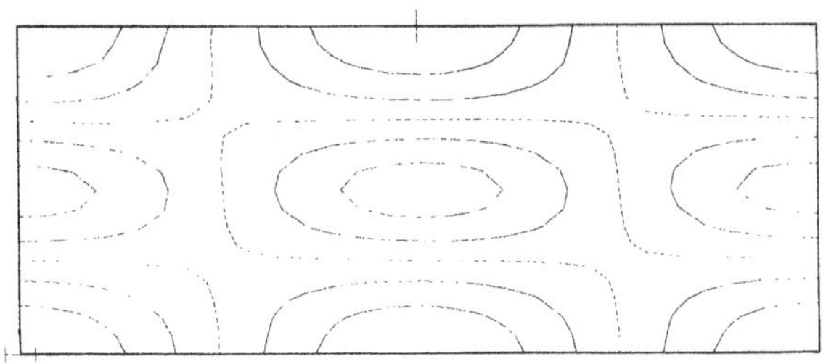

FIGURE 1.d residual map : MAP(AAD') - 2 * MAP(DIEM)

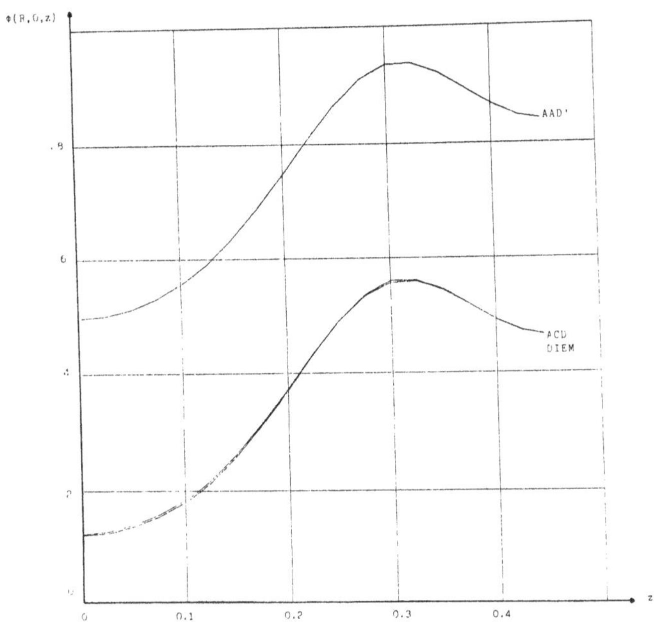

FIGURE 2. Discrepancy between different solutions of the forward potential problem on the surface $\rho = R$ of a finite cylinder for an enclosed horizontal centric dipole oriented along the x-axis and located at a distance of 0.300 from the bottom of the cylinder.
The figure shows Φ (R,0,z)

Normally, substituting $\Phi(\bar{r})$ obtained by the AAD' solution, in this equation should give an identity. One obtains however : $\bar{P} = (2p_x, 2p_y, p_z)^\tau$.
We have proven mathematically (4) that the AAD' solution introduces higher order components inside the finite cylinder which are not present in the postulated source (fig 1.d). It is important to be aware of the fact that the error in the still general accepted AAD' solution is not a constant scale factor or offset. In (4) we describe where and how the error occurs in the reasoning which leads to the AAD' solution.

3. REDERIVATION OF THE AAD SOLUTION (4)

Our approach consists of summing a general solution of the Laplace equation to a solution of the Poisson problem corresponding to the applied monopolar source and matching the unknown coefficients to the Neumann-boundary conditions at $\rho = R$. We obtain for the infinite cylinder :

$$\Phi_m = \frac{I}{4\pi\sigma}\frac{1}{|\bar{r}-\bar{r}'_m|} - \frac{I}{2\pi^2\sigma}\int_0^\infty \sum_{n=0}^{\infty}(2-\delta_{n0})\cos n(\vartheta-\vartheta'_m)\,I_n(k\rho'_m)\cos k(z-z'_m)\,I_n(k\rho)\frac{K'_n(kR)}{I'_n(kR)}\,dk \tag{1}$$

The correct analytical solution for arbitrary dipolar sources(AAD) is the gradient with respect to the coordinates of the source point $\bar{r}'$.

$$\Phi_d = \frac{\bar{P}^\tau}{4\pi\sigma}\frac{(\bar{r}-\bar{r}'_d)}{|\bar{r}-\bar{r}'_d|^3} - \frac{\bar{P}^\tau}{2\pi^2\sigma}\int_0^\infty \sum_{n=0}^{\infty}(2-\delta_{n0})\begin{pmatrix} k\cos n(\vartheta-\vartheta'_d)\,I'_n(k\rho'_d)\cos k(z-z'_d) \\ \frac{n}{\rho'_d}\sin n(\vartheta-\vartheta'_d)\,I_n(k\rho'_d)\cos k(z-z'_d) \\ k\cos n(\vartheta-\vartheta'_d)\,I_n(k\rho'_d)\sin k(z-z'_d)\end{pmatrix} I_n(k\rho)\frac{K'_n(kR)}{I'_n(kR)}\,dk \tag{2}$$

To match the boundary conditions at the top and bottom of the cylinder, the method of images has to be applied.

4. NUMERICAL IMPLEMENTATION OF THE AAD SOLUTION (4)

The correct AAD equations may be used to derive general properties of the potential distribution on a homogeneous cylindrical conductor. Attempts to evaluate these equations numerically however, prove that they are totally inadequate for numerical computations. This is always due to the behaviour of the modified Bessel functions for small arguments :

- The equations (1) and (2) have obviously the form of a two-dimensional continuous-discrete Fourier (co)sine transform of a function F(k,n). In (6) solutions for cylindrical forward problems through an FFT based algorithm

are proposed. When such a discrete fourier method is designed for equations (1) and (2), problems arise : sometimes it is necessary to select very small sampling intervals in the k-domain, which results in very long series to be transformed, sometimes the factor consisting of Bessel functions is unbounded and the DFT method can simply not be applied.
For eccentric sources, a rapid loss of accuracy is observed for increasing n-values when recursion formulas are used for the evaluation of the higher-order Bessel functions.
Finally it can be shown that when the eccentricity is important, the factors in the general term rapidly reach their over- and underflow values, while the general term itself converges slowly.

5. DISCUSSION

In electrophysiology, conductors under study often have approximately a cylindrical shape (nerve and muscle fibres, limbs, the human or animal torso,...). Until now, no valid analytical solution of the forward potential problem was proposed for a finite cylindrical conductor containing eccentric current sources. As such analytical solutions are often used to check the correctness of numerical procedures, we decided to identify the nature of the incorrectness of the existing solution (3) and to design a new correct one (4).

REFERENCES

1. A.C.L.Barnard, I.M.Duck, and M.S.Lynn : "The application of electromagnetic theory to electrocardiology - numerical solution of the integral equations". Biophysical Journal, vol. 7, pp. 463-491, 1967.
2. H.C.Burger, H.A. Tolhoek, and F.G. Backbier : "The potential distribution on the body surface caused by a heart vector". Am. Heart Journal, vol. 48, pp. 249-263, 1954.
3. R.H. Okada : "Potential produced by an eccentric current dipole in a finite-length circular conducting cilinder". IRE Trans. Med. Electron., vol. 7, p. 14, 1956.
4. J. Cornelis, E. Nyssen : "Potentials produced by arbitrary current sources in an infinite - and finite - length circular conducting cylinder". IEEE Trans. Biomed. Engineering - accepted for publication.
5. D.B. Geselowitz : "Multipole representation for an equivalent cardiac generator". Proc. IRE, vol. 48, pp. 75-79, 1960.
6. A.Heringa, D.F.Stegeman, G.J.H.Uijen and J.P.C.De Weerd : "Solution methods of electrical field problems in physiology". IEEE Trans. Biomed. Engineering, vol BME-29, no 1, pp. 34-42, January 1982.

Chapter 36

3-DIMENSIONAL PROPAGATION MODEL FOR SIMULATION OF THE VENTRICULAR DEPOLARIZATION AND REPOLARIZATION PROCESSES AND INDUCED BODY SURFACE POTENTIALS

M. AOKI, Y. OKAMOTO, T. MUSHA, K. HARUMI

INTRODUCTION

We have some knowledge about how the depolarization front propagates down from the sinus node to the ventricles and how its front behaves when it meets myocardial infarction or block of bundle branches. But, the so-called inverse problem, in which electric activities of the heart is estimated from the body surface potential, does not use such knowledge and too heavy load is given to mathematics. Therefore, details of the propagation of the depolarization front and the repolarization cannot be obtained. To overcome this difficulty we have tried computer simulation for propagation of depolarization and repolarization in the myocardium based on a model involving local propagation mechanisms of the action potential.

Much work [1]-[6] has been done to clarify depolarization and repolarization processes which yield the QRS complex and T wave. However, nobody to our knowledge has ever tried a computer simulation which can derive the T wave as well as the QRS complex, in which natural propagation of the excitation front is considered.

We have constructed a precise heart model which takes into account action potential waveforms of individual cell units, and derive the QRS complex and the T wave under an arbitrary heart condition such as myocardial infarction and bundle branch block. In this paper, the standard 12 lead ECGs, the VCG, and the body surface potential map will be given for the normal heart, the complete left bundle branch block and the myocardial infarction. This model is also applicable to compound heart diseases.

METHOD

1. Depolarization process

The heart model is composed of about 50,000 cell units whose size is about 1.5 mm as shown in Fig.1. The model has been constructed from the cross sections of the human heart which were observed by Durrer et al.[7]. The depolarization is initiated in the atrio-ventricular node and the depolarization front propagates from the bundle branches to the Purkinje fibers, where it spreads isotropically into the neighboring ventricular muscles. The conduction velocity in the bundle branches and the Purkinje fibers is 5 times faster than that in the ventricular muscles.

Electric dipoles are developed across a boundary between depolarized units and polarized ones, and an electric uniform dipole layer is formed along the boundary. Electric currents flow in the forward direction, this is the first phase of the action potential waveform.

The heart model is placed in a homogeneous torso volume conductor, on which 344 nodes are arranged and are connected by 684 triangles. The body surface potential distributions are calculated by the boundary element method [8] in which nodal points can be settled on the body surface independently of the configuration of the excitation front.

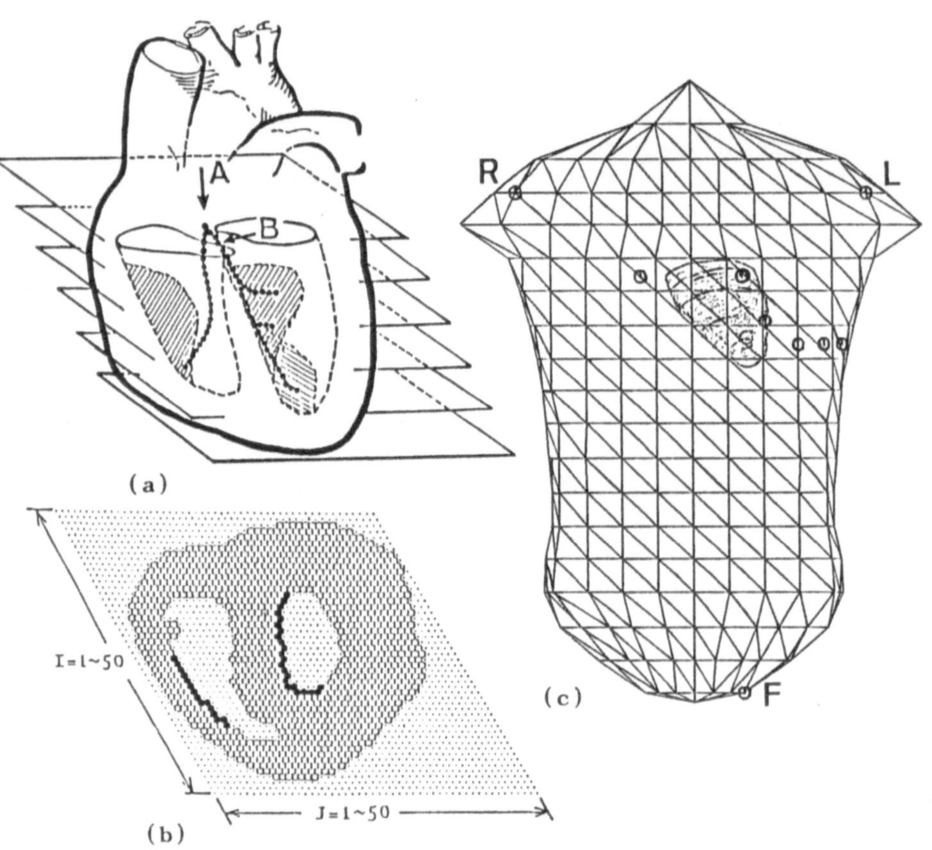

FIGURE.1 (a). A heart model established in a parallelepiped. The first stimulus causes at the unit shown with an arrow A in the normal heart; a bundle branch is denoted by dark circles and shaded regions represent the distribution of the Purkinje fibers. The conduction is interrupted at the point B for the CLBBB. (b). The horizontal cross section of the heart model; dark circles denote the Purkinje fibers. (c). A human torso model; small circles denote electrode positions.

2. Repolarization process

For simulation of the T-wave, it is necessary to assign the activation time and the action potential waveform to each unit in the heart model. The activation time is obtained by the previous excitation propagation simulation. The normal human QRS period is 70 to 90 msec and simulation of this process needs 27 time steps for the depolarization front to finish its propagation in the normal ventricles, this time step corresponds to 3 msec.

If all the units have identical waveform of the action potential, the T wave would have opposite polarity to the QRS complex, which does not agree with observations. Hence, it is required that the waveform, especially the duration, must differ from unit to unit. It has been found that the depolarization period of a dog heart becomes shorter towards the epicardium from the endocardium, and that is shorter near the base than near the apex of the ventricle [9]. Duration of the depolarization was distributed continuously in the heart. Fig.2 shows the distribution of the duration thus obtained. The electric motive force is proportional to the spatial gradient of the action potential. The body surface potential distribution generated by this electric motive force distribution is calculated by means of the boundary element method as mentioned before.

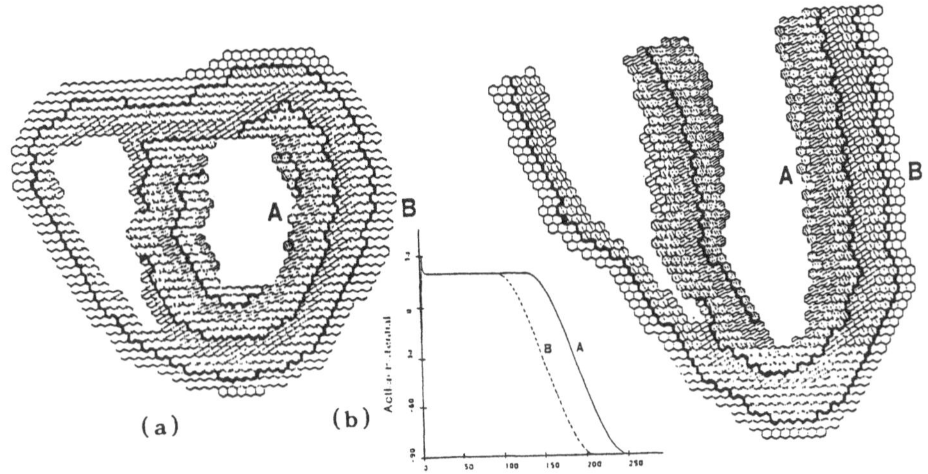

FIGURE.2 (a). The distribution of action potential duration (APD); the APD of the endocardial unit neighboring a epicardial unit is always longer 4 msec. (b). Action potential model adopted in the present model. The endocardial action potential A and the epicardial action potential B are shown. The depolarization periods are different each other.

RESULTS

1. Propagation of the excitation front

Horizontal (K=20) cross sections of the human heart, in which

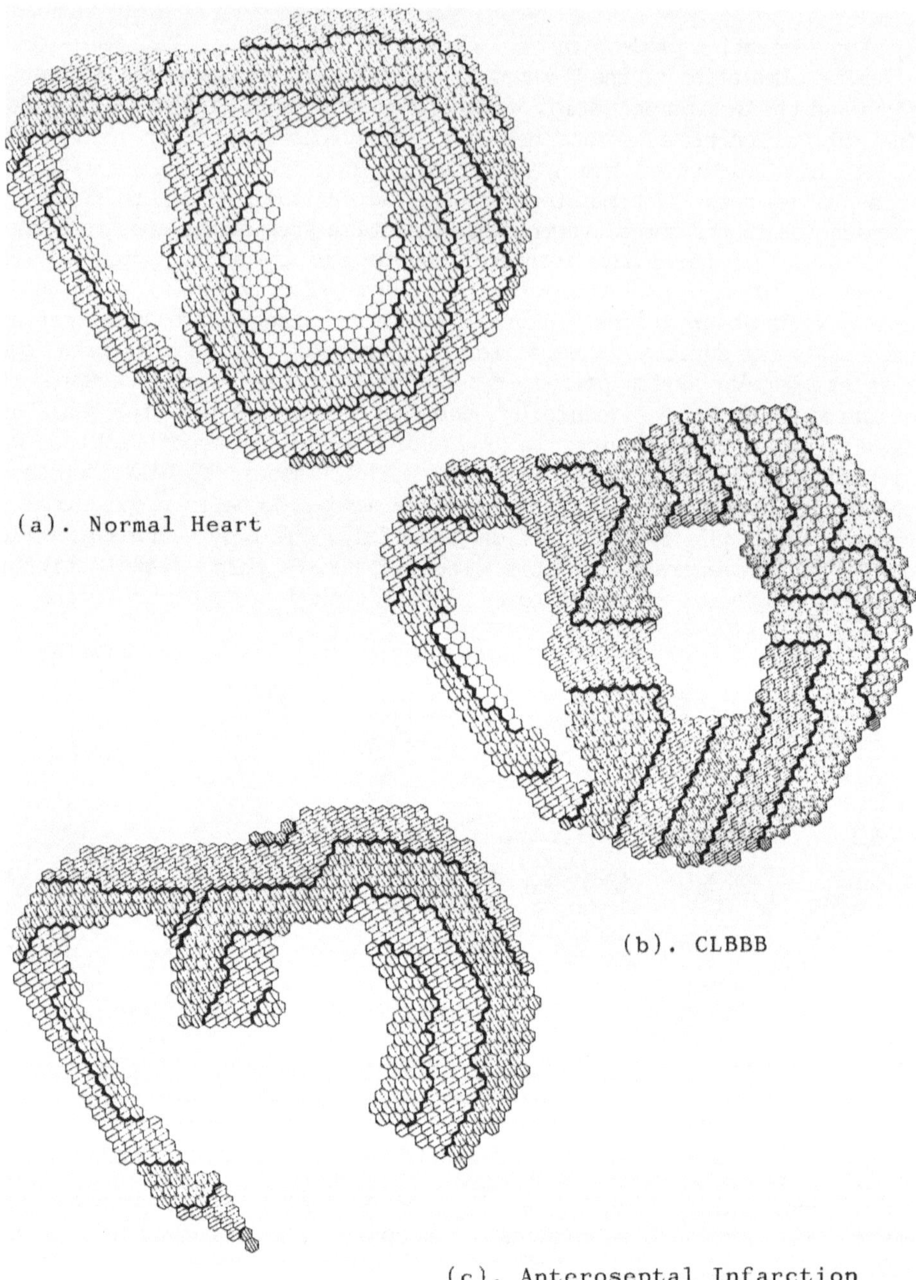

FIGURE.3 Horizontal cross sections of the heart model in which are illustrated excitation fronts at every 4 time steps; brighter regions are earlier in time. (a). Normal heart, (b). Left bundle branch block and (c). Anteroseptal infarction are shown.

propagation of the depolarization wave front is described, are illustrated in Fig.3. Fig.3(a) refers to a normal heart where a depolarization front propagates from bundle branches to the Purkinje fibers on the septum, the left and the right endocardium, and then spreads very rapidly over the ventricular wall, reaching the epicardium. These results are in good agreement with the observations made by Durrer et al.[7] for a human heart. It took 27 time steps for the depolarization front to travel through the ventricular units within a CPU time of 90 sec on computer HITAC M-180 with 3 MPS.

Similarly, Fig.3(b) refers to the complete left bundle branch block(CLBBB). Depolarizaton starts at the same spot on the right ventricular free wall as that in the normal case, and propagates towards the left ventricle where the Purkinje fibers on the left ventricular side do not participate in the propagation. It took 50 time steps for the depolarization front to travel through all ventricular units under the CLBBB. Arrival of the depolarization front at some vetricular units becomes very late, which greatly modifies the QRS complex and the T wave in CLBBB. The result of simulation qualitatively agrees with observations of van Dam [10] for canine and human hearts.

Fig.3(c) refers to the anteroseptal infarction. Depolarization starts in the same way as that in the normal heart. But, the excitation front goes around the site of infarction, and the area of infarction does not have the electric motive force.

2. Standard 12 leads ECG

Fig.4 shows standard 12 leads ECG´s resulting from the simulation of the ventricular depolarization and repolarization: (a), (b), and (c) refer to the normal case, CLBBB, and anteroseptal infarction. The potential values have been normalized to that of the normal case. V1 to V6 are the chest 6 leads on the torso illustrated in Fig.1(c), and I, II, and III are bipolar leads. Here Wilson´s central terminal potential is equated to the mean potential at electrodes R, L, and F. aVr, aVl, and aVf refer to potential values at electrodes R, L, and F after subtracting this central terminal value. The characteristics of the ECGs thus obtained are the following.

(a) Normal Heart : Duration of the QRS complex is 81 msec. The electrical axis of QRS complex is about 70 deg. The transitional zone lies between V3 and V4. The T wave has a possitive potential except for aVr and the maximal T wave is observed at V2.

(b) Complete left bundle branch block : Duration of the QRS complex is more than 120 msec. RR´ is observed at V5 and V6. rS is observed at V1, and a deep S and a possitive T wave are observed from V1 to V4.

(c) Anteroseptal infarction : Duration of the QRS complex is 81 msec. QS is observed from V1 to V3, and a negative T wave is observed from V2 to V4.

3. Vectrcardiogram

Electric dipoles appear on the depolarization front in the QRS period and on the repolarization zone in the T period. Their vector sum was evaluated at every time step during the QRST period. Horizontal, frontal, and sagittal projection of the vector components are illustrated in Figs.5(a), (b), and (c), where rotation of the vector component is indicated by an arrow.

(a) Normal heart : The QRS loop rotates counter-clockwise on the

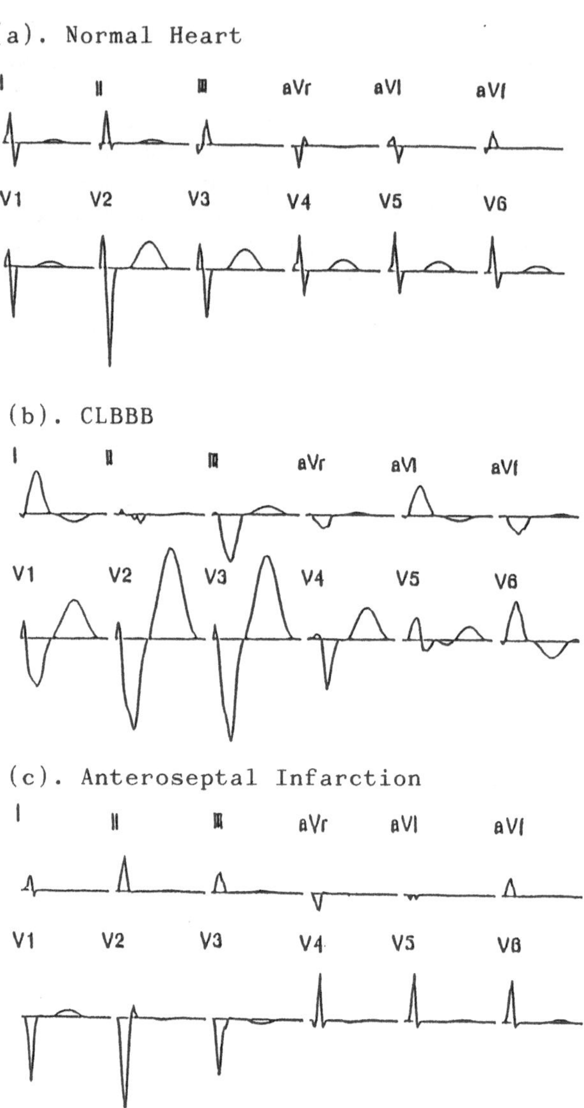

FIGURE.4 Standard 12 lead electrocardiograms eveluated in the present model.

horizontal plane. Initially it rotates counter-clockwise, and a maximum is reached at - 70 deg; a part of the loop lies in the second quadrant which is sometimes the case for a normal subject. The T loop also turns counter-clockwise and a maximum appears at 60 deg, which is beyond the limit of normal VCG, too. The similar results are obtained in frontal and sagittal planes as well as in horizontal plane.

(b) Complete left bundle branch block : The QRS loop and the T loop rotate counter-clockwise; the T loop is more oblong and narrower than in the normal case. These results agree with observations of M.Gardberg et al.[11].

(c) Anteroseptal infarction : The QRS loop and the T loop rotate counter-clockwise on horizontal plane. Initially the QRS loop turns to left-backward, and lacks the Q loop in horizontal plane.

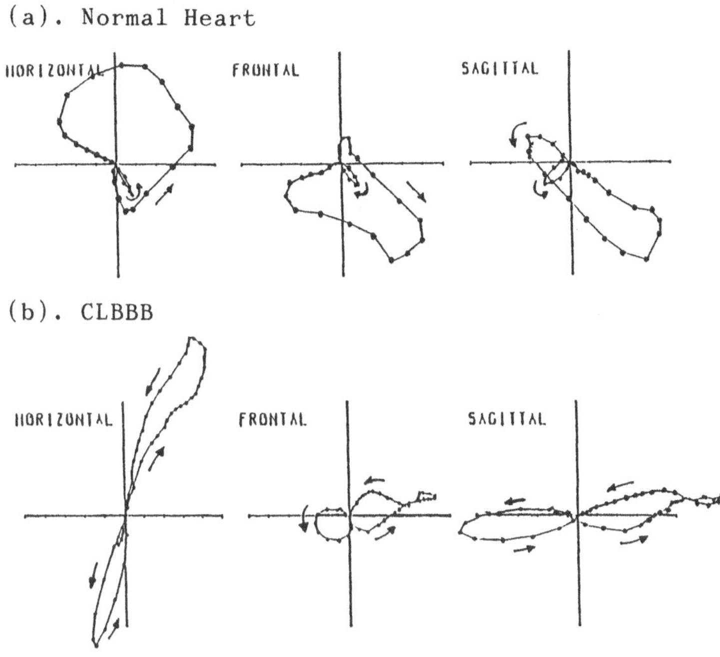

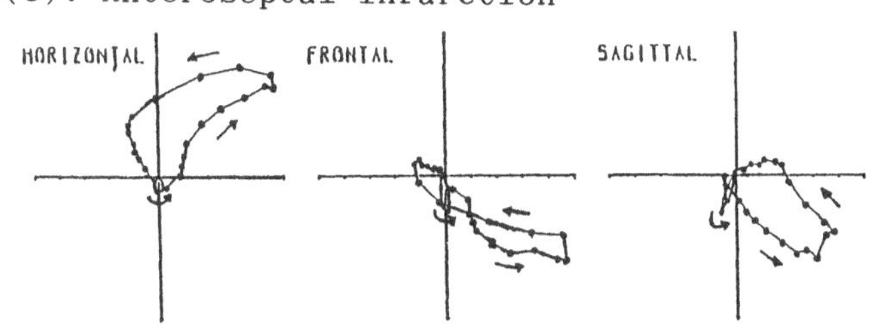

FIGURE.5 Vectorcardiograms evaluated in the present model.

4. Body Surface Potential Map

Time evolution of the body surface potential distributions is obtained and the results are illustrated in Fig.6 during the QRS and T periods, where the left and right halves refer to the chest and the back. The time is counted from starting of the depolarization. Potential values have been normalized to the normal case. Potential distributions showing the maximal T wave are arranged on the rightmost.

(a) Normal Heart : In the first stage, a maximum potential appears at the chest front, and then the minimum potential comes down from the right-arm side, where a maximum potential moves to the back. From the middle to the last stage in the QRS complex, the minimum stays at the chest front. Maximal potential appears at 36 msec. The maximal potential of T wave rises and falls at chest-frontal.

(b) Complete left bundle branch block : The maximum potential value which appears in the initial stage of the QRS complex is smaller than that in the normal one. At about 90 msec a deep negative region appears at the precordial; the depth becomes gradually shallower. After this period the potential distribution remains almost invariant.

(c) Anteroseptal infarction : Initially a minimum potential appears

(a). Normal Heart

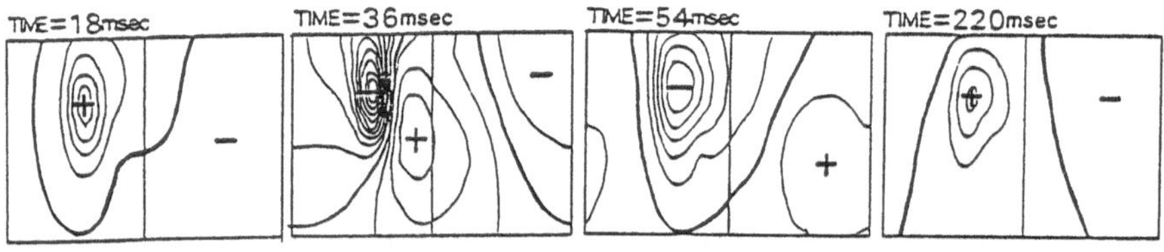

(b). CLBBB

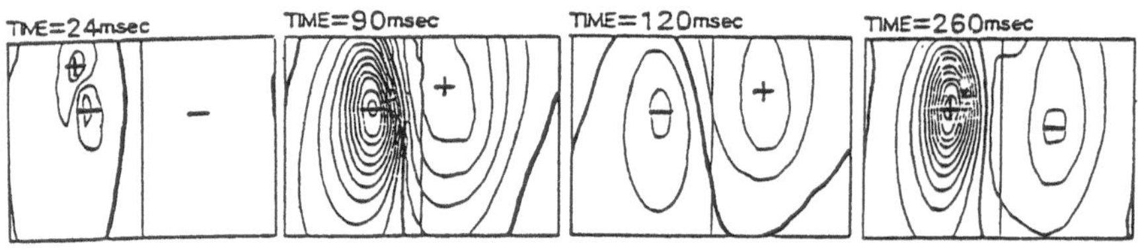

(c). Anteroseptal Infarction

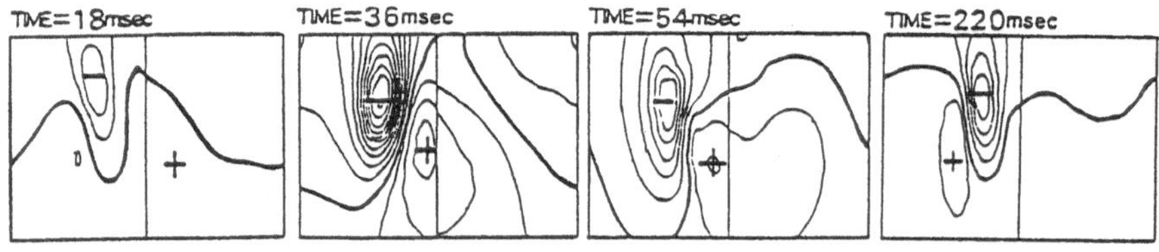

FIGURE.6 Body surface potential distributions evaluated by the present model.

locally at the chest front. Until the last stage of the QRS complex, a negative potential remains at the right chest front. And the mininum potential of T wave rises and falls locally at chest-frontal.

DISCUSSION

The present work is aimed at constructing a precise computer simulation program which can clarify a relationship between electric activities of the heart and the body surface potential distribution throughout the QRST period under an arbitrary heart condition. The rectangular model of Inoue et al. [5] or the left ventricular model of Horan et al. [6] cannot explain the observation. To correctly simulate the QRST wave under an arbitrary heart condition, depolarization and repolarization processes in the right and left ventricles must be taken into account in the program such that they simulate the real processes as much as possible. Miller and Geselowitz [3] used Durrer´s measured data [7], and hence their treatment does not cover abnormal heart conditions where depolarization process will be different from Durrer´s observation. Under myocardium infarction the a depolarization front goes around the site of infarction. To simulate the T wave a suitable waveform of the action potential must be given to each of the units in the ventricles. Sekiya et al. [9] examined the action potential duration in a canine left ventricle. They suggested that the duration is longer near the endocardium than near the epicardium and is longer near the apex than near the base. We found that many layers of different depolarization periods must be assumed to have the repolarization front propagating from outside towards inside of the ventricle.

Characteristics of the present simulation which are not included in the previous works [1]-[6] are the following.

(1) Geometry of the heart and the torso is very similar to the real ones.

(2) The special conduction systems have been taken into account.

(3) Propagation of the depolarization front is included in the model and the propagation under an arbitrary defect is correctly described.

(4) Proper action potential waveform is assigned to each unit in the right and left ventricles.

(5) The 12 leads ECG, the VCG, and the body surface potential map during QRS-T periods are calculated automatically under an arbitrary heart condition.

Details in the cardiac condition cannot in principle be estimated from the body surface potential distribution unless as much physiological knowledge we have as possible is utilized. In this sense the inverse problem is not so promissing. To overcome this difficulty we have tried to establish a precise computer model on electric activities of the heart. We have obtained a satisfactory computer program in Fortran 77. This is useful for detailed diagnosis of the heart disease by comparing the time evolution of the body surface potential distributions which is obtained under various heart conditions; at the same time this program is useful for education purposes.

REFERENCES

1. M. Okajima, T. Fujino, T. Kobayashi, and K. Yamada, "Computer simulation of the propagation process in excitation of the ventricles," Circ. Res., vol.23,pp.203-211,1968.
2. J. C. Solomon, and R. H. Silvester, "Simulation of measured activation sequence in the human heart," Amer. Heart J., vol.85,pp.518-524,1973.
3. W. T. Miller,III, and D. B. Geselowitz, "Simulation studies of the electrocardiogram I. The normal heart," Circ. Res., vol.43,pp.301-315, 1978.
4. R. L. Cohn, S. Rush, and E. Lepeschkin, "Theoretical analyses and computer simulation of ECG ventricular gradient and recovery waveforms," IEEE Trans. Biomed. Eng., vol.29,pp.413-423, 1982.
5. M. Inoue, H. Inada, N. Hoki, M. Fukushima, M. Hori, H. Kusuoka, H. Abe, F. Kajiya, T. Furukawa, and S. Takasugi, "A simulation of QRS-T wave based on the transmembrane action potential of myocardial cell," Jpn. J. Med. Electron. Biol. Eng., vol.15, pp.121-128,1977.
6. L. G. Horan, R. C. Hand, J. C. Johnson, M. R. Sridharan, T. B. Rankin, and N. C. Flowers, "A theoretical examination of ventricular repolarization and the secondary T wave," Circ. Res., vol.42,pp.750-757,1978.
7. D. Durrer, R. Th. Van Dam, M. G. Freud, M. J. Janse, F. L. Meijler, and R. C. Arzbaecher, "Total excitation of the heart," Circulation, vol.41,pp.899-912, 1970.
8. C. A. Brebbia, The boundary element method for engineers, Pentech Press,1980.
9. S. Sekiya, S. Ichikawa, T. Tsutsumi, and K. Harumi, "Distribution of action potential durations in the canine left ventricle," Jpn. Heart J., vol.25, pp.181-194, 1984.
10. Van Dam R Th, Ventricular activation in human and canine bundle branch block., In the conduction system of the heart, Eds. Lie Wellens, Lea Janse, Febiger, Philadelphia, 1976.
11. M. Gardberg, and I. L. Rosen, "The electrocardiogram and vectorcardiogram in various degrees of left bundle branch block," Amer. J. Cardio., pp.592-596,1958.

Chapter 37

MOVING DIPOLE ANALYSIS IN NORMAL AND MYOCARDIAL INFARCTION

K. HARUMI, H. TSUNAKAWA, S. KANESAKA, G. NISHIYAMA

1. INTRODUCTION

The body surface potential mapping has been considered to provide more detailed information on the ventricular depolarization process in various cardiac deseases. Recent advances in mathematical techniques and inverse solution make it possible to analyze the nature of the instantaneous dipole during the ventricular depolarization in patients with myocardial infarction (MI). In this study, the single moving dipole approximation was performed in patients with old MI and compared with normal subjects.

2. METHOD

Twenty seven normal adult males, 25 patients with old anterior, 18 patients with posterior and 3 patients with lateral infarction were studied. The location and the size of infarction were defined by thallum^{201}, myocardial scintigrams. Body surface potentials were recorded simultaneously at intervals of 2 ms from 64 sites on the anterior chest wall. The position and the moment of the cardiac dipole were calculated using Okamoto's method described previously (1,2). In brief, an infinite boundary plane is assumed as a body surface and the calculated potential on the boundary plane is obtained, assuming an electrical dipole in a uniform volume conductor.
An instantaneous equivalent dipole is determined as that dipole which optimally represents the observed potential distribution. The proximity function is minimized as shown in figure 1. To express the non-dipolarity, the term residue is introduced as a parameter of body surface potential not represented by single moving dipole. The root mean square (RMS) of the measured potential is calculated to represent the magnitude of obtained potential.

1) Instantaneous Dipole Moment from Body Surface Potential

$$S(\vec{r}, \vec{d}) = \Sigma_{i=1}^{N} (\varphi\text{meas.}i - \varphi\text{cal.}i)^2$$

S: Proximity function ($\vec{r}$: Position, $\vec{d}$: Component)

φmeas. i: measured potential at i position

φcal. i: caluculated potential at i position

2) Ratio of Non-dipolar Component (Residue)

$$\sqrt{\frac{\Sigma(\varphi\text{meas.}i - \varphi\text{cal.}i)^2}{\Sigma\varphi\text{ meas.}i^2}}$$

3) Root Mean Square (RMS)

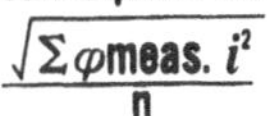

$$\frac{\sqrt{\Sigma\varphi\text{meas. }i^2}}{n}$$

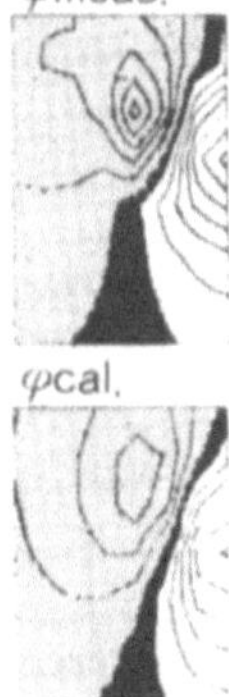

Fig. 1

3. RESULT

1. Normal subjects (3): The residue and RMS calculated at 2 ms intervals of a representative subject were shown in figure 2. The RMS curve increased smoothly and small notch was present at 20 ms. A second small notch was noted at 40 ms after the peak of RMS curve. Two peaks indicated by arrows 2 and 3 corresponded to each notch on the RMS curve during the QRS. During ST-T the residue was lower and more stable than that of QRS. The residue value, the time of appearance of notches on the RMS curve and the characteristic patterns of the isopotential maps corresponding to the times of peak residue are summarized in table 1. In all 27 normal subjects the mean residue of whole QRS was 24.0±3.5%. The mean residue of the latter half was higher than that of the initial half of QRS in 23(85%) of a total of 27 cases. The residue showed two high peaks. The first peak appeared at 24.4±6.7 ms from the onset of QRS in 11 cases and the second at 46.4±8.1 ms in 25 cases. These corresponded with a notch on the RMS curve and with more non-dipolar distributions of isopotential maps.

2. Old anterior infarction (4): Figure 3 shows an example of the alteration of the residue and RMS curves and isopotential maps in old anterior infarction. The patients with anterior infarction with the perfusion defect of 32% of the left ventricle exhibited higher residue during the initial QRS than the normals.

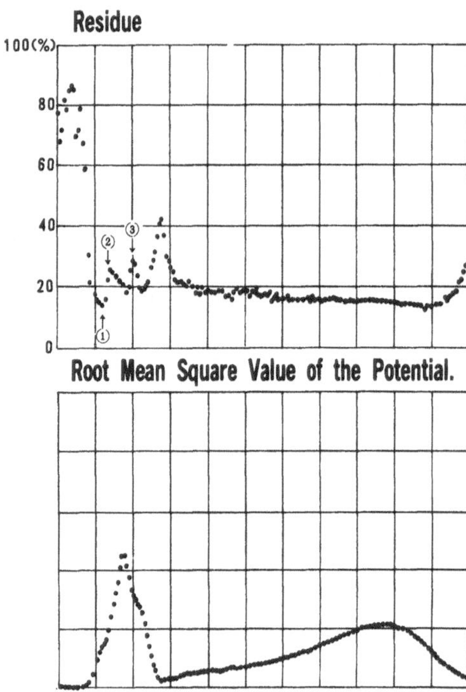

Fig. 2

Residue, RMS and Characteristic Patterns of Isopotential Maps of 27 normal Cases —QRS—

Case	Residue (%) QRS					Notch in RMS curve	Isopotential Map
	mean of initiai half	mean of later half	mean of QRS	peak residue	(msec from the onset of QRS)	(msec from the onset of QRS)	pseudopod irregularity of negative area
Group 1 (11 cases)	20.1±2.7	25.7±2.6	23.1±2.3	27.6±5.6 (24.4±6.7)	33.6±5.6 (48.5±5.9)	(20.5±3.3) (48.6±4.9)	+5/11 + 8/11
Group 2 (14 cases)	22.5±4.4	27.6±6.1	25.1±4.1		40.7±11.3 (44.7±9.4)	(46.6±4.5)	+ 9/14
Group 3 (2 cases)	19.0±1.4	23 ±4.2	21.0±2.8				
Mean±1SD (Total 27 cases)	21.3±3.8	26.5±4.9	24.0±3.5	27.6±5.1 (24.4±6.7)	37.6±9.7 (46.4±8.1)	(20.5±3.3) (47.5±4.7)	+5/11 +17/25

Table 1

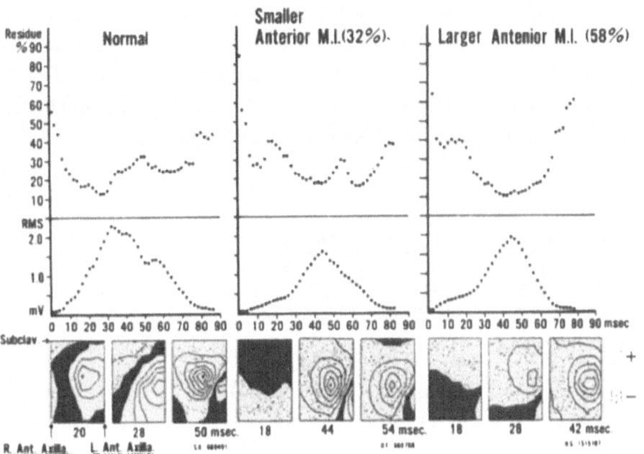

Fig. 3

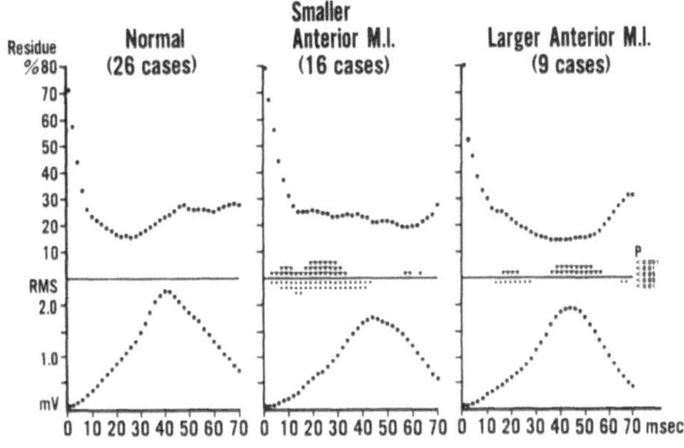

Fig. 4

Whereas the residue became lower during the mid QRS in extensive anterior MI as shown in the right panel. The residue value between 18 and 28 ms was significantly smaller than that of normals ($p<0.001$) in 16 cases with anterior MI (Fig. 4). In 9 cases with extensive anterior MI, the residue between 41 and 53 ms was significantly smaller than that of the normals ($p<0.001$). When the instantaneous residue during QRS of all 25 patients with anterior MI was compared with the size of MI defined as the ratio of cold area to the left ventricle on thallium^{201} myocardial scintigram, there was a negative correlation between the size of infarction and the residue value at 38 ms as shown in figure 5.

3. Old posterior, lateral infarction (5): Residue and RMS curves in representative subjects are shown in figure 6. In an example of posterior infarction, the high residue value was obtained during the late QRS. On the other hand, the residue showed high value during the mid QRS in an example of lateral infarction.

Figure 7 shows the appearance time of the peak of residue in patients with posterior or lateral infarction. In 18 patients with posterior MI, the second peak appeared at 50±7 ms, significantly later than that of normal subjects. Compared with the instantaneous residue curve in normals, no significant difference was shown on the mean residue curve in 18 patients with posterior and 3 patients with lateral MI except the initial QRS in posterior MI (Fig. 8). The RMS showed significantly smaller value during the mid and late QRS in posterior infarction than in the normals.

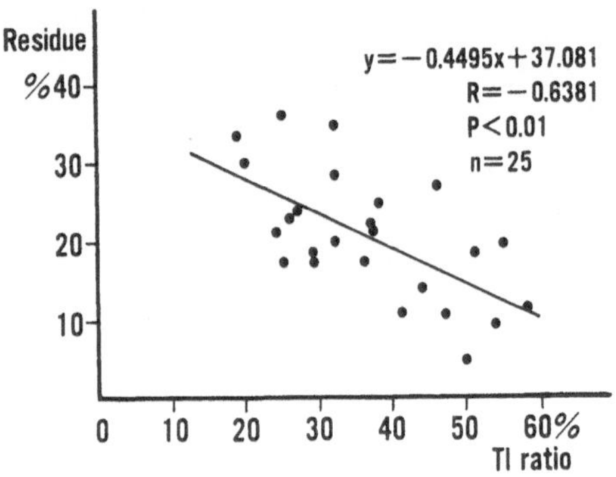

Fig. 5

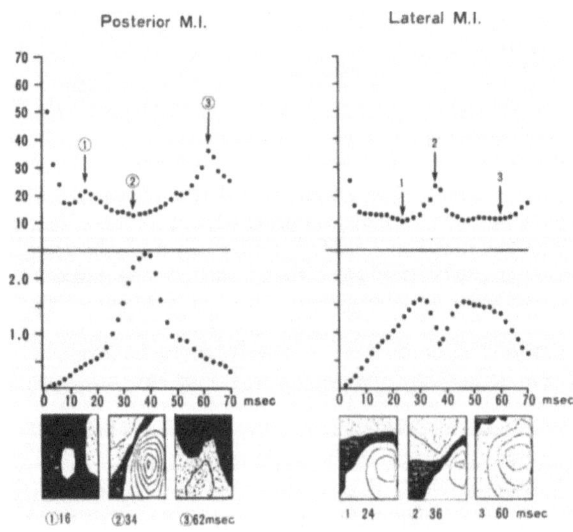

Fig. 6

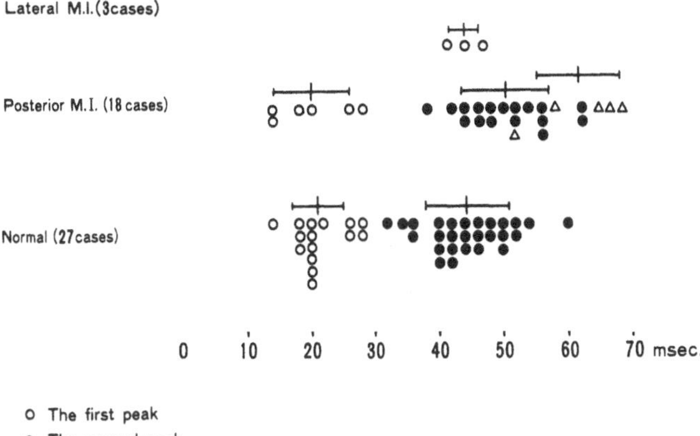

Fig. 7

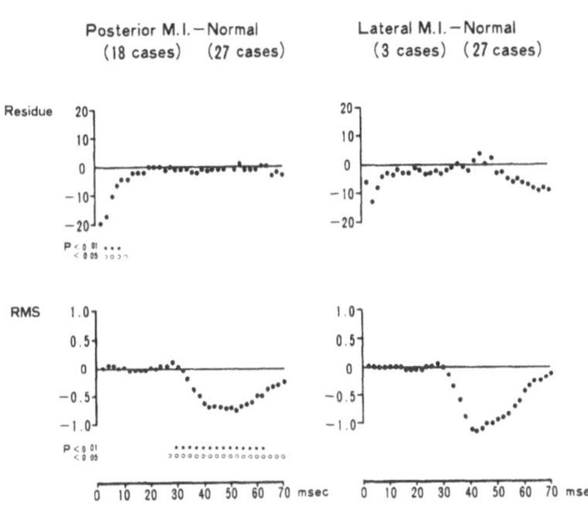

Fig. 8

4. DISCUSSION

In a recent study based on the calculation of multiple nonfixed dipoles, the information of the residue which could not be accounted for by single moving dipole was mainly present at approximately 25 and 45 ms during the normal QRS. These periods correspond to multiple activation fronts resulting from right ventricular breakthrough and geometrically separated activation fronts in the left ventricular base and interventricular septum or right ventricle in the normal cardiac cycle.

The major findings from this study are that the alteration of the electromotive force in MI can be readily analysed and the size of infarction of anterior MI could be predicted by the present method. These findings would be related to the alteration of the ventricular activation sequence induced by the infarcted area which may be more or less complex and the multiple fronts or single front would be expected to depend upon the size of infarction. Therefore, despite some limitations, the analysis of dipole would be a promising method for further understanding of the patients with various cardiac deseases.

REFERENCES

1. Okamoto Y, et al: Motion of equivalent electric dipole to cardiac activity estimated from body surface potentials. Jpn. Heart J. 21: 761, 1980
2. Okamoto Y, et al: Moving multiple dipole model for cardiac activity. Jpn. Heart J. 23: 293, 1982
3. Tsunakawa H, et al: Dipolarity and Dipole Location during QRS and T waves in normal men estimated from body surface potential distribution. Jpn. Heart J. 26: 319, 1985
4. Kanesaka S. : Cardiac dipolarity of ventricular excitation sequence calculated from body surface potential maps: Old anterior myocardial infarction. J. Jpn. Soc. Inter Med. 74: 16, 1985
5. Nishiyama G, et al: Dipole behavior of posterior myocardial infarction. Comparison with the three dimensional infarction model. Jpn. Heart J. to be published.

DISCUSSION

Introduction

At the end of the symposium a discussion session was held which was attended by almost all participants. The session lasted a good three hours. The main line of the discussion will be summarized here. The length of this session prohibits a full documentation of all points raised by the various participants. However, several full quotes will be included. The contributants will be identified by using their surnames only. Their full names and addresses may be found elsewhere in this book.

The discussion covered the following six topics:
1. standardization of recording and display of maps.
2. proven and promising applications of mapping.
3. exchange of data
4. the value of low level potentials
5. ECG independent evavaluation
6. international cooperation.

This report on this discussion session closely follows these topics. The main attention was focused on the first two topics.

1) Standardization

This topic was introduced by Taccardi.

Taccardi:
I think we should conclude our meeting with a few simple statements about what we are thinking we might do in order to make body surface maps widely accepted as a clinical method.
Every laboratory is at present recording body surface maps according to a different standard. I am afraid this is a serious drawback which prevents maps from being accepted. This had been the case, I remember, for vectorcardiography for many years until one single method was proposed, which was essentially Frank's method. After that electrocardiography became standardized and has developed for many years in a well organized way. At present there are surface mapping systems with 16 leads, with 32, 64 and so on, but this is not the main difficulty. The difficulty is that the area explored is different and so the amount of information is different and not transferable.

The need for standardization of the area explored and for including a proper reference to anatomical landmarks which will enable the transfer of map data between research groups was formulated by Selvester.

Selvester:
One of the advantages of being my age is that you do remember certain things that happened way back and I can remember quite well the old CF leads and I can remember quite well the New York Heart Association's big brawl about where the leads ought to be and Goldberger influencing everybody when they finally decided to set up a recommendation that became the world standard. And I can remember the literature before that happened, everybody having his leads everywhere else and nobody able to tell whether what he was finding meant anything compared with what other people were finding. I think that, while Goldberger used all the wrong reasons, the NYHA accepted them and for all the wrong reasons they decided where the leads ought to be. The standardization of agreeing to put them in the 4th intercostal space, in the midclavicular line, in the anterior axillary line, in the 5th intercostal space etc. was in fact what made the difference between being able to share the data and only when that happened did the accumulated data begin to bringing into focus the value of ECG. I think that's a fair statement and so I think that one of the obligations for this group is to agree on some common locations for putting the leads in such ways that you can transform your data from one laboratory to another and not haggle with each other about where you put the leads. I think you have to agree on that. I don't see any reason not to, is what I am saying, I don't see any advantage to be so provincional about it. Anyone of us I've got 192 leads and I can wiggle them around. 196 I guess it means a few centimeters here or there. They don't matter that much. You have got so much redundancy what difference does it make and you've got 240, or whatever it is. It just seems like that when we start talking about changes across maps, we ought to know where the top of the map is, where the bottom of the map is, where the middle of the map is and where the leads are. So, whenever we report data to each other we ought to be able to transform the data from one group to the other without any argument about what it is really meaning. That's why the standardization of the lead location is as simple minded as it was back in the forties when the New York Heart Association made that recommendation. That's what it accomplished for the community. It accomplished the advantage to be able to talk sensibly to each from one lab to the other, to pool data. Then the literature began to pool data for us automatically.

The meeting agreed that a proposal for the standardization of the area explored should be worked out, in which a clear reference to anatomical landmarks and to the position of the standard ECG and VCG electrodes will be included. This task will be undertaken by Musso.

A major part of the discussion was devoted to the problem of deciding on the number of leads. It started off from the suggestion that a minimum number of leads should be decided on from which the standard ECG leads should be a subset. Although almost everybody seemed to agree that this number should be no less than 32, there was no sympathy for the suggestion that any specific number should be put forward as a recommendation at this stage.

Rudy:
I think that the necessary number of electrodes really depends on the goal of what you want to do with the data and there is not one single number that is useful for all those goals. The 24 leads that Duke has been using or the 32 which Bob Lux has been using are numbers of leads which are being used to reconstruct the maps so that they can be used for observation and for making comparisons and for finding correlations and so on. I am convinced that for good inverse problem solutions you need many more. So it really depends on what goal you have in mind when you decide on the number of electrodes.

Gulrayani:
One of the questions the number of leads is also related to the location. For example, if you use 32 leads you have to position them irregularly. Now most people who start would like to start with a regular positioning so that sort of implies you need more than 32 to begin with. I think the question of location also has to be addressed together with the number of leads.

Kozmann:
If you use only 32 electrodes, you have to use sophisticated interpolation of estimation methods. And certainly the whole system will be noise-sensitive so if one or two of the 32 is noisy, the reconstructed field will be noisy as well. So I have the feeling that as a minimum one should take about 60-64, which contains already some redundancy and you can profit from this redundancy.

Kornreich:
I think the logical way would be to start with the common data base with a maximum number of leads and then test out whatever number of leads people are using: 100, or 50 or 32 or 24, and compare the results before settling on a given number. It depends on the goals which people are trying to achieve. If everybody

records in his place whatever number of leads he wants and if we settle on a common number of 32. let it be 32, I still don't see how we are going to assess whether that is really the right thing to do. Unless we start from a common data base.

The need for some kind of standardization was stressed by

Green:
I am going to speak by virtue of the 2 years experience in the US, trying to get funding for clinical research with body surface mapping. Bob Lux and I and others in our group spent almost 2 years continuously writing grant applications, so far unsuccessfully. I am not speaking from an advocacy of any system that would make the point that based on our experience with study sections in NIH. If there is not concrete evidence of the clinical utility of body surface mapping in providing information of clinical significance that other types of cardiac imaging don't provide within a fairly short time span, we are not gonna be planning another meeting, at least not with much participation from our country. The funding is just not gonna be there.

Taccardi:
If I understand the point which you and others are making is, what we need to do in order to get funds and go on with our work is to demonstrate the utility. Now everybody here is also interested in research and for research we are going to use whatever system we like, but to get funds for this work, we have to demonstrate the utility of maps. We can demonstrate the utility of maps with the different systems. We are trying to do so and I think we succeed and so are you and Jerry Liebman with many electrodes and so are many others. But if we go on in this way, we shall only have small statistics, because every lab has 100-200 patients, which looks like a big number, but it is not if you consider all the variability in normals, and age. So, in order to demonstrate the utility we probably need larger statistics. So, the question I'm asking now (while everybody must go on with as many leads as he can afford) is: "Can we in addition found some common standard, which would enable us to establish a common data base and finally within a few years come up with sufficiently large learning sets and test sets which will demonstrate the utility of mapping?" We have interesting data with 20 patients with angina and we can detect angina with normal ECG's, but just in 20 patients; what about 2000? How often does it occur in a population? I think we need a large population of cases and are we able to dilute a little bit of our desire

for perfection in getting a large data bases, or are we not? I think we should leave this session with a statement on whether we want larger data base, and on whether we can provide the demonstration of the utility without data bases.

Harumi:
One of the reasons for the proposed standardization is that so many institutes use different numbers of electrodes and different location. We proposed a processed map made from each original map and this processed maps can be used for the exchange of the data.

The idea that any lead system should have the standard leads as a subset received much acclaim.

Arnaud:
An important problem is the acceptability of the methods to the cardiologist in practice. In such a way I think we need to have the standard ECG as the subset of the body maps.

Brohet:
The situation is very similar to the problem that we have when we want to compare the diagnostic accuracy of standard 12 lead electrocardiography and Frank vectorcardiography. It was very difficult to answer that question because we didn't have a common data base where we could use optimal methods of analyzing both 12 lead and VCG on the same patients. I would strongly advise that at the same time as you record any number of electrodes for body surface maps, that you have a subset of ECG and VCG and also that you should record that ECG and VCG in digital form and in such a way that these methods could be allowed to perform in optimal conditions. It's not enough to compare quantitative knowledge on body surface maps with the Minnesota code. You should use sophisticated methods like multivariate statistical analysis for the ECG and the VCG as well as for the body surface maps.

Taccardi:
I think what we can try to change in what we are doing in our lab in this sense is that we will be going on with our 219 leads but that we will make sure that we know were the six precordial leads are and probably also where the 32 leads are located with respect to ours. They may have the same location or they may be somewhere in between, which can be easily interpolated.

Yet, some of the participants were not so convinced:

Horacek:
So far we didn't discuss any estimation of interpolation methods which will be sort of certified. We went to the ridiculous extreme that we cause Bruno Taccardi to put V1 to V6 into his lead system, but he can predict, safely interpolate, whatever there is to be known. By simple linear interpolation you can get lead V1 to V6 but it is not so sure, and also Bob Lux can not be sure, that he can reconstruct all the possible positions. At least not in all diagnostic categories, but it is ridiculous to talk about incorporating V1 to V6. The key word here is interpolation or estimation.

Savard:
You just remarked on something that I was going to say but I may add one more thing on the electrode placement. In the standard ecg system you can misplace those electrodes and this can have a great effect on your diagnostic. We've had that experience in WPW for example where the body surface potential maps were more robust. If the entire pattern is shifted by one centimeter, it still is the same pattern, but if you look at the individual leads, there might be some differences. So I'm not so sure, I'm not so convinced about incorporating the standard ecg leads into the body surface area and one of the reasons again is that the most of us use strips or vests or other kind having fixed distances between the electrodes while the body shape, the intercostal space is not always the same between one person and the other.

However, a final conclusion was reached, as summed up by Taccardi.

Taccardi:
When we say we are willing to change our system, in fact we said we are willing to do what is possible. Since our strips are fixed we certainly cannot change the position of the electrodes. But we can establish where the six leads, the six precordial leads are located in our grid and in many cases it will coincide with some position in our system and when it doesn't, interpolation will be straightforward and resolve our problems. Another point which can be taken as a conclusion is that everybody continues studying the maps providing that the area explored is the same and then every point on the chest map has a potential value, whether by measurement or interpolation and these values can be compared. The only problem I have is: how are we going to exchange data. Everybody has a

different system and I am not sure that we can arrive today to a conclusion on how we can exchange data. Nevertheless I do think that if we don't exchange data then our statistics will be insufficient, I just propose that we go home and think about the way of exchanging data, for instance by interpolating and having maps and the maps can be exchanged as images or as local variation of potential whether interpolated or not. We may try to establish where the 32 points of the Salt Lake City system, which has the largest data on magtape, are located on our grid and everybody can do the same and see whether this comparison gives good results. So when we go back home I am going to think about this and make a proposal about practical interchange because this should be the conclusion of this meeting that we should arrive at an exchange of data. We are not ready to say how, but we should do that. All of us can not change our lead system because there are years of investment in hardware and software, but we can make it comparable. We can, without formal committees, think and write to those who have to formulate the proposal for the comparison, as we are going to do in Parma. We can go on along this line and exchange a few letters so as to propose a general way to exchanging data. This is the way I would like to make a conclusion on the first part of this discussion which is on the area explored and on lead systems.

Taccardi:
Practically, Esio Musso and I will write to everybody asking landmarks of their grids and we will put all the grids together and consult Bob Lux and also other volunteers to establish how to pass from one system to the other. This will be undertaken.

2 Proven and promising applications of mapping

Since all participants had been invited by the scientific committee of this symposium on the basis of their active involvement with the mapping technique it seemed to be a good idea to make an inventory of their ideas on the usefulness of these mapping techniques. The outcome of this will be listed here. This will merely be a survey of the opinions of contributants. For more solid evidence of their statements the reader is referred to the original work of these people, some of which may be traced by their contributions to this book.

Proven

* basic research tool:
  high stability of interpretation of recorded potentials; amenable to inverse procedures; all basic electrical disorders; epicardial mapping.
  (Harumi, Horacek, Rudy, Nadeau)

* Myocardial Infarction
  general; location; extent
  (Kornreich, van Dam)

* Myocardial infarction in combination with left Bundle Branch Block.
  (Harumi, Musso)

* Right Bundle Branch Block
  (Liebman)

* Partial Right Bundle Branch Block
  versus Right Ventricular Hypertrophy with terminal conduction delay
  (Liebman, Musso)

* Myocardial Infarction without Q-waves
  (Rudy)

* acute Myocardial Infarction
  size; location; extension; apex
  (Okta, van Dam)

* Coronary Artery Disease
  extension and size; at rest
  (Horacek, Musso)

* induced Ischemia; pacing and exercize test
  (Mirvis)

* WPW:
  more precise localisation; non-invasive; MAP better than cath lab. studies
  (Selvester, Nadeau, Sippens Groenewegen)

* Premature Ventricular Beats
  Ventricular Tachycardia; origin
  (Rudy, Nadeau, Savard)

* Right atrial enlargement
  (Musso)

* Follow-up of P.T.C.A.
  (Green)

Promising (further study required).

* Coronary Artery Disease
  (Musso, Mirvis)

* serial comparison
  (Kornreich)

* arrhythmia's; conduction disturbances
  (Taccardi, Nadeau, Rudy, Green)

* hypertrophy; obstructive cardiomyopathy
  (Green, Brohet)

* low level potentials U-waves; late potentials
  (Taccardi, Rudy, Teramachi)

During this discussion the general indication for applying diagnostic mapping, and of its cost effectiveness were raised. Several people pointed out that apart from comparing the performance of the mapping technique with other diagnostic methods there are situations where mapping is the sole technique available since the disturbances are of an electrical nature and cannot be studied by any other means.

The need for worrying too much about the cost of the mapping technique was brushed aside by Horacek.

> Horacek:
> I think we should emphasize that mapping is an important basic research area for electrocardiography. There are, I don't know exactly the numbers I had, some staggering numbers that 100 million electrocardiograms are taken every year on North American continent alone. If it costs 10 dollars to record one ecg and if effectiveness, cost-effectiveness of that procedure is improved by 10%, that means 100 million bucks a year in savings. This is what any undergraduate student of economics would calculate and one has to look at it from the point of view that basic research actually can bring, (again I have it from literature) one dollar invested in basic research can bring $40 back.
>
> I just give it as an example that it's like in cancer research. If you just are too authoritarian, you don't get anywhere. You have to just look at it and this is why we are here, I think that it is basic research in electrocardiography, that's the business we are in and that's how it should be called. It's not strictly mapping or some infatuation with gadgets and utility of putting lots of electrodes on the patients. It is just collecting basic knowledge in the field of electrocardiography.

Taccardi stressed the need, though, for being aware of the following problem:

Taccardi:
We know that maps are superior to ECG in the area of arrhythmia, we need some more statistics but we know that this is the case, but how useful is it to have that information? How cost effective is it to have this. This is provocative, we know that is is useful but somebody might challenge or discuss it. Isn't it easier just to make an exercise test with ordinary ECG and have the same information, I believe this it is not the case, but it is just a provocative question. Or, by just making echocardiogram, can't we have the same information at lower cost or by making radionuclide imaging?

3 Exchange of data

Apart from the problem related to differences in lead systems between groups as discussed before (subsection 2) the exchange of data between groups is hampered at present by differences in the FORMAT in which these data are recorded. In particular the general information related to technical points like sampling rate, lead placement; recording conditions and applied filtering are at present non standard. Chapters 20 and 21 deal with this problem. During the discussion it was emphasized that it was this FORMAT specification which was the main problem rather than the actual hardware (tape, disk) on which this information was stored.

Horacek:
I was in favor of 9 track magnetic tape. Nine track magnetic tape with 800 density can hold 40 Mega bytes of data and so it is cheap and economical, it's easy to work with, but I want to caution now. We should not get married to this kind of technical things, what is the medium, it's not I'm not married to this IBM 9 track magnetic tape, I think a floppy disc, or whether it is 8 inch whether it is 5 1/2 inch, whatever the medium is not as important as what we put on it.

Selvester:
I want to make one other suggestion and that is that it's not enough to put a number in there as how this data was calibrated. I think the raw calibration signal coming through the system all the way from the patient to the final digitized data is something that really if you gonna process data you need to know. I suppose you know this, but there are commercial systems on the market that all the nice neat little square waves positions that's what the switch position is set to.

And I think we need to know that it does not view the performance of the system all the way through. It does not measure the action of normal calibration going into that hardware and that sounds prosaic but if there are just plenty of glitches between the front and the back of our systems, I think we need to know that as basic data that's right up in the header formation in the front of every system.

Nijssen:
I think that where it is possible, data perhaps measurement data, but at least header data, should be stored as text and for example in ASCI code. That would have much advantages, for example, one can very easily, when there are problems in the data, one can easily pinpoint where the problems are, texts can be edited on most computer systems and so on, so I think that is an important general characteristic that data should have.

At the end of this discussion it was agreed that Teramachi and Horacek will start working on a definite proposal for the organisation of a proper tape (disc) header for mapping procedures.

4. The value of low level potentials

As a prelude to the discussion the entire audience agreed that it is essential to include at least a few electrodes at the back. During the discussion on low level potentials the following major points were raised.

Musso:
We thought that it was almost impossible to say on body surface mapping in normal people how precise were the topographical aspects of body surface mapping during the PQ-wave and STT but even during the P-wave. So, if you don't know how things are normally, I think you can not tell how things will be with people who are abnormal. So we decided to start the investigation in order to have, as much as we could, a good representation of body surface mapping during these low level intervals. We have just collected data in people with angiographical documented coronary artery disease and in some of these people, I would say most of these people, if you look at the first two hundred milli-seconds of the STT-interval, or if you look at the potential maximum, it's just in a normal position as far as the location is concerned, but the potential values are usually 100 microvolt lower in ischaemic people as compared to normals.

Horacek:
What we use in Halifax is a logarithmic scale and now when we talk about low level potentials, I realize that this is a very important issue which is related to this. I have been mapping PR-segment potentials as low as 5,6,7 microvolts and we use our standard plotting programs which simply adjust themselves to these low levels. I have seen maps here that have to few contour lines, under 200 microvolts. Sometimes you don't see any contour lines under 200 microvolts and then you miss all those features. 200 Microvolt is a huge signal in a good quality ecg. On the other hand you see maps with a ridiculously large number of contours when you are at the peak of QRS.

Kornreich:
You're mentioning special purposes. You don't have to go that far for usual purposes. For separating normals from MI's, you're using potent discriminators that are of the order of magnitude of 60 μV in one group and 200 μV in the other group.

van Oosterom:
In my opinion that means that any expansion, should not only state the RMS-error but should definitely also include the maximal absolute error occurring in the expansion and possibly express that as a relative error.

Teramachi:
The resolution of the AD converter and its skew (time) must be considered, otherwise the low level potentials will all be in error, they will be meaningless I think.

5 ECG independent evaluation

This topic is related to any study in which the diagnostic performance of the mapping technique is compared to that of the standard ECG or the VCG.
The discussion was opened by Van Dam.

van Dam:
Don't you think that the best independent evidence we can have about myocardial perfusion in case of infarctions is in the form of scintigraphic data and secondly by the data on left ventricular wall motion by angiography, ventriculography in particular and by echo or any other means. Are there other means which we should include? ((Audience: CATscan)).
CATscan (very expensive). Alright. Unfortunately. We all are aware that the criteria for the 12 lead electrocardiogram all have been verified as far as

infarctions go against post mortem studies but they are going out of fashion, so I think we should not count too much on that method.

Selvester:
I think the one thing that you need to be sure of when you get into that mix - when you're talking about contrast ventriculography - preferably biplane ventriculography, is biplane ventriculograms with clearcut akinesis. There's all the data now, from the Duke group in particular, which shows that hypokinesis has a 50% chance of having no infarction at all, so if we're gonna use the gold standard we really have to stick to both biplane images and akinesis rather than hypokinesis. That's sort of the standard, I think, in the industry at the moment and does relate pretty well to pathology. We haven't given up on quantitating pathology but there are only 4-5 people in the world doing it, so it's hard to get a large data base.

Harumi:
In our country we have a special group which is studying the comparison of the body surface maps and autopsy. They are getting the data. And also I would like to comment on what dr. Taccardi said. You mentioned the atrium and also there is some group in Japan now that is studying the U-wave.

Nadeau:
Just a word about validation. Ventriculography is much more the validation I think we should use for body surface mapping and not scintigraphy because perfusion refers to vessels and I think the body surface maps are more related to the muscle function. In the very limited series that we did we had a very good correlation with ventriculography, but a much poorer one with scintigraphy and coronary angiography.

Green:
Anybody that works in a cath lab, knows that the presence of a 75% coronary occlusion doesn't tell a thing about perfusion and in the age of angiography a 75% coronary lesion has as much chance as not any chance at all of having a pressure gradient across it and body surface mapping may well play a role in determining the physiologic significance of coronary lesions. You've got a real problem there in terms of what are you going to compare the map to as a gold standard. About the only thing that is available is pressure gradient across the lesion that is available with angiography catheters. We've been trying to do a little bit of that now that angioplasties have been going on in our institution, and that may be one other item of information that you wanna have. It is

possible, they are admittedly not terribly accurate, they are certainly not as accurate as microsphere techniques in experimental animals, but there are techniques available for sampling coronary sinus blood flow in man in a variety of ways other than looking at lactate-excretion for trying to assess the significance of coronary lesions. I think there is a possible role for BSM. May be one has to put it on the "promising" list of using maps as a tool to determine the potential physiologic significance of coronary lesions.

Mirvis:
I think Larry Green's point is very valid. We just completed our study in dogs using aneroid constrictors to produce incomplete coronary occlusion but normal resting myocardial blood flow. When paced, these dogs get myocardial underperfusion and get ST-segment shifts on body surface maps that look just like positive exercise tests in people, and using regional myocardial microsphere techniques for regional blood flow measurements there's a very clear cut-off in endo-cardial/epicardial perfusion ratio's when the dog gets ST-depression and when he doesn't. That's about 0.6 as compared to a normal, or a little bit over 0.1, so I think there is a real potential for potential maps to provide good correlation with flow measurements.
Dr. Harumi has brought up another problem in the same area of defining control groups as well as defining the anatomic or functional abnormalities. If we include as a criterium for normality a normal 12 lead electrocardiogram we are including an internal inconsistency in our terms of defining what is abnormal. We're excluding a lot of abnormals, we're including anyone as abnormal who may be normal i.e. normal anatomically, but abnormal by some electrical mechanism in the cell or whatever. This is a particular problem. I think, in terms of coronary disease, particularly with resting but also with stress induced changes. Does this person have coronary disease anatomically but not functionally? His ECG aberration is a difficult problem for example. He may be a person who was born with an abnormal cardiogram and then he gets coronary disease at age 50 and now has both, but they're truly not related. It's an old medical board question. My own feeling is that if you are going to evaluate an anatomic variable, then your control group has to have everything but that anatomic variable, not other constraints. And a control group really probably should be people who are anatomically normal or clinically normal without the additional constraint of a normal cardiogram. That obviously gives problems as what I told you before in terms of defining normal. It's almost like the study appearing in the Journal of Irreproducible Results of several years ago about the

incidence, the very high incidence of breast cancer in women who have breast cancer; the incidence is extremely high. Interesting but absurd, of defining a normal group as well extremely carefully. My own feeling of this is that we're probably better off with a small but rigorously defined control group, than with a larger, loosely defined one. How to do that? I think it's difficult, but I think it is possible. I can tell you about one hospital in Memphis that has about 900 normal CATs, so the numbers are there, but my own bias would be towards a rigorous definition of a smaller group rather than a looser definition of a large one.

Brohet:
Just a very short additional comment on what is normal. I think that we should also collect 2 different types of normals. Normal patients, I mean patients who have been catheterized and in whom no coronary lesion has been found and on the other hand normals from the street, I mean normal volunteers without any complaint. This is because the clinical characteristics of the two groups of these normals may be very different and the specificity of any diagnostic method may be different in the two groups.

Selvester:
We wrestled with that question in the market users group just as a starter, just got a bunch of cardiologists together, and actually agreed - if you can believe this - in a couple of hours on a non-ECG basis for establishing a normal data base. I have added that as an addendum to my paper just because I think that's an important first step. Those of you who really are thinking about establishing a normal data base may at least look at what this group decided since it might be a basis for establishing non-ECG criteria for a normal data base. And I think we do have to avoid somehow contaminating that with our preconception about how normal a normal 12 lead ECG is. I think we put that in because you leave yourself wide open for all kind of criticism for the data base later on.

6 International Cooperation

At the end of this symposium the participants agreed in the founding of the ISCPM being "the International Society of Cardiac Potential Mapping".

The purpose of this society is the coordination and stimulation of all kinds of activity related to the study of the potential distribution generated by the heart. This interest includes both body surface potentials and the potentials of the exposed heart as observed during surgery.
The society will organize regular meetings, for instance in the form of satallite symposia of the major international meetings on electrocardiology. Its further activities will entail the promotion of the exchange of data between research groups and the formulation of standard procedures for the facilitation of such exchanges.
Prof.Dr B. Taccardi was elected as the first president of this society. Dr E. Musso will act as its secretary. Further suggestions for the future development of the society will be worked out by them.

AUTHORS INDEX:

ADDRESSES OF FIRST AUTHORS

Ambroggi, L. de
Istituto Simes di Cardiologia Sperimentale
Via C. Colombi 18
20161 MILANO
Italy

Aoki, M.
Tokyo Institute of Technology
Nagatsuta Midoriku Yokohama
Japan 227

Arnaud, P.
Institut National de la Santé et de la Récherche Médicale
Hôpital Cardio-Vasculaire
BP Lyon Monichai
69394 LYON Cedex 3
La France

Block, P.
Departments of Cardiology and Nuclear Medicine unit "Heart"
Free University Brussels
School of Medicine
BRUSSELS
Belgium

Brohet, C.R.
Cliniques Universitaires St. Luc
Université Catholique de Lourain (UCL)
Box 5550
Avenue Hippocrate 55
B 1200 BRUSSELS
Belgium

Dam, R.Th. van
Dept. of Cardiology
University of Nijmegen
Geert Grooteplein Zuid 8
6525 GA NIJMEGEN
The Netherlands

Green, L.S.
University of Utah
Nora Eccles Harrison Cardiovascular Research & Training Institute
Nora Eccles Harrison Building, University of Utah
SALT LAKE CITY, Utah 84112
U.S.A.

Gulrajani, R.
Centre de Récherche
Hôpital du Sacré-Coeur
5400 Ouest, Boul. Gouin
MONTRéAL, Québec
Canada H41 1C5

Harumi, K.
Showa University Fujigaoka Hospital
1-30 Fujigaoka, Midori-ku
YOKOHAMA 227
Japan

Hayashi, H.
Aichi Prefectural Center for Health Care
3-z-1, Sannomaru, NAKA-KU
NAGOYA 460
Japan

Klersy, C.
Department of Cardiology
University of Pavia
PAVIA
Italy

Kornreich, F.
Free University Brussels
School of Medicine
Departments of Cardiology and Nuclear Medicine; unit "Hart"
BRUSSELS
Belgium

Kozmann, G.
Central Research Institute for Physics
P.O.B. 49
H-1525 BUDAPEST
Hungary

Liebman, J.
Department of Pediatrics and Department of Biomedical Engineering
Case Western Reserve University
CLEVELAND, Ohio 44106
U.S.A.

Lux, R.L.
Nora Eccles Harrison Cardiovascular Research and Training Institute
Nora Eccles Harrison Building
SALT LAKE CITY, Utah 84112
U.S.A.

Macchi, E.
Istituto per le Applicazioni del Calcolo
C.N.R.
Viale del Policlinico n. 137
ROMA
Italy

Marangoni, E.
Department of Cardiology
University of Pavia
PAVIA
Italy

Mirvis, D.M.
Section of Medical Physics
University of Tennessee
Center for the Health Sciences
956 Court Avenue
Room 2 F 18
MEMPHIS, Tennessee 38163
U.S.A.

Musso, E.
Instituto di Fisiologia Generale e Centro Simes di Studi Elettrofisiologici
Università di Parma
Via Gransci 14
43100 PARMA
Italy

Nadeau, R.
Institut de génie biomédical
Case Postale 6128, succursale A
MONTRéAL, Québec H3C 3J7
Canada

Nyssen, E.
Faculteit Geneeskunde ; Vrije Universiteit Brussel
Eenheid "Hart"
Laarbeeklaan 103
B 1090 BRUSSELS
Belgium

Ohta, T.
Aichi Prefectural Center for Health Care
3-z-1, Sannomaru, NAKA-KU
NAGOYA 460
Japan

Preda, I.
Second Medical Clinic of Postgraduate Medical School
H-1389
P.O.B. 112
BUDAPEST
Hungary

Rudy, Y.
Department of Pediatrics, Department of Biomedical Engineering
Case Western Reserve University
CLEVELAND, Ohio 44106
U.S.A.

Savard, P.
Hôpital Sacre-Coeur / Genie Biomedical
5400 Govin Ouest
MONTREAL H4J 1C5
Canada

Schoffa, G.
Lehrgebiet Biophysik, Universität Karlsruhe
Engesserstr. 7
D 7500 KARLSRUHE 1
B.R.D.

Selvester, R.
University of Southern California
Rancho Los Amigos Hospital
7601 East Imperial Highway
DOWNEY, Calif. 90242
U.S.A.

Spekhorst, H.H.M.
Dept. of Cardiology
Academic Medical Centre
Meibergdreef 9
1105 AZ Amsterdam

Taccardi, B.
Istituto di Fisiologia Generale e Centro Simes di Studi Ellectrofisiologici
Università di Parma
1-43100 PARMA
Italy

Tanaka, H.
Institute of Medical Electronic
Faculty of Medicine, Univ. of Tokyo
7-3-1 Hongo, Bunkyo-ku
TOKYO
Japan 113

Teramachi, Y.
Tokyo Institute of Technology
Nagatsuta, Midoriku Yokohama,
Japan 227

Uijen, G.
Dept. of Cardiology
University of Nijmegen
Geert Grooteplein Zuid 18
6525 GA NIJMEGEN
The Netherlands

Van Dam, R.Th.
Dept. of Cardiology
University of Nijmegen
Geert Grooteplein Zuid 18
6525 GA NIJMEGEN
The Netherlands

Yamashita, Y.
Dept. of Biomed. Engineering
Tokai University, School of Medicine
Bosheidai, Isehara
KANAGAWA
Japan